PAIN TREATMENT FRAUD

A PRESCRIPTION FOR DISASTER

William E. Ackerman MD

PAIN TREATMENT FRAUD

Copyright © 2017 by William E. Ackerman MD

All rights reserved. No part of this book may be reproduced or transmitted in any form or by any means without written permission of the author.

Table of Contents

1. MEDICAL FRAUD 1
2. PAIN TREATMENT FRAUD 9
3. PAIN DEFINED..15
4. PAIN CLINIC SCAMS..25
5. PAIN CAUSATION 33
6. PAIN COSTS..41
7. PAIN RELIEF...47
8. PAIN ASSESSMENT 53
9. DIAGNOSTIC TESTS..61
10. QUALIFICATIONS TO PRACTICE PAIN MANAGEMENT 69
11. OPIOIDS..77
12. ADDICTION 85
13. ANTI INFLAMMATORY MEDICATIONS..............................93
14. MUSCLE RELAXANTS 99
15. NEUROPATHY 107
16. MYOFASCIAL PAIN 117
17. TOPICAL ANALGESICS 125
18. ANTIDEPRESSANTS 137
19. ALTERNATIVE TREATMENTS 147
20. CHIROPRACTIC 159
21. PHYSICAL THERAPY..167
22. NECK PAIN 177
23. LOW BACK PAIN..189
24. WORKMAN'S COMPENSATION 201

25. FIBROMYALGIA	207
26. HEADACHES	213
27. INJECTIONS	223
28. INFLAMMATION	233
29. ACUTE PAIN	241
30. URINE DRUG TESTING	247
31. OSTEOPOROSIS	253
32. TMJ	259
33. SHINGLES	269
34. HIV	277
35. BIG PHARMA	285
36. PILL MILLS	291
37. HOSPITAL PAIN MANAGEMENT	299
38. PALATIVE CARE	307
39. RSD	313
40. ELDERLY PAIN MANAGEMENT	321
41. VASCULAR PAIN	329
42. CANCER PAIN	335
43. ABDOMINAL PAIN	345
44. THORACIC PAIN	357

1. MEDICAL FRAUD

Medicare fraud and healthcare fraud in general is illegal. The US Office of Management and Budget says "improper payments" made by Medicare in 2010 amounted to more than $47.8 billion. That represents almost 10% of the $528 billion total Medicare spend that year. Fraud, waste, and abuse pose major risks for the healthcare system.

Fraud means an intentional deception or misrepresentation made by a person with the knowledge that the deception could result in some unauthorized benefit to himself or some other person." "Abuse means provider practices that are inconsistent with sound fiscal, business, or medical practices, and result in an unnecessary cost to the Insurance provider or in reimbursement for services that are not medically necessary or that fail to meet professionally recognized standards for health care."

Although health care fraud has many cons, they can be broken down into three major categories: Phantom Billing. In this scenario, the provider bills Medicare for procedures which are either unnecessary or not performed at all. Durable medical equipment false billings fall into this category as well. An example would be billing Medicare for a wheelchair or homecare hospital bed which is either unneeded or undelivered.

False patient billing is often carried out in areas with large numbers of senior citizens, such as Florida, and the patient may be duplicitous. For instance, for a kickback, a Medicare-eligible patient may provide his Medicare number and allow a provider to bill Medicare for tests and procedure either unneeded or unfulfilled.

Up coding and up billing seek to receive additional and unwarranted and illegal Medicare funds by using a code that may not be merited but results in the need for further services and tests, and, therefore higher reimbursements.

Providers who engage in fraud and abuse are subject to sanctions under a number of Federal and State laws. Sanctions under Federal law, for example, can take the form of administrative, civil, and criminal penalties. These penalties range from monetary fines and damages to prison time and exclusion from the Federal healthcare programs. Becoming familiar with common types of fraud, waste, and abuse, will better position providers to ensure they or their patients are not involved in such conduct.

Although the following examples involve violation of Federal laws, many states have similar laws against fraud, waste, and abuse. Medical Identity Theft involves the misuse of a person's medical identity to wrongfully obtain health care goods, services, or funds. Medical identity theft has been defined as "the appropriation or misuse of a patient's or a provider's unique medical identifying information to obtain or bill public or private payers for fraudulent medical goods or services."

Be aware that stolen physician identifiers can be used to fill fraudulent prescriptions, refer patients for unnecessary additional services or supplies, or bill for services that were never provided.

Some people use beneficiary medical identifiers to fraudulently bill services or items not provided, or to enable an ineligible person to receive services by impersonating a beneficiary. Billing for Unnecessary Services or Items by physicians also occurs. Providers are responsible for ensuring authorized services meet the definition of medical necessity in the States where they practice. To be covered by insurance the billed service or supply must be provided.

Some providers bill Medicaid for a covered service or item but do not deliver the service or item. These providers may create false records in an attempt to justify the bills. For example, a physician might sign charts and submit bills for examinations and tests that never took place. Providers should only bill for the medically necessary or otherwise authorized services or items provided to the beneficiaries.

Up coding is a term that is generally understood as billing for services at a higher level of complexity than the service actually provided. For example, a pain physician might bill for a steroid injection with X ray but no X ray machine was used. The physician payment is more when the procedure is done with an X ray machine.

Unbundling is the practice of submitting bills in a fragmented fashion in order to maximize the reimbursement for various tests or procedures that are required to be billed together at a reduced cost. For example, a physician may order a urine drug screen panel which tests for many substances in a patient's urine to ascertain patient compliance. Instead of billing for the whole panel, the laboratory might attempt to increase income by billing for each test separately.

Kickbacks can be defined as offering, soliciting, paying, or receiving remuneration to induce, or in return for referral of patients or the generation of business involving any item or service for which payment may be made under Federal health care programs. For example, it would be illegal for a physician to accept payments from a medical imaging facility for referring patients.

A patient should learn some of the basic health care provider schemes and how to deter them from taking some easy money such as: billing for services not rendered, Billing for a non-covered service as a covered, service Misrepresenting dates of service, Misrepresenting locations of service, Misrepresenting provider of service, Waiving of deductibles and/or co-payments, Incorrect reporting of diagnoses or procedures, Overutilization of services, Corruption (kickbacks and bribery), False or unnecessary issuance of prescription drugs.

Billings for services and care not rendered are not uncommon. Providers might make more money by reporting they visited with or and treated the same patient on two separate days rather than one day. Each office visit is usually considered a separate billable service.

It is not uncommon that somebody may impersonate a physician and bill for treatment. Medical doctors sign insurance claim forms showing that they had provided care but in reality, lesser-educated health professionals actually conducted the treatment.

Most government health care plans and insurance companies don't allow medical providers or facilities to waive patients' deductibles or co-payments. The rationale may be that if patients have to pay something to see doctors, they'll only seek care if they really need it.

Regardless, some providers do waive patients' deductibles or co-payments and then submit other false claims to insurance companies to make up the dollar difference. Truly unscrupulous providers also will add a bunch of other false services to the claim forms to increase their illegal gains knowing that the patients are unlikely to complain because their co-payments and deductibles were waived.

Listing an incorrect diagnosis or procedure is fraudulent. Unscrupulous providers can bill for extra services if they report procedures performed. Like all industries, the potential for corruption in the health care industry is great. Providers have been known to unlawfully pay for and/or receive payment for referrals. Obviously, that practice can lend itself to abuse when referrals are made for services that aren't even needed, such as X-rays, MRIs, prescription drugs, etc.

Prescription drug abuse is sometimes defined as taking prescription medication for reasons beyond physicians' intentions. Painkillers are the most commonly abused prescription. These drugs' street value is almost 10 times the legal prescription value. Media around the country often report that thieves have robbed pharmacies at gunpoint to get painkillers. Crime prevention tips often suggest that homeowners should ensure don't have unneeded access to the occupants' prescription drugs.

Some patients doctor shop to obtain drug prescriptions. The doctors usually have no idea that the patients have already visited other physicians to obtain the same or other drugs. Impostors can easily recover the cost of the doctors' visits and filling of prescriptions by selling some or all of the drugs on the street. Some patients and medical facility employees have taken prescription paper pads and forged prescriptions and provider signatures on them. Others make pen-and-ink changes to the quantity and/or authorized refill numbers on the paper prescriptions. (Electronic prescriptions from providers to pharmacists are helping prevent this fraud.)

A pharmacist previously stole large quantities of painkillers from his employer's inventory and then electronically submitted false claims to insurance companies using names of other beneficiaries' and their insurance policy numbers, which he obtained from his employer's computer. A pharmacist could also alter the quantity listed on legitimately received prescriptions for drugs, and manipulate the patients' paperwork and receipts or make co-payments like the above pharmacist and steal the extra drugs for himself.

Joint investigation by the FBI, DEA, U.S. Department of Health and Human Services-Office of Inspector General and Blue Cross Blue Shield of Michigan revealed that patients were getting prescriptions for narcotics for no medical purpose from a pain management clinic.. Patients were recruited to come to the office and agree to diagnostic tests. In return, they would receive cash or prescriptions for Vicodin, Oxycontin, or Opana ER. Some patients agreed to get prescriptions for narcotics and then immediately turn them over to a recruiter. The recruiters were filling the prescriptions for resale on the streets.

In a typical visit, a patient would agree to medical tests such as blood tests, breathing tests, EKGs, EEGs, ultrasounds, X-rays, and psychological testing, no matter what their supposed medical problems were. The testing was all done before being seen by the doctor. All these tests were being billed to Blue Cross Blue Shield of Michigan and Medicare. The investigation revealed that for some of the tests that the clinic billed, the equipment was broken or the clinic did not even own the necessary equipment.

In addition to the prescription of narcotics, a large part of the practice conducted at the clinics was to provide patients with injections of lidocaine combined with steroids which at times provided temporary relief of various joint and muscle pain. Although the injections given to the patients were superficial, they were billed falsely to the insurance companies as facet joint injections, paravertebral injections, sacroiliac nerve injections, sciatic nerve injections, and various nerve block injections.

The pain management practice at the clinics grew quickly during the time period of the conspiracy. The doctors went from seeing an average of 50-60 patients per day in 1998 to more than 100 per day beginning in 2003 with a high of 279 on Jan. 6, 2005. From 1998 through 2002, one of the doctors saw pain patients at the clinics in addition to her own allergy patients. This doctor sustained a modest allergy practice, and would sign patient procedure forms and superbills, falsely indicating that she had administered facet joint injections or other paravertebral injections when in reality she did not.

Nearly every patient was prescribed one or more controlled substances and put on a regimen of shots every two weeks. The patients were required to sign the medical progress and procedure notes in their patient chart to prove they were at the clinic and received the shots. One doctor tried to convince all patients to have shots at every visit, but many of the patients did not want the shots every two weeks. For those patients who ultimately refused the shots, this doctor regularly required the patients to sign the progress and procedure notes even though they received only a prescription for controlled substances and did not receive any injections.

By the beginning of 2000, one of the doctors was having certain patients sign blank procedure/progress notes and then use the forms to generate a superbill in order to bill the insurance companies for injection procedures on days when the patient was not in the clinic.

One of the doctors in question hired several foreign medical graduates (FMGs) over the course of the conspiracy to assist in the movement of patients through the clinics. Several of the FMGs helped add fictitious patient examination information to the blank progress/procedure notes after one doctor had added non-existent medical procedures to the blank forms so that insurance companies could be billed as if the person had been in the clinic when in reality they had not. The ultimate purpose was to bill insurance companies for procedures that never occurred.

These doctors' records indicated that more than 100 patients allegedly received injections on 708 different days during this conspiracy.

Furthermore, these doctors' billings showed that as many as 279 patients allegedly received injections on one day alone. Health economists have reported the annual cost of chronic pain in the United States is as high as $635 billion a year, which is more than the yearly costs for cancer, heart disease and diabetes. (Darrell J. Gaskin, Patrick Richard. The Economic Costs of Pain in the United States. The Journal of Pain, 2012; 13 (8): 715 DOI: 10.1016/j.jpain.2012.03.009).

The results of this study showed that mean health care expenditures for adults were $4,475. Prevalence estimates for pain conditions were 10 percent for moderate pain, 11 percent for severe pain, 33 percent for joint pain, 25 percent for arthritis, and 12 percent for functional disability. Persons with moderate pain had health care expenditures $4,516 higher than someone with no pain, and individuals with severe pain had costs $3,210 higher than those with moderate pain. Similar differences were found for other pain conditions: $4,048 higher for joint pain, $5,838 for arthritis, and $9,680 for functional disabilities.

Based on their analysis of the data, the authors determined that that the total cost for pain in the United States ranged from $560 to $635 billion. Total incremental costs of health care due to pain ranged from $261 to $300 billion, and the value of lost productivity ranged from $299 to $334 billion. About 100 million adults in the United States were affected by chronic pain, including joint pain or arthritis. Pain is costly to the nation because it requires medical treatment and complicates treatment for other ailments.

Pain is costly to the nation because it requires medical treatment and complicates treatment for other ailments. Nonmalignant chronic pain (NMCP) is a public health concern. Information about costs and use of pain medications is valuable for the practitioner making individual patient care decisions. The total costs of prescription medications prescribed for pain were $17.8 billion annually in the United States.

Pain management is a branch of medicine employing an interdisciplinary approach for easing the suffering and improving the quality of life of those living with chronic pain. Treatment approaches to chronic pain include pharmacological measures, such as analgesics, antidepressants and anticonvulsants, interventional procedures, physical therapy, physical exercise, application of ice and/or heat, and psychological measures, such as biofeedback and cognitive behavioral therapy.

Interventional procedures typically used for chronic back pain - include epidural steroid injections, facet joint injections, neurolytic blocks, spinal cord stimulators and intrathecal drug delivery system implants.

Pain physicians are medical or osteopathic doctors and often fellowship trained and board certified anesthesiologists, neurologists, physiatrists or psychiatrists. Palliative care doctors are also specialists in pain. The cost of cancer pan treatment is an aspect of growing importance in the conversation between healthcare providers and patients as drug prices continue to rise across the world.

Low back pain (LBP) has a major economic impact in the United States, with total costs related to this condition exceeding $100 billion per year. In the United States, patients with musculoskeletal conditions incur total annual medical care costs of approximately $240 billion. The reasons for long-lasting pain are many, from cancer and multiple sclerosis to back pain and arthritis. Adults with low back pain are often in worse physical and mental health than people who do not have low back pain.

A study cited by WebMD, the average estimated annual medical expenditures for adults with back pain in 2005 was $6,096, while the estimated annual medical expenditures for those without pain was $3,516. Treating spine problems in the United States costs $85.9 billion a year, while cancer treatment, which costs $89 billion.

One doctor in Texas served prison time for health-care fraud. Another has been disciplined by regulators five times, on charges including dangerous overuse of anesthesia. A third devotes his practice to a controversial therapy that Medicare won't cover.

Researchers have found that up to 42 percent of Medicare patients experience unnecessary treatment. Is this criminal behavior? White collar crimes are characterized by "deceit, concealment, or violation of trust and are not dependent upon the application or threat of physical force or violence. Health care fraud is a form of white collar crime that may be committed by health care providers, consumers, companies providing medical supplies or services, and health care organizations.

The common types of fraud committed by physicians include billing for services that were never rendered, providing unnecessary treatments or tests, up coding (billing for a more expensive diagnosis or procedure), falsifying or exaggerating the severity of the medical illness to justify coding, and accepting kickbacks for referral.

The FBI has functioned as the primary investigative agency for health care fraud in both the public and private health systems. The Financial Crimes Section of the FBI was created in the 1980s. It comprises three units, one of which is devoted to health care fraud. The FBI has developed several national initiatives including the Internet Pharmacy Fraud Initiative, the Auto Accident Insurance Fraud Initiative, and the Outpatient Surgery Center Initiative.

The FBI has emphasized the investigation of medical professionals who engage in schemes that can directly harm patients. Such schemes include performing unnecessary surgeries, diluting medication for profit, and inappropriate prescribing practices

The FBI previously announced indictments against 53 persons in Detroit and Miami accused of conspiring to submit more than $50 million in false Medicare claims. It was alleged that at least nine Medicare provider companies as well as company executives, doctors, therapists, medical recruiters, medical assistants, and Medicare consumers participated in these schemes, which involved billing for physical therapy, occupational therapy, and infusion therapy that had not been provided

Law enforcement is beginning to use technology to monitor discrepancies in billing as a means of preventing and identifying health care fraud. The Medicaid Anti-Kickback Statute prohibits knowingly and willfully paying or receiving any remuneration directly or indirectly, overtly or covertly, in cash or in kind in exchange for or to induce referrals of program-related business including prescribing, purchasing, or recommending any service, treatment, or item for which payment will be made by Medicare, Medicaid, or any other federally funded health care program.

Physicians may perform unnecessary procedures to increase reimbursement, compromising patient safety. When medical providers bill for services never rendered, they create a false medical history for patients that may later cause them difficulty in obtaining disability or life insurance policies.

When physicians bill the government for medical services that are not needed by the patient, they violate the trust placed in them by their patients and the government to provide only medically necessary care. The FDA describes health fraud as "articles of unproven effectiveness that are promoted to improve health, wellbeing or appearance." The articles can be drugs, devices, foods, or cosmetics for human or animal use.

Twenty-eight defendants, from the Dallas-Fort Worth Metroplex, have been previously charged with various crimes related to their roles in a massive health care fraud scheme that involved bribes, unnecessary medical treatment, fraudulent billing, and the falsification of medical documents to fraudulently bill the federal government, through the Department of Labor's (DOL) Office of Worker Compensation Programs (OWCP), more than $9.5 million.

Individuals claims of an "innovation," "miracle cure," "exclusive product," or "new discovery" or "magical" are highly suspect as being potentially fraudulent. The purpose of this book is to educate patients, insurance companies, government officials etc. that pain management is potentially full of fraudulent practices and practitioners and it hoped that this book can help identify these individuals because sham treatments can be detrimental to a person's health and defer proper treatment. When in doubt about a particular treatment it is prudent to get a second opinion.

2. PAIN TREATMENT FRAUD

The purpose of this book is to inform the reader about pain management fraud. However, one needs to be aware that health care fraud is prominent throughout the entire healthcare industry. Health care fraud includes health insurance fraud, drug fraud, and medical fraud. Medical fraud not only occurs in pain management, it also occurs in healthcare in general.

One should be aware that some pain clinics use a "hook em, stick em and boot em" pain management philosophy. In other words the goal is to get a patient dependent on pain pills and then do injections until the patient's insurance declines any further injections and once this happens the clinic will discharge the patient for some reason.

For example, in 2011, $2.27 trillion was spent on health care and more than four billion health insurance claims were processed in the United States. It is an undisputed reality that some of these health insurance claims are fraudulent. Although they constitute only a small fraction, those fraudulent claims carry a very high price tag.

The National Health Care Anti-Fraud Association (NHCAA) estimates that the financial losses due to health care fraud are in the tens of billions of dollars each year. The FBI is the primary agency for exposing and investigating health care fraud, with jurisdiction over both federal and private insurance programs. The Bureau also maintains significant liaison with private insurance national groups, such as the National Health Care Anti-Fraud Association, the National Insurance Crime Bureau, and private insurance investigative units.

Whether you have employer-sponsored health insurance or you purchase your own insurance policy, health care fraud inevitably translates into higher premiums and out-of-pocket expenses for consumers, as well as reduced benefits or coverage. For employers-private and government alike-health care fraud increases the cost of providing insurance benefits to employees and, in turn, increases the overall cost of doing business.

For many Americans, the increased expense resulting from fraud could mean the difference between making health insurance a reality or not. Some of the most common methods used by criminals to fraudulently obtain patient insurance information include: Obtaining patient information when patients obtain a free screening, a method frequently seen at health fairs or . inducing medical personnel with access to patient insurance information to copy the material and provide it to those involved in fraud schemes.

Fraud drives up the costs for everyone in the health care system, in addition to hurting the long term solvency of the Federal health care programs, like Medicare and Medicaid, upon which millions of Americans depend. Individual victims of health care fraud are those are people who are exploited and subjected to unnecessary or unsafe medical procedures or whose medical records are compromised or whose legitimate insurance information is used to submit falsified claims.

The majority of health care fraud is committed by a very small minority of dishonest health care providers. Unfortunately, the stock in trade of fraud-doers is to take advantage of the confidence that has been entrusted to them in order to commit ongoing fraud on a very broad scale. And in conceiving fraud schemes, this group has the luxury of being creative because it has access to a vast range of variables with which to conceive all sorts of wrongdoing.

Health care fraud affects the entire population of our nation's patients. The entire range of potential medical conditions and treatments on which to base false claims and the ability to spread false billings among many insurers simultaneously, including public programs such as Medicare and Medicaid, increasing fraud proceeds while lessening their chances of being detected by any a single insurer.

The most common types of fraud committed by dishonest providers include: billing for services that were never rendered-either by using genuine patient information, sometimes obtained through identity theft, to fabricate entire claims or by padding claims with charges for procedures or services that did not take place.

Another scam involves billing for more expensive services or procedures than were actually provided or performed, commonly known as "upcoding" i.e., falsely billing for a higher-priced treatment than was actually provided (which often requires the accompanying "inflation" of the patient's diagnosis code to a more serious condition consistent with the false procedure code).

Performing medically unnecessary services solely for the purpose of generating insurance payments is seen very often in nerve-conduction and other diagnostic-testing schemes. Misrepresenting non-covered treatments as medically necessary covered treatments for purposes of obtaining insurance payments-widely seen in cosmetic-surgery schemes, in which non-covered cosmetic procedures such as "nose jobs" are billed to patients' insurers as deviated-septum repairs.

Falsifying a patient's diagnosis like calling a back strain a ruptured disc to justify tests, surgeries or other procedures that aren't medically necessary occurs frequently in some offices. Unbundling is common in urine drug screen tests. For example a n insurance company will pay for tests that are bundled into one cost. Some laboratories will bill for each test done creating a higher charge by billing each step of a procedure as if it were a separate procedure for each substance to be tested.

Some clinics bill a patient more than the co-pay amount for services that were prepaid or paid in full by the benefit plan under the terms of a managed care contract. Accepting kickbacks for patient referrals is fraud. For example, a surgeon cannot pay a family physician for referring a patient for surgery. Waiving patient co-pays or deductibles for medical or dental care and over-billing the insurance carrier or benefit plan is not legal.

Health care fraud, like any fraud, demands that false information be represented as truth. An all too common health care fraud scheme involves perpetrators who exploit patients by entering into their medical records false diagnoses of medical conditions they do not have, or of more severe conditions than they actually do have. This is done so that bogus insurance claims can be submitted for payment.

Unless and until this discovery is made, the phony or inflated diagnoses become part of the patient's documented medical history, at least in the health insurer's records. A Boston-area psychiatrist, forfeited $1.3 million and was sentenced to several years in federal prison following his late-1990s conviction on 136 counts of mail fraud, money laundering and witness intimidation related to his fraudulent billing of several health insurers for psychiatric therapy sessions that never took place-using the names and insurance information of many people whom he actually had never met, let alone treated.

In fabricating the claims, the psychiatrist also fabricated diagnoses for those "patients". Unfortunately many of the patients were adolescents. The phony conditions he assigned to them included "depressive psychosis," "suicidal ideation," "sexual identity problems" and "behavioral problems in school."

Patients who have private health insurance often have lifetime caps or other limits on benefits under their policies. So every time a false claim is paid in a patient's name, the dollar amount counts toward that patient's lifetime or other limits. This means that when a patient legitimately needs his or her insurance benefits the most, they may have already been exhausted.

As a consumer, you should be aware of the hazards of identity theft and the devastating affects it can have on your financial health- jeopardizing bank accounts, credit ratings and your ability to borrow. You need to furthermore be familiar with the risks posed by medical identity theft. You must be aware that 250,000 to 500,000 individuals have been victims of this type of crime.

When a person's name or other identifying information is used without that person's knowledge or consent to obtain medical services or goods, or to submit false insurance claims for payment, this behavior is called medical identity theft. Medical identity theft frequently results in erroneous information being added to a person's medical record, or even the creation of an entirely fictitious medical record in the victim's name.

Victims of medical identity theft may receive the wrong medical treatment or find that their health insurance benefits have been exhausted, and could become uninsurable for both life and health insurance coverage. A medical identity theft victim may unexpectedly fail a physical exam for employment because a disease or condition for which he's never been diagnosed or received treatment has been unknowingly documented in his health record. The effects of this crime can plague a victim's medical and financial status for years to come. Furthermore, there have been many cases where patients have been subjected to unnecessary or dangerous medical procedures simply because of greed.

In June, 2002, for example, a Chicago cardiologist was sentenced to 12-1/2 years in federal prison and was ordered to pay $16.5 million in fines and restitution after pleading guilty to performing 750 medically unnecessary heart catheterizations, along with unnecessary angioplasties and other tests as part of a 10-year fraud scheme. Three other physicians and a hospital administrator also pleaded guilty and received prison sentences for their part in the scheme, which resulted in the deaths of at least two patients.

The physicians and hospital induced hundreds of homeless persons, substance abusers, and elderly men and women to feign symptoms and be admitted to the hospital for the unnecessary procedures by offering them incentives such as food, cash and cigarettes. "There were 750 people who had needles stuck into their hearts purely for profit

Health care fraud is not just committed by dishonest health care providers. So enticing an invitation is our nation's ever-growing pool of health care money that in certain areas - Florida, for example law enforcement agencies and health insurers have witnessed in recent years the migration of some criminals from illegal drug trafficking into the safer and far more lucrative business of perpetrating fraud schemes against Medicare, Medicaid and private health insurance companies.

In South Florida alone, government programs and private insurers have lost hundreds of millions of dollars in recent years to criminal rings. These individuals fabricate claims from non-existent clinics, using genuine patient-insurance and provider-billing information that the perpetrators have bought and/or stolen for that purpose. When the bogus claims are paid, the mailing address in most instances belongs to a freight forwarder that bundles up the mail and ships it off shore.

In response to these realities, Congress-through the Health Insurance Portability and Accountability Act of 1996 (HIPAA)- specifically established health care fraud as a federal criminal offense, with the basic crime carrying a federal prison term of up to 10 years in addition to significant financial penalties. The federal law also provides that should a perpetrator's fraud result in the injury of a patient, the prison term can double, to 20 years; and should it result in a patient's death, a perpetrator can be sentenced to life in federal prison.

Congress also mandated the establishment of a nationwide "Coordinated Fraud and Abuse Control Program," to coordinate federal, state and local law enforcement efforts against health care fraud and to include "the coordination and sharing of data" with private health insurers. Many states have responded since the early 1990s, not only by strengthening their insurance fraud laws and penalties, but also by requiring health insurers to meet certain standards of fraud detection, investigation and referral as a condition of maintaining their insurance or HMO licenses.

Founded in 1985 by a handful of private insurers and law enforcement personnel, the National Health Care Anti-Fraud Association is a private-public non-profit organization focused solely on improving the private and public sectors' ability to detect, investigate, prosecute and, ultimately, prevent fraud against our private and public health insurance systems.

Today NHCAA represents the combined efforts of the anti-fraud units of the majority of our country's private health payers and the entire spectrum of federal and some state law enforcement agencies that have jurisdiction over the crime, along with hundreds of individual members from the private health insurance sector and from federal, state and local law enforcement.

The NHCAA pursues its mission by nurturing private-public cooperation against health care fraud at both the case and policymaking levels, by facilitating the sharing of investigative information among health insurers and law enforcement agencies and by providing information on health care fraud to all interested parties. The NHCAA Institute for Health Care Fraud Prevention, a non-profit educational foundation, provides professional education and training to industry and government anti-fraud investigators and other personnel.

Protect yourself from health care fraud. Safeguard your health insurance ID card like you would a credit card. In the wrong hands, a health insurance card is a license to steal. Don't give out insurance policy numbers to door-to-door salespeople, telephone solicitors or over the Internet. Be careful about disclosing your insurance information and if you lose your insurance ID card, report it to your insurance company immediately. Report any suspected fraud as well.

Call your insurance company immediately if you suspect you may be a victim of health insurance fraud. Many insurers now offer the opportunity to report suspected fraud online through their Website. Be informed about the health care services you receive, keep good records of your medical care, and closely review all medical bills you receive. Read your policy and benefits statements before seeking care.

Read your insurance policy including the Explanation of Benefits statements and any paperwork you receive from your insurance company. Make sure you actually received the treatments for which your insurance was charged, and question suspicious expenses. Are the dates of service documented on the forms correct? Were the services identified and billed for actually performed? Furthermore, beware of "free" offers. Offers of free health care services, tests or treatments are often fraud schemes designed to bill you and your insurance company illegally for thousands of dollars of treatments you never received.

Health care fraud is a serious crime that affects everyone and should concern everyone-government officials and taxpayers, insurers and premium-payers, health care providers and patients-and it is a costly reality that none of us can afford to overlook.

3. PAIN DEFINED

Almost everyone experiences pain at some time. Pain can be a natural response to injury and disease in some instances. With the advent of pain medicine as a medical specialty, patients no longer need to suffer. Suffering is how our lives are affected. Patients who suffer have significant reductions in the normal joys of their lives. They cannot enjoy their families or enjoy recreational activities etc. Their pain affects them emotionally.

Animal models have enhanced our understanding of pain mechanisms and make forward-looking statements as to our proximity to the development of effective mechanism-based treatments. Animal pain models have failed in some aspects as animal models cannot always be extrapolated to humans.

Pain is an unpleasant sensory and emotional experience following tissue injury. Your pain management can be expensive as well as ineffective if you do not communicate truthfully with you doctor. Different specialties in medicine practice pain medicine. Chiropractors practice pain management as well. Anesthesiologists manage your pain with injections. Physiatrists manage pain with heat, cold, etc. and do needle studies on you to see if you have nerve damage.

Orthopedic and neurosurgeons can perform surgery on you. A neurosurgeon can place a spinal morphine pump that directs morphine into your spinal fluid. All of these specialists can prescribe drugs to you for pain management. A multidisciplinary pain clinic will have physicians, physical therapists, and psychologists who can collectively treat your pain. The effectiveness of psychosocial interventions for back pain in primary care has been established.

Pain is a complex, idiosyncratic experience. When pain is the primary complaint for seeking medical attention, understanding of multiple factors is essential in guiding successful treatment. Behavioral medicine, a branch of psychology, has been an integral part of interdisciplinary/multidisciplinary care of pain patients.

Prominent and distressing emotions, cognitions, and behaviors frequently accompany chronic pain. In many cases, these psychological symptoms will be sufficiently severe to qualify the patient for a diagnosis of a mental disorder.

For thousands of years, doctors have been helping to relieve their patients' pain with a variety of medications and treatments. Like other areas of medicine, a new subset of doctors has become specialists in treating pain. The question that you should ask yourself is if any of the modalities such as heat, cold, injections, drugs etc. will actually stop your pain. The answer is no if your pain is chronic.

Chronic pain is a disease. Your doctor will strive to provide you with a quality of life. If your pain is acute such as post-surgical pain, or after a fall on your hip you should expect significant pain relief. Chronic pain is that pain that persists after your body has healed. Nothing unfortunately will completely eliminate your pain.

The goal of pain management is to decrease your pain so that you can maintain your normal activities of daily living. This means that your pain should not interfere with your work, family or recreation. As a result, if you have chronic pain your goal and your doctor's goal should be to decrease your pain to a tolerable level. Pain management is expensive. Because nothing will completely stop your chronic pain, you will need to follow up frequently with your health care provider. Different treatments will be tried until you begin to have a reduction in your pain.

When you see a specialist or go to a hospital or surgery center, if you have insurance, you will have to pay a co-payment to have a procedure or an examination performed. Because many pain treatments will not benefit you, it is necessary for you to become an informed consumer.

You can do this by trying to understand what is causing your pain and what alternative modalities (such as chiropractic, herbs etc.) are available to you. If you complain of pain to your primary care physician, your doctor may refer you to someone who only treats pain. This individual may have no or minimal training or may have extensive training.

Remember that these treating individuals have expenses such as MRI machines, X ray machines to do steroid injections on you, physical therapy equipment etc. This equipment must be paid for. You, the patient will ultimately pay for the equipment. You must therefore, become knowledgeable as to what treatment is necessary to treat your painful condition so that you will not receive treatments that you do not need. This is why communication between you and your doctor is important.

You must be aware that pain management can be an environment where essentially a practitioner in some situations needs only minimal credentials such as a medical license to do potentially harmful procedures to unsuspecting individuals suffering from excruciating pain. This can be a world where most procedures can be done in out-patient surgery centers to avoid the peer review scrutiny of a hospital medical staff. You must therefore, inquire if your practitioner is trained and certified in pain medicine. Approximately forty-eight million Americans suffer from chronic pain.

Americans spend over one hundred billion dollars annually on pain care. One-third of all adult Americans suffer from chronic pain. Over the counter annual analgesic costs amount to three billion dollars. Your pain treatment can bankrupt you. You must be able to identify the ethical pain treatment physicians and clinics as well as the "get rich" schemers.

The cost of medical care is rapidly escalating. Employers may not be able to afford health insurance for their employees. The cost of pain management is contributing to the increase in health care costs and amounts to hundreds of thousands of dollars. As a result, there is considerable profit to be made by unethical health care providers that include hospitals as well as physicians.

Unfortunately, along with many reputable excellent pain clinics many pain management centers have sprouted up like weeds throughout the United States staffed by individuals with little or no formal training. One may look in the Yellow Pages of any telephone book in most communities to find an establishment that will manage chronic pain syndromes including cancer pain.

Unfortunately, there are no state regulatory bodies, which govern the way these clinics or physicians practice pain management. Patient influence and persuasion to go to a specific pain clinic is noted in many pain treatment center advertisements, which become unethical if anything is done to interfere with patient free choice through intentional deception or distortion. These abuses are becoming sufficiently common and flagrant.

Physicians who themselves do not practice pain medicine such as orthopedic surgeons might refer patients to medical centers that they own to have MRI's and multiple injections done by pain specialists to be performed in an operating room setting. The reader must realize that the facility owner must pay for the MRI scanner, X ray machine, the building and the personnel that it takes to staff the facility. This cost can be millions of dollars annually. However, physicians with shares in these facilities realize handsome profits from ownership in these facilities.

Patients who are unable to pay are frequently excluded from treatment. If the treatment is as good as advertised in the newspaper, on television or on the radio, why are some patients denied care? The sad fact is that this behavior is legal. Consumer protection legislation and patient education will play an increasingly significant role when one decides to choose a pain treatment center and/or physician.

Many pain clinics hire marketing firms to promote their services. Very few advertisements that this author has reviewed in ten large cities, mention the credentials of their physicians. Most advertisements mention only the treatment of many painful entities. These advertisements fail to mention that they will only do invasive care in a facility that they own to enjoy a bigger payday.

You as a patient and consumer should have the choice of the facility where your procedure will be done. In fact, you should insist on it. You need to be aware that many hospital administrators and physicians in the 1990's realized after considerable market research that they could enjoy large profits from pain management. Hospitals could charge fees by having nerve injections performed in the hospital instead of in a physician's office.

Health care costs due to chronic pain are particular high during the first year after pain onset, and remain high compared with health care costs before pain onset. The majority of chronic pain patients incur the costs of alternative treatments. Chronic pain causes production losses at work, as well as impairment of your non-work activities.

Chronic pain patients must realize that the majority of pain procedures can be done in the physician's office. You or your insurance company will save approximately $1200.00=$1500.00 per procedure. Medicare realizes this and encourages office based pain management. Private insurance carriers now realize that they are literally being fleeced by some pain block facilities.

Medical equipment companies in the 1990's also saw the potential to make considerable sums of money by selling devices that could burn nerves, freeze nerves, place salt solutions on nerves or "melt" disc structures in the back. Unfortunately many of these devices have no scientific merit. Medical instrument companies also manufactured electric catheters to be placed in the backs of patients that were intended to diminish pain. There may be medical evidence that these devices diminish pain in a number of select patients with specific pathological entities.

Three companies at the time of the writing of this book sell a light scope that is placed into your spine from above the rectum. Allegedly, a physician can identify where one should place a steroid. Unfortunately, some patients have been blinded by this procedure. One company did manufacture a pump device, which does deliver morphine or morphine like drugs into the spinal fluid of cancer patients.

This device did provide significant pain relief and did increase the quality of life in many cancer patients. This company then used their technology to provide pain relief in noncancerous pain patients. Unfortunately, they and the other companies required no training by physicians for the implantation of any of these devices. Outside of the medical field, this activity would attract widespread media attention.

Most medical specialties other than pain management require extra training (usually a minimum of 12 months) in a subspecialty of medicine before a physician may refer to themselves as a specialist. However, in pain medicine if an individual is not trained in a procedure the sales representative will come into the operating room (usually without a patient's consent) and instruct a physician on how to do a potentially dangerous procedure or a physician may go to a weekend course sponsored by the manufacturer and practice on a cadaver and subsequently be "certified" as an expert in the performance of a procedure.

You should be aware that pharmaceutical representatives may have access to the prescribing habits of physicians. Physicians are frequently enticed into prescribing a certain medication with luncheons, dinners and at one time lavish trips provided by a pharmaceutical company. This practice has been recently documented on a television news story. You should be aware that many of these medications are not safer, better or cheaper than existing medicines.

You should also be aware that the American Board of Medical Specialties has a list of specialties recognized as true medical specialties or subspecialties in the United States. Pain management itself is not included in this list. However, the American Board of Anesthesiology added qualification in pain medicine is recognized.

hysicians other than anesthesiologists such as physical medicine and rehabilitation, neurologists etc. can become board certified. This should tell you "Buyer beware!" Many patients use the Internet to access information regarding pain management. In my practice, less than ten percent of patients obtain medical information from an academic source such as the National Library of Congress from computer sources.

The purpose of this book is to inform you that outstanding pain centers do exist throughout the United States but that the "buyer must beware" mentality must be considered with respect to some "injection mills" staffed by some profit only driven individuals with minimal training. The reader must furthermore, be aware that a small number of pain clinics will prescribe potent narcotic medications until an individual becomes addicted. This behavior is not unlike the drug dealer on the street.

At the time of your addiction, you must agree to have expensive injection procedures that must be done biweekly with the threat that if a patient is noncompliant which means if the patient refuses injections he/she will have their narcotic prescriptions discontinued. This practice is called "hookem, stickem, and bootem".

The street drug hustler is incarcerated when caught. Nothing happens to the physician who intentionally causes a patient to become addicted to narcotics. On occasion a state medical board will investigate unscrupulous practices. An unscrupulous physician can legally get by with causing a patient's death or in many instances mutilation. The reader of this book will be aware that there is no rationale to ever having any "series" of injections done unless benefit is noted with each preceding injection.

Individuals must be aware that some physicians on occasion will entice a patient to have more than one procedure even if the first procedure was ineffective. Usually the physician will recommend three procedures. If the first procedure was properly done why have two more procedures? Two more procedures will make the physician's house payment but probably will not have any effect on your chronic pain.

Small pain centers, which have few patients, will entice patients to have three or more injections in a weekly or biweekly series only to increase facility and physician revenues. You will need to learn to distinguish the physician who practices science-based medicine from the physician who is a charlatan.

After completing this book, you should be able to discern what modalities can benefit you and which modalities benefit only the physician. This book may save the person who is suffering from chronic pain, significant time and money by learning what modalities can actually help an individual suffering from chronic pain. If a nerve block is done in the physician's office there is no facility charge. This will save you a facility co-payment.

Did you know that the doctor doing your injection may have trained at a weekend course or may have learned on the job? The weekend courses are cadaver courses. Do you want to be that doctor's first patient? You might be. There are no regulations on pain injectionists.

Doctors who manage pain are frequently anesthesiologists. Anesthesiologists ensure that you are safe, pain-free and comfortable during and immediately following surgery. But not everyone realizes that decades of research and work done by anesthesiologists have led to the development of newer, more effective treatments for patients who have pain unrelated to surgery. Many techniques used to make surgery and childbirth virtually painless is now being used to relieve other types of pain. In fact, the work pioneered by anesthesiologists has led to treatments for pain control outside the operating room.

Frequently an anesthesiologist heads a team of other specialists and doctors who work together to help you manage your pain. Pain medicine doctors are experts at diagnosing why you are having pain as well as treating the pain itself. Some of the more common pain problems they manage include: arthritis, back and neck pain, cancer pain, nerve pain, migraine headaches, shingles, phantom limb pain for amputees and pain caused by AIDS. Pain medicine doctors are experts at diagnosing why you are having pain as well as treating your pain.

Like other physicians, anesthesiologists have completed four years of medical school. They spent four more years learning anesthesiology and pain medicine during residency training. Many anesthesiologists who specialize in pain medicine receive an additional year of fellowship training to become an expert in treating pain. Some also have done research, and many have special certification in pain medicine through the American Board of Anesthesiology.

This board is the only organization recognized by the American Board of Medical Specialties to offer special credentials in pain medicine. Medical specialty certification in the United States is a voluntary process. While medical licensure sets the minimum competency requirements to diagnose and treat patients, it is not specialty specific. Board certification demonstrates a physician's expertise in a particular specialty and/or subspecialty of medical practice. Pain medicine is a subspecialty of anesthesiology.

The American Board of Medical Specialties member boards (24) are responsible for setting the standards for quality practice in a particular medical specialty. Each Member Board has a board of trustees or directors, all of whom are certified in that Board's medical specialty.

Individual Member Boards evaluate physician candidates to ascertain if the candidate completed the appropriate residency requirements and if he or she has an institutional or valid license to practice medicine. If a physician meets these basic admission standards, the Member Board will evaluate the candidate using written and oral examinations. Because specialties differ so widely, the criteria that inform these tests are quite different. What makes someone a good anesthesiologist does not necessarily make him or her a competent cardiologist.

Ultimately, the measure of physician specialists is not merely that they have been certified, but that they keep current in their specialty. The American Board of Medical Specialties requires maintenance of certification that is a formal means of measuring a physician's continued competency in his or her certified specialty and/or subspecialty.

To become recertified a physician must: hold a valid, unrestricted medical license, meet educational and self-assessment programs determined by the particular Board, demonstrate specialty-specific skills and knowledge, demonstrate the use of best evidence and practices compared to peers and national benchmarks.

Unfortunately, a physician needs no credentials to practice pain management other than a medical or osteopathic medicine degree and a state medical license. As a result, there are no guidelines as to who can call themselves a pain medicine "specialist". There are no local, state or national standards with respect to pain management.

The American Academy of Pain Medicine, the American Academy of Pain Management, and the American Board of Anesthesiologists administer written examinations to certify pain management doctors. These organizations provide continuing education courses annually. Some physicians do not certify through one of these organizations but classify themselves as pain physicians.

They may go to a weekend cadaver course to be able to do a certain procedure. You should ascertain that you are not the first live patient that one of these doctors practices on after finishing a weekend cadaver course. Other professionals (plumbers, nurses, teachers, policemen, etc.) must have formal training to practice their profession. Pain doctors in many instances do not! Does this frighten you? It should!! I recommend that you investigate your prospective pain physician before you receive treatments that will not benefit you or may actually harm you.

Ask to see your physician's credentials. Hospitals in many instances may want anyone who will show up and has a medical degree to do potentially mutilating procedures on patients who have insurance.

You should ascertain if your pain doctor has completed a fellowship (specialized training in pain medicine) or has sufficient experience through residency training to do a procedure on you. With these facts in mind, you must do your homework when choosing a pain medicine physician. Most university pain centers require that pain medicine physicians have a formal fellowship before they can begin to treat patients.

It is your duty to find the best-trained physician. Your insurance plan will list doctors approved by their plan. Some companies have strict criteria before admitting physicians to their plan. The American Association of health plans lists a Web site with a doctor finder at www.aahp.org. Click on to this site and follow the instructions to help locate a physician.

A background information check can be done on every physician. Go to ama-assn.org/aps/amahg.htm. Has your physician ever been disciplined by a state medical board? Find out by going to the Web site ama-assn.org/ama/pubcategory/2645.html to find out if your doctor is a health hazard. If your doctor has been disciplined find out the reason.

A physician should have some certification from a medical specialty like anesthesiology, physical medicine etc. to do pain medicine in addition to completion of a fellowship. Ideally, the pain medicine physician should have further training in pain medicine. If your physician has no certification in any specialty you should eliminate that physician from your list of potential treating physicians. There may be some qualified doctors who have not taken a certification test but it would be extremely difficult identifying those individuals who are truly competent. You should ask your physician if he or she has credentials in pain medicine including research publications etc. To ascertain if your physician is certified by the American Board of Medical Specialties, go to the website www.ABMS.org.

This book will enable you to gain a basic knowledge of the pathophysiology (the cause of your pain) and treatment of various chronic pain entities. This will enable you to become a team member with your doctor. This knowledge should help prevent you from becoming a potential victim by avoiding the incompetence of certain physicians who claim to be "pain medicine specialists" and by avoiding procedures that are possibly dangerous or have absolutely no scientific merit.

For those individuals who do not wish or have the time to read this book or a similar book you may be leaving your overall wellbeing to the "luck of the draw". You must be aware that many referring physicians have minimal knowledge as to what constitutes ethical pain medicine as pain management is not taught in most medical schools. This book is written for the layperson suffering from chronic pain. It is hoped that you will derive an understanding of various painful conditions that may affect you or a family member and to relate to you what potentially effective treatments are available to you.

Years ago, Voltaire summarized the medical situation of his time with respect to the practice of medicine: "Doctors pour drugs, of which they know little, for disease, of which they know less, into patients, of which they know nothing." With respect to pain management, has time changed anything?

4. PAIN CLINIC SCAMS

Pain management clinics specialize in treating chronic pain patients. Treatments involve therapy, injections, implantable devices and oral pain medications. Legitimate pain clinics have a trained certified clinician. Multiple fraudulent pain man management clinics exist and in some cases have become problematic. Pain patients need to investigate a clinic before they go to one because of fraudulent practices and practitioners in some clinics.

Over a trillion dollars has been spent on healthcare and more than 4 billion health insurance claims were processed in the United States in 2011. Some of these health insurance claims were noted to be fraudulent. These fraudulent claims however result in higher premiums and out-of-pocket expenses for consumers. Healthcare fraud is committed by a small minority of healthcare providers.

Healthcare fraud consists of billing for services which were never rendered or billing for expensive procedures that were never provided. Furthermore performing medically unnecessary services to generate to insurance payments is another form of fraud as well. Falsification of a patient's diagnosis to justify surgeries, procedures or tests that aren't medically necessary also is fraudulent. Accepting kickbacks for patient referrals constitutes fraud and waving patient copayments also constitutes fraud under Medicare.

Healthcare fraud also involves making a false diagnosis of a medical condition that a patient does not have or describing more severe conditions then the patient actually has as well. Identity theft is also fraudulent. Doing unnecessary procedures also constitutes medical fraud. There are fraud and abuse allegations in interventional pain management practices as well.

Furthermore, state investigators and state prosecutors have been targeting medical establishments that they believe may be operating as pill mills. It should be in noted that some pain physicians bill for patients that they have never seen even though prescriptions were written for narcotic medications.

Patients should be aware that some urine drug testing companies provide kickbacks to physicians who send urine drug screens to them. This is a serious offense and does some are draw attention from the federal government with respect to fraud.

Most pain clinics staff and are reputable and caring. However, many are not. For example, in 2009, insurance Corporate and Financial Investigations departments and law enforcement began receiving complaints about a doctor who claimed to specialize in pain management. One health insurance member in Michigan reported that his stolen insurance card had been used at the clinic by an individual trying to get narcotics. Another member said his wife had been contacted by a recruiter and told that she could get prescriptions for narcotics from this doctor.

Other tenants at the medical office building where the practice was located complained to police about the crowds that were gathering in the parking lot and hallways of the building while individuals waited for hours to be seen by this doctor.

Joint investigation by the FBI, DEA, U.S. Department of Health and Human Services-Office of Inspector General and Blue Cross Blue Shield of Michigan revealed that patients were getting prescriptions for narcotics for no medical purpose. Patients were recruited to come to the office and agreed to diagnostic tests. In return, they would receive cash or prescriptions for hydrocodone, Oxycontin, or Opana ER. Other patients agreed to get prescriptions for narcotics and then immediately turn them over to the recruiter. The recruiters were filling the prescriptions for resale on the streets.

In a typical visit, a patient would agree to medical tests such as blood tests, breathing tests, EKGs, EEGs, ultrasounds, X-rays, and psychological testing, no matter what their supposed medical problems were. All these tests were being billed to Blue Cross Blue Shield of Michigan and Medicare. The investigation revealed that for some of the tests that the clinic billed, the equipment was broken or the clinic did not even own the necessary equipment.

The doctor was initially charged in federal court with health care fraud. In a plea agreement, the doctor pled guilty to the charge of paying kickbacks. He was sentenced to 1 ½ years in jail and his medical license was suspended. At the time of his arrest, the government seized $883,452 in assets from the doctor which he has since forfeited.

Patients who take Schedule II drugs are subject to random urine drug screens to valuate drug compliance and to ascertain that an individual is not taking a non-prescribed scheduled medication. If a patient takes a drug as prescribed, that drug will be present in the urine as his/her kidneys excrete the drug from the body. In Baltimore, Maryland a federal grand jury indicted five defendants on charges arising from a scheme whereby physicians and administrative personnel associated with a

Maryland pain management practice agreed to refer urine specimens to a testing lab for evaluation in return for $1.37 million in kickbacks:

Federal investigators said Thursday that a pharmaceutical sales manager helped organize a kickback scheme that paid tens of thousands of dollars in illicit fees to medical professionals in Connecticut and elsewhere who prescribed a powerful painkiller his employer manufactured.

The payoff scheme probably cost the Medicare program millions of dollars by inducing physicians and other medical professionals to prescribe the painkiller to patients who were not eligible for the treatment under federal heath guidelines, authorities said.

FBI agents arrested a district sales manager for Arizona-based Insys Therapeutics, for paying kickbacks in relation to a federal health care program. His charges carry a sentence of up to five years. Pearlman, 49, of Edgewood, N.J., is accused of collecting a $95,000 quarterly bonus in 2013 based on his success selling Subsys, a powerful, fentanyl-based oral spray approved by the FDA to manage breakthrough pain experienced by cancer patients.

Insys and Subsys were not mentioned by name in legal filings associated with the arrest, but multiple officials confirmed the identities.

This individual was accused in an FBI affidavit of arranging for $83,000 in kickbacks to just one Connecticut nurse who was authorized to write prescriptions by her ex-employer, the Comprehensive Pain and Headache Treatment Center of Derby. This individual an advanced practice nurse, is cooperating with federal investigators and was among the highest Subsys prescribers in the country.

Another individual, has been charged with taking cancer drug kickbacks. Federal authorities said several of this physician's patients, who are Medicare Part D beneficiaries and who were prescribed the drug, did not have cancer, but were taking Subsys for chronic pain. Medicare and most private insurers will not pay for the drug unless the patient has an active cancer diagnosis and an explanation that the drug is needed to manage the patient's cancer pain.

Federal prosecutors said that a company executive arranged hundreds of "sham" speakers programs to pay off doctors and others qualified nurses for prescribing Subsys. The programs were ostensibly education gatherings to inform health professionals about pain management. In reality, federal officials said the programs were social gatherings at which Pearlman picked up the bill for food and drink and paid prescribers to attend.

The FBI said one drug company managers sales territory was Connecticut, Rhode island, New Jersey and New York and he arranged hundreds of speakers programs across the country. People involved in the investigation said it is continuing and that additional arrests are expected.

FBI agents arrested, a district sales manager for an Arizona-based Insys Therapeutics, for paying kickbacks in relation to a federal health care program. His charges carry a sentence of up to five years. One pharmaceutical company executive was accused of collecting a $95,000 quarterly bonus in 2013 based on his success selling Subsys, a powerful, fentanyl-based oral spray approved by the FDA to manage breakthrough pain experienced by cancer patients. The sales manager was accused in an FBI affidavit of arranging for $83,000 in kickbacks to one Connecticut nurse who was authorized to write prescriptions by her ex-employer.

A former Insys sales representative in Alabama also pleaded guilty to a conspiracy to violate the antikickback statute by paying two doctors to prescribe the drug. Illinois has filed claims against Insys related to pushing Subsys for unapproved uses.

The chief financial officer of a group of pain management clinics located in central Maryland was indicted. The group's clinics required its patients who have been prescribed pain relief medications to submit urine samples for testing in order to monitor the levels of pain medication or other narcotics in their bodies. The group's clinics generated hundreds of urine samples each month, which were sent to an outside lab for testing.

In March 2011, others at the group's clinics decided to shift the group's testing business to a laboratory testing company in New Jersey, after learning that the lab testing company was willing to pay a kickback for every urine sample that the group of clinics submitted for testing. The chief financial officer negotiated the arrangement, whereby the lab company promised to pay kickbacks equal to half of its profit, after accounting for expenses, for every urine sample that the group of clinics submitted for testing.

The group of clinics submitted urine samples for testing to the lab company from approximately March 2011 to August 2012. During this time, the lab company received total reimbursement payments of $4,033.846.70 from private insurers, Medicare and the Federal Employees Health Benefit Program for lab tests ordered by the group of clinics.

Between the time the kickback payments commenced in July 2011 and the end of the scheme in July 2012, the lab company paid the group of clinics a total of $1,376,540.85 in kickbacks. Out of this amount, chief financial officer received approximately $459,245.

A New Jersey doctor admitted to hiding more than $3.6 million in income to avoid paying taxes and using the money to bribe other medical professionals for illegal pain referrals. He made up phony payroll expenses and hid money from his pain management business in private accounts, according to the state Division of Criminal Justice. This type of corruption in the health care industry, which causes patients to receive unnecessary services and raises costs for all healthcare consumers.

Pain management clinic specialize in treating chronic pain patients. Treatments involve therapy, injections, implantable devices and oral pain medications. Legitimate pain clinics have a trained board certified clinician in charge of the clinic as previously mentioned . Multiple fraudulent pain man management clinics have occurred and now exist and in some cases have become problematic. Pain patients need to investigate a clinic before going to a pain clinic because of fraudulent practices and practitioners.

Over one trillion dollars has been spent on healthcare and more than 4 billion health insurance claims were processed in the United States in 2011. Some of these health insurance claims were noted to be fraudulent. These fraudulent claims however carry an extremely high financial cost. Healthcare fraud results in higher premiums and out-of-pocket expenses for consumers. Healthcare fraud is committed by a small minority of healthcare providers.

Healthcare fraud consists of billing for services they were never rendered or billing for expensive procedures that were never provided. Furthermore performing medically unnecessary services to generate to insurance payments is another form of fraud as well. Falsification of a patient's diagnosis to justify surgeries, procedures, or tests that are not medically necessary also constitutes fraud.

Accepting kickbacks for patient referrals in most instances constitutes fraud. Furthermore, waving patient copayments to entice a patient into an office also constitutes fraud under Medicare.

Healthcare fraud also involves making false diagnoses of a medical condition that a patient does not have or describing more severe conditions then the patient actually has as well. Identity theft is also fraudulent. A medical identity theft victim may unexpectedly be denied employment after a physical examination for potential employment because of a disease for which the person has never been diagnosed. Doing unnecessary procedures also constitutes medical fraud. There are fraud and abuse allegations in interventional pain management practices as well.

Furthermore, state investigators and prosecutors have been targeting medical establishments that they believe may be operating as pill mills. This occurs where patients with no pathology pay cash for narcotic prescriptions. It should be that some pain physicians bill for patients that they have never seen even though prescriptions were written for narcotic medications.

A patient should be aware that some urine drug testing companies provide kickbacks to physicians as well who send urine drug screens up to them for drug analysis. This is a serious offense and does some are draw attention from the federal government with respect to fraud.

Pain doctors can charge more money if a pain procedure is done under X-ray or ultrasound needle guidance. There have been cases where patients have been placed under or in a "plain box" and were charged for x-ray utilization for pain block procedures when an x-ray machine or an ultrasound device was not actually used.

It is not illegal for a physician to prescribe narcotic drugs to patients that have no disease nor have no reason to have pain. This occurs when patients take prescriptions, get narcotics, and give the prescribing physician certain sums of money in return. he patient in many instances then sells the drugs on the street.

Health care fraud is a crime that involves the filing of dissed honest healthcare claims for profit. It essentially involves the filing of unneeded procedures her medications. The FBI, the US Postal Service and the office of the inspector general are all involved in investigating healthcare fraud. Some physicians submit bills for procedures that were never done as well as submitting bills for office or hospital examinations that never took place.

The US Office of Management and Budget says "improper payments" made by Medicare in 2010 amounted to more than $47.8 billion. That represents almost 10% of the $528 billion total Medicare spend that year. In the current era of shrinking budgets and unbalanced budgets, the US simply cannot afford to allow this level of fraud.

Physician service "billing up coding "is not uncommon. A physician will bill for services at a higher level of complexity then the service actually provided. For example a provider may bill an insurance company for a motorized wheelchair when only providing a regular wheelchair without a motor.

Healthcare fraud cost American taxpayers $80 billion a year. Excessive services occur when Medicare for example is billed for something greater than what the actual care requires. For example, a patient may have wrist pain. An X ray would identify a patient's pathology in most instances. However, a dishonest physician who has an invested interest in a MRI unit will order an MRI of the wrist to make more profit.

Insurance codes are used by health plans to make decisions about how much to pay a doctor for his/her services to a patient. A patient should know something about these codes. The explanation of health benefits can be hard to understand with respect to these codes. These codes are used to reimburse the services performed by the healthcare provider as well as a patient's diagnosis.

One example of a code is a CPT code. This is used for medical billers. Certain codes reimburse physicians for higher amounts of money. Fraud occurs when medical providers give codes to insurance companies that are in error to make more money instead of the code that is supposed to be used for a specific medical condition.

There is a coding system called the International Classifications of Diseases or the ICD code. The code is assigned to identify the patient's specific health condition. These codes are used in combination with CPT codes to make sure that a patient's health condition and the services that a patient received match. The wrong code can result in an overpayment to a physician.

The health system reform law that President Obama and Congress passed closes the door on new physician-owned hospitals by prohibiting them from obtaining a Medicare provider number. Since 2003, several efforts have been mounted in Congress to ban or limit physician ownership. In general, health insurers strongly support the provision in the health reform law that bans self-referrals to new physician-owned hospitals because that practice drives up health costs by increasing utilization.

The US Office of Management and Budget says "improper payments" made by Medicare in 2010 amounted to more than $47.8 billion. That represents almost 10% of the $528 billion total Medicare spend that year. In the current era of shrinking budgets and unbalanced budgets, the US simply cannot afford to allow this level of fraud.

Recent changes to US whistleblower laws allow healthcare professionals to collect a significant financial reward (often millions of dollars) for reporting fraud against the government in the healthcare industry. US laws now allow individuals reporting Medicare fraud to receive full protection from retaliation and collect up to 30% of the fines that the government collects. The US government has paid out hundreds of millions of dollars to whistleblowers that come forward with information about healthcare fraud, with some individual whistleblowers receiving a reward worth tens of millions of dollars.

Medicare fraud whistleblowers are almost always healthcare professionals. They are commonly employed as hospital administrators, nurses, hospice or nursing home workers, ambulance drivers, pharmacists, or as any other type of healthcare professionals. The False Claims Act is often touted as the most effective tool the government and its citizens have to recover monies stolen by fraudulent and false claims lodged by government suppliers.

5. PAIN CAUSATION

Pain is complex, so there are many treatment options including medications, therapies, and mind-body techniques. A patient must initially know what pain is and subsequently learn the benefits and risks of each treatment, including addiction. A patient should understand the cause of his/her pain in order to decrease the incidence of unnecessary pain treatments. For example, muscle pain is less expensive to treat than ruptured disc pain. This knowledge may prevent you from having unnecessary spine surgery.

The word "pain" is derived from the Latin word poena that means punishment. St. Augustine wrote in the 5th century that all diseases afflicting Christians were derived from demons. Ancient tribal concepts of pain were based on beliefs that evil spirits were sent as punishment from their gods to invade one's body and cause severe pain. In the book of Genesis, Eve was condemned to pain during childbirth as a result of her encounter with the devil in the Garden of Eden. It has been reported that a shaman could suck an evil spirit from a wound to decrease one's pain.

The ancient Greeks such as Aristotle were the first individuals who believed that pain was derived from various nerves in the body. The exact cause of pain was unknown to them. Unfortunately, not unlike ancient times, the diagnosis and treatment of many chronic painful conditions today remains mostly guesswork. Pain medicine is for the most part subjectively based, because pain is a subjective symptom while other medical specialties are based upon objective medical evidence.

Pain in general is not bad. Pain is a protective mechanism that warns you that your body has something wrong at some location. The sensation of pain tells you to stop activity or to at least slow down your activity. For example if you sprain your ankle, your pain is a warning for you not to put weight on that leg. The International Association for the Study of Pain defines pain as" an unpleasant sensory and emotional experience associated with tissue injury as a result of trauma (e.g. bone fracture) or disease (e.g. cancer, shingles).

Pain has psychological effects in some instances especially when pain is severe. Pain may cause anxiety and depression. Acute pain is associated with injury, bone fractures, surgery or sprains and strains. Once these entities have healed sometimes, the pain continues. Arthritis is another example of chronic pain. Arthritic pain is caused by continuous joint destruction. However, once the pain becomes chronic, your pain it becomes a problem. Not only does pain become a personal problem but pain can become a social problem with creation of family problems, loss of self-esteem and lost wages. Fibromyalgia patients have alterations in CNS anatomy, physiology, and chemistry that potentially contribute to the symptoms experienced by these patients

The purpose of this chapter is to present you with the basic anatomy and physiology of painful sensations. Pain impulses are in essence, electrical signals that travel from various areas of your body such as the extremities, heart, appendix etc. to the spinal cord and eventually reach the brain where the pain signals are processed like data in a computer. The brain is like a computer hard drive, which stores painful experiences that ultimately results in the suffering associated with chronic pain. Pain is produced by unpleasant stimuli to nerve endings throughout the body which include chemical, extreme heat cold and mechanical injury. These nerve endings are silent until mechanical, heat or cold injures tissue. In order to experience pain we need these pain receptors and the nerve fibers that transmit pain to the spinal cord and then to the brain.

Nerves, which conduct pain impulses to the spinal cord, are composed of neurons (nerve cells) that make up nerve fibers that form neurons. Two common pain fibers are the C fibers and the A-delta fibers. A-delta fibers conduct fast onset sharp pain impulses. The C fibers conduct slow onset dull, aching or burning pain. If you hit your finger with a hammer, you will experience a sudden pain response followed by a dull pain response.

Other types of fibers that transmit touch and vibration exist do not cause pain in most instances. However, these fibers can become hypersensitive and may contribute to your total pain experience. A neuron is an electrically excitable cell in the nervous system that processes and transmits information. Neurons are the significant core components of your brain and spinal cord as well as your peripheral nerves. Neurons are typically composed of a cell body, a dendrite and an axon.. Neurons receive input from dendrites and transmit output via the axon.

Neurons are the building blocks of nerves. In other words, multitudes of neurons are necessary to form a nerve. Nerves that exist outside of your central nervous system are called a ganglion. Your stellate ganglion in your neck is an example. An injection into this ganglion may relieve pain associated with Reflex Sympathetic Dystrophy (now called

Complex the Regional Pain Syndrome). Various ganglia may form a plexus. An example of a plexus is your celiac plexus. Sometimes this plexus is blocked with numbing medicine or phenol or alcohol to relieve severe abdominal pain.

Action potentials generated by the neuron initiate pain signals. If your skin is pinched a mechanical pain receptor begins and action potential. An action potential begins after a depolarization (a change in the electrical activity within the neuron) such that it could cause a membrane transitory modification, turning prevalently permeable to sodium ions more than to potassium ions. Sodium permeability can cause an action potential.

Neuropathy generates a local accumulation of sodium channels, with a consequent increase of density. This remodel seems to be the basis of neuro hyperexecitably. Calcium channels have also an important role in cell working. Intracellular calcium increase contributes to depolarization processes, through kinase and determines the phosphorylation of membrane proteins that can make powerful the efficacy of the channels themselves.

Following an acute injury, AMPA receptors are stimulated which cause sharp pain. Receptors (areas in the body where biochemicals or drugs attach) are present in the spinal cord are called NMDA (N-methyl-D-aspartate) receptors and cause chronic pain.. When these NMDA receptors are stimulated, pain becomes more severe and this severe pain is maintained which implies that the pain does not decrease. The brain is responsible for the suffering associated with pain.

Pain results in bodily responses especially with respect to the cardiovascular system (heart rate increases, blood pressure increases, renal arteries constrict etc.). When pain is severe, the brain can cause the body to increase both the heart rate and blood pressure. Severe pain can also result in profuse sweating as well as nausea and vomiting. There are different types of nerve endings throughout the body. The pain nerve endings become hyper excitable when stimulated by injury, inflammation or a tumor. Occasionally the nerve endings remain irritable even after the painful stimulus has been removed. Pain signals from areas in the body reach the brain by four processes (transduction, transmission, modulation and perception).

The following illustration demonstrates by the arrows that pain signals enter the back of your spinal cord. They cross over to the other side. The pain impulses will then proceed upwards to go to your brain. It is important to know that pain signals can be dampened by structures and chemicals that exist in your spinal cord. Pain signals as mentioned previously are transmitted from the site of injury as action potentials. Electrical and/or chemical activity between the neuron dendrites and axons propagate the axon potentials.

Axons carry pain fibers away from your neuron and direct them to the dendrites of the next neuron until they terminate in your brain or spinal cord. Remember that the axons and dendrites do not touch. They form synapses or clefts between the axon and dendrite. The synapse has chemicals in the axon nerve ending. These chemicals allow communication between the neurons. Drugs are chemicals that can interrupt the communication between the neurons.

You need to understand that pain signals cross to the opposite side from the injury and therefore travel to the opposite side of your brain.It is important to understand these processes in order to understand how your pain can be treated effectively. Transduction is a process where electrical signals originate in the nerve endings throughout your body. These impulses are chemically, mechanically and/or thermally mediated and transmitted to your spinal cord where they can be modulated and then sent to your brain. Tissue injury or disease (including arthritis) cause the body to release biochemicals called prostaglandins.

Prostaglandins themselves do not cause pain. Prostaglandins do however sensitize pain receptors to other chemicals in the body, which facilitate the transmission of pain impulses. Nonsteroidal drugs like ibuprofen decrease the number of prostaglandins produced in your body and may in a decrease in your pain perception. Topical creams such as Ben Gay can decrease the process of transduction at the nerve endings.

Transmission is a process where pain signals are transported to the spinal cord. Nerves in body tissues transmit impulses to the spinal cord. Nerve blocks with anesthetics like Novicaine can interrupt the transmission of pain impulses to the spinal cord. Once pain impulses reach the spinal cord they are modulated or changed by chemicals and nerves that inhibit or lessen the number of pain impulses from going up the spinal cord to your brain. Fibers called internuncial fibers are present within the spinal cord that can decrease pain transmission. The brain can send impulses back to these pain control fibers within the spinal cord to decrease the number of impulses that reach the pain perception center of the brain. This is the basis of hypnosis.

Severe pain however, overwhelms the nerve fibers and they essentially become ineffective. Most pain impulses cross over into the opposite side of the spinal cord from where they entered the spinal cord.

The spinal cord acts like a transformer to intensify or decrease the intensity of pain impulses. Narcotics and anticonvulsants can modulate pain impulses within the spinal cord. Finally, pain impulses reach the brain where you perceive pain. Be aware that pain signals enter the posterior part of your spinal cord (figure 1) and then cross to the other side and travel upwards to the pain processing of your brain.

Narcotics can "numb" your brain to decrease the effects of the pain impulses on your brain by decreasing the intensity of these impulses. Higher brain centers determine how we respond to a painful stimulus. This explains why an individual can respond differently to a painful stimulus from other individuals (eg. "cry baby, whiner, vs macho man etc.). A chapter describing the anatomy and physiology of pain is not complete without an explanation of the Gate Theory of pain. Melzak and Wall described this theory in 1965. Different types of nerve fibers (both pain and non-pain fibers) enter the spinal cord at the same time. Non-pain fibers essentially dilute out the number of pain impulses that enter the spinal cord.

An example of the Gate Control Theory is given by the following analogy. If you can imagine severe pain impulses represented by of multiple black balls going down a sink (analogy to spinal cord). If one adds multiple white balls (neutral non-pain transmitting entities), the number of black balls (pain impulses) is diluted. Therefore less severe impulses reach the spinal cord and the brain. The white balls are non-pain balls and can close the gate (drain) to the number of black balls that go down the sink. To open the gate to more pain impulses, one only needs to decrease the number of white balls going to the hole in the sink.

At this time, there are more black balls (pain impulses) available. The gate is now open. As you can see, pain perception in the human body is complex. Because there are many different chemical transmitters and anatomic structures that contribute to chronic pain syndromes, each patient's treatment must be individualized. This is where the art of pain medicine is separated from pure science.

In order to understand pain transmission concepts, you must first become familiar with several biochemicals that are stored in your body that affect your pain signals. In order for you to hurt, pain-producing chemicals in your body tissue must stimulate pain fibers (Alpha-delta and C fibers). In general, the greater the tissue trauma, the more pain transmitting chemicals are produced and the worse the pain.

In medical terminology, a stimulus (pin prick) produces a response (pain perception). When a stimulus such as heat produces, tissue injury chemicals are released at the site of nerve injury, which cause pain fibers to become hyperactive. These chemicals include bradykinin, histamine, substance p, acetylcholine, serotonin and histamine. These chemicals act at the nerve endings and ultimately travel to the spinal cord and brain.

The nerves that conduct pain go to the spinal cord that allows pain signals to ultimately reach the brain. Areas of your body that have many pain receptors include the skin, the outer aspect of bone called the periosteum, ligaments, joints, teeth and gums and the cornea of the eye. Muscle also contains pain fibers but not as many per square meter (a measure of area) as the previously mentioned structures.

Where the nerves from your body enter your spinal cord, aspartic and glutamic acid are produced. These acids increase pain impulse generation. NMDA may also be produced. GABA (gamma-aminobutyric acid) in the spinal cord on the other hand, decreases the number of pain impulses that reach the brain. GABA inhibits pain impulse transmission. Norepinepherine and serotonin are two more chemicals in the spinal cord which attenuate the number of pain impulses which reach your brain.

The brain and spinal cord regulate pain by the production of naturally occurring narcotic-like substances that decrease pain transmission in specific areas of the brain. These narcotic-like drugs are called enkephalins, dynorphins and beta-endorphins. Some of these substances also decrease pain transmission in the spinal cord. Enkephalins are located in areas of the brain related to pain modulation.

Enkephalins inhibit pain at the spinal cord level. Enkephalins bind to narcotic receptors. When the narcotic receptors are activated, they inhibit pain signals. Dynorphins exist in both the brain and spinal cord but are more prevalent in the brain. Like enkephalins these substances bind to narcotic receptors in the brain and spinal cord. Pain impulses that enter your spinal cord cross over to the other side and then progress upward to your brain.

The natural beta-endorphins in your body exhibit morphine-like activity. They work like morphine to decrease your pain. Following injury or stress these endorphins are released into the blood stream. The effects of beta-endorphins are similar to morphine. Beta-endorphins like narcotics can cause respiratory depression, constipation, euphoria, tolerance and physical dependence. The exact biochemical actions of all of the substances mentioned are complex.

For a more detailed explanation of the actions of these substances one should consult a pain medicine textbook. The purpose of this chapter is to emphasize the multiple substances that can generate the transmission of pain signals. This is furthermore the reason why there are so many medications available for the management of your pain. This is also the reason why your physician may prescribe multiple medications for the management of your chronic pain.

With respect to tissue and nerve ending biochemicals, neurotransmitters and pain transduction, your physician may recommend a skin (topical) cream to decrease the transmission of pain signals to your brain. Red pepper cream decreases the pain generator called substance P. An example is Zostrix cream. Menthol containing creams (Ben Gay) also decrease pain over muscles and joints. Non-steroidal anti-inflammatory drugs (NSAIDS) decrease the production of prostaglandin that can sensitize your body to pain mediators. Examples include Advil and Celebrex.

Remember that prostaglandins sensitize pain nerve endings to pain producing tissue chemicals. Antidepressant drugs like Elavil or Prozac decrease pain by increasing norepinephrine and serotonin in the spinal cord. As previously mentioned, these two substances decrease the number of pain impulses that reach the pain perception areas of the brain.

Anticonvulsant drugs like Gabitril (tiagabine) affect GABA and by enhancing GABA blood levels which in turn decreases the number of pain signals in your spinal cord that can go to your brain. Narcotic drugs also decrease pain impulse conduction in both the spinal cord and brain. Injections of numbing medicine (local anesthetics with steroids) can decrease pain in muscle and nerves in the arms, legs and the trunk of the body.

Epidural steroid injections can decrease pain in nerves that are buried deep within the spine. As you see there are multiple biochemical sources of pain and in many instances your physician may elect to prescribe multiple medications with good reason. Remember that each of these medications can have side effects that will be discussed in a later chapter. There is an area of your brain that represents an area where you process pain signals.

This area detects tissue injury and is a protective mechanism to alert you that something is wrong. A burn of the palm of your hand alerts your brain that tissue injury is occurring and initiates a reflex in your spinal cord to have you immediately remove your hand from the hot object. Without pain interpretation in your brain, you could sustain multiple bodily trauma and have no knowledge of its occurrence.

The different dimensions of pain perception have been shown to depend on different areas of your brain. In contrast, much less is known about the neural basis of pathological chronic pain. Patients may report combinations of spontaneous pain and allodynia/hyperalgesia-abnormal pain evoked by stimuli that normally induce no/little sensation of pain. Modern neuroimaging methods (positron emission tomography (PET) and functional MRI (fMRI)) have been used to determine whether different neuropathic pain symptoms involve similar brain structures.

PET scan studies have suggested that spontaneous neuropathic pain is associated principally with changes in thalamic activity and the medial pain system, which is preferentially involved in the emotional dimension of pain. Not only are there areas of your brain where you perceive pain but there are areas that are responsible for suffering as well. An area of your brain called the amygloid is associated with fear.

Animals who have had their amygloid areas excised do not exhibit fear. Fear, suffering and pain are in different areas of your brain but these areas are connected to each other. These interconnections ultimately can communicate with areas of your brain that control your heart rate and respiratory rate as well. If you have severe pain you may sweat profusely in addition to having increases in your heart and respiratory rates. As you can see, severe pain can have adverse physiologic effects on your body.

6. PAIN COSTS

Approximately forty-eight million Americans suffer from chronic pain. According to a previous Wall Street article, Americans spend over 100 billion dollars on pain care. Over one third of all adult Americans suffer from chronic pain. Over the counter annual analgesic costs amount to three billion dollars. Chronic pain is a prevalent and costly problem. One must assess the clinical effectiveness and cost-effectiveness of the most common treatments for patients with chronic pain.

Untreated or under treated chronic pain costs health plans and their purchasers much money. It afflicts 40 million or more Americans, with a cost of nearly $100 billion a year in direct medical costs and indirect costs, such as lost productivity and workers' compensation, according to the American Pain Society. Most primary care physicians are not adequately treating pain, primarily because they are not trained to do so and because they are afraid of litigation and regulatory restrictions.

Chronic pain with conservative care such as medications, physical therapy, chiropractic etc. costs North American adults an estimated $10,000 to $15,000 per person per year. Furthermore, estimates of the cost of pain do not include the nearly 30,000 people that die in North America each year due to non-steroidal anti-inflammatory drug-induced gastric lesions.

Because patients usually have to pay a significant portion of their bill for fees charged for procedures done on them as well as for medications prescribed, representative published studies that evaluate the clinical effectiveness of pharmacological treatments, conservative (standard) care, surgery, nerve blocks and pain rehabilitation programs must be examined and compared. When you're in pain, the last thing you want to think about is the cost of getting the relief you deserve.

Your physician can help. The cost-effectiveness of various treatment approaches must also be considered. Outcome criteria of a particular treatment should include the prevalence of pain reduction. Patients prior to consenting to any treatment modality should evaluate medication use and health care consumption. In addition to clinical effectiveness, the cost-effectiveness of conservative care, surgery and nerve blocks must be compared.

There are limitations to the success of all available treatments. Chronic pain programs are in many instances in need of rehabilitation.

Although hard statistics regarding such programs are difficult to obtain, one frequently hears of programs closing down or modifying their treatment protocols to meet their own survival needs rather than meeting the needs of the patients they serve.

After rapid growth during the 1980s and through the mid-1990s, the number of inpatient chronic pain management programs actually declined. Concurrent with the decline in intensive programs is the rise of procedural interventions and medications, which receive a great deal of support from hospitals and pharmaceutical companies. The use of muscle relaxants for patients appears to be increasingly prevalent when compared with teaching relaxation techniques, and implanting a device is more lucrative than giving patient's guidance or advice.

Healthcare specialists have to determine whether this apparent shift in treatment emphasis away from rehabilitation is a healthy development for the patients they serve. Many hospitals encourage physicians with minimal or no training to open pain clinics in their facilities. They can charge facility fees of $1000.00 or more for a procedure like an epidural steroid injection. Your physician doing the procedure may own shares in the center or hospital. As a result, every time that a physician schedules a procedure in the hospital he or she makes a share of the profit. The sad fact is that this behavior is legal.

Medical procedures, such as trigger-point injections, sympathetic nerve blocks, and epidural steroid injections, are rated as significantly less helpful, less invasive modalities; despite their considerably higher average cost. Research is needed to identify which patients are most likely to benefit from the available treatments and to study combinations of the available treatments since none of them appears capable of eliminating pain or significantly improving functional outcomes for all treated. The cost of chronic benign (non-cancer pain) spinal pain is large and is increasing.

The costs of interventional treatment for spinal pain were at a minimum of $13 billion (U.S. dollars) in 1990, and the costs are growing at least 7% per year. The interventional medical treatment of chronic pain costs $9000 to $19,000 per person per year. It should be understood that only a small percentage of patients receive long-term relief with these procedures. You should inquire about the cost of any treatment before agreeing to have the procedure done. You also need to contact your insurance carrier and ascertain if your treatment is covered under your insurance plan.

Before consenting to a potential expensive therapy do research. Check the Internet for a description of the procedure and if it is effective. Ask your physician what the cost is for the treatment in question. Is there a surgery center charge in addition to the physician fee? You should ask your physician if there is an extra fee for sedation if you have to have a nerve block. Some centers bundle this fee with the facility charge.

Your treatment for your back pain may only cost $3.00 for a bottle of aspirin. However, you need to calculate and add your chiropractor fees or the costs of a massage. What about the housekeeper you had to hire to do the housework that you can't do while you were disabled? What about the heating pad? What does it cost you if you need to cut down on the hours you work, or quit your job because of your pain? Pain costs can affect your family if your spouse has to take off work to help you.

Pain treatment can be expensive for you but a question arises concerning the cost of you not receiving pain management. Pain patients frequently miss work because their pain is too severe to allow them to work. As a result business productivity can be decreased. Lost workdays also cost businesses money. The overall cost of pain amounts to over sixty billion dollars per year. When deciding on whether or not to get pain treatment the following are recommended: call your medical insurance company and find out what treatments your insurer will cover.

You need to ascertain if you have to pay co-payments and how much those costs are. You also need to know whether the balance of the charge beyond the co-payment will be billed to your insurer, or whether you have to pay in full when the service is provided and then request reimbursement from your insurer. You should also ask your insurance company if it will pay for alternative medicine therapies like acupuncture.

If you could look at your past 12 months and calculate how much time that you lost from work because of your pain and compare these figures to your cost of receiving care, you can estimate the actual cost of your treatment. For example, if an epidural steroid injection costs $500.00 but saves you 3 days of lost work time at $200.00/day, you actually save $100.00. If an injection keeps your activities of daily living normal, then one would expect the treatment to be cost effective if the treatment itself is effective.

Professional fees charged by physicians may differ from doctor to doctor. In some areas of the United States, physicians will post their professional service fees somewhere in their office so that you are informed of the costs before you consent to a procedure. Before you seek medical care, you should call several pain management offices to ascertain professional fees. Your primary care physician will then refer you to a physician that you chose.

Physicians and pharmacists are entrusted to make decisions that are medically necessary and that are in the best interest of their patients, not for their own personal financial gain. According to the indictment and documents filed in court a physician specializing in physical medicine and rehabilitation. She was a participating provider in Medicare and Medicaid. Most of her patients were Medicare and Medicaid beneficiaries. This doctor was the sole owner and CEO of a physical medicine practice.

According to the indictment and documents filed in court, from at least February 2011 through December 2014, this doctor conspired with others to fraudulently bill Medicare and Medicaid for topical pain-relief creams that she prescribed. The defendant referred virtually every patient prescribed topical pain-relief cream to a single pharmacy, which prepared and dispensed the topical pain-relief creams.

According to the indictment and documents filed in court, the manager and part-owner of the pharmacy was charged separately by information, and a pharmacist was also charged separately by information, he compounded pain creams using bulk-powder forms of the various ingredients called for by the prescriptions and dispensed in the pain creams to customers.

The pharmacy then submitted claims for reimbursement to Medicare and Medicaid that falsely represented that the pain creams had been made using tablet, capsule or liquid forms of the various ingredients in the pain creams. The physician received more than $40,000 in kickbacks.

According to the indictment and documents filed in court, the physician also knowingly wrote prescriptions, on at least one occasion, for morphine and oxycodone in the absence of a legitimate medical purpose and outside the course of usual professional practice.

According to evidence presented at the eight day trial, from at least January 2011 through May 2014, the pain management physician defrauded federal health benefit programs including: Medicare, Medicaid, TRICARE, Federal Employees Health Benefits Program and the Office of Workers' Compensation Programs. This physician filed claims for procedures that were not performed. Specifically, the physician performed less expensive procedures but falsely billed for procedures that provided higher reimbursement amounts. Finally, the physician submitted claims for procedures that had not been performed at all.

For example, the physician submitted claims that he had performed nerve block injections with the use of an imaging guidance machine, when in fact he neither owned nor used such a machine. The physician also falsely documented patient files to indicate that an imaging guidance machine had been used to verify needle placement and caused the alteration or destruction of patient files to conceal the scheme from auditors and law enforcement.

In 2015 alone, the U.S. government recovered over $3.6 billion in either settlements or judgments in cases brought under the False Claims Act. In another case, the U.S. Attorney for the District of Vermont alleged that a physician knowingly presented, or caused to be presented, hundreds of false claims for payment to the Medicare and Medicaid programs for 'trigger point injections' that were not reasonable and medically necessary and which did not comply with applicable Medicare and Medicaid laws, regulations, and program requirements."

The case was investigated by the Medicaid Fraud and Residential Abuse Unit of the Attorney General's Office, the United States Attorney's Office, and the Office of the Inspector General of the Department of Health and Human Services.

The government alleged that the trigger point injections performed by the physician in question The "medication" consisted only of saline or saline-based "anthroposophic injectates," which did not have any health benefits, and were not considered reasonable or medically necessary under Medicare and Medicaid regulations.

Unfortunately 42 percent of Medicare patients experience unnecessary treatment. A 2012 report said Medicare and Medicaid, the government insurance program for the poor, waste up to $87 billion annually on "care rooted in outmoded habits, supply-driven behaviors and ignoring science."

The Office of Inspector General (OIG), Department of Health and Human Services (HHS), in a 2009 report, showed that unqualified nonphysicians performed 21% of the services. These nonphysicians did not possess the necessary licenses, certifications, credentials, or training to perform the services. Since the time the medical profession was founded, advances in treatments and technology, as well as educational and training standards, have promoted a desire to go forward beyond the basic scope of a physician pain practice.

Supporters of interventional pain management disagree on multiple aspects for various reasons while detractors claim that interventional pain management should not exist as a specialty. Issues to be addressed with respect to the practice of pain management include appropriate use of evidence-based medicine overuse, overutilization, and abuse.

7. PAIN RELIEF

This chapter presents a general overview of modalities available to treat your pain. These modalities will be discussed individually in later chapters in this book. The ability to relieve pain is very variable and unpredictable, depending on the source or location of pain and whether it is acute or chronic. Pain mechanisms are complex and have peripheral and central nervous system aspects. Therapies should be tailored to the specifics of the pain process or processes in the individual patient.

Modalities are specialized therapeutic techniques, agents or devices often integrated into the comprehensive treatment program. Modalities utilize sound waves, heat, mechanical, electrical, and light energy to create changes in tissues for therapeutic purposes. Modalities utilize sound waves, heat, mechanical, electrical, and light energy to create changes in tissues for therapeutic purposes.

A patient evaluation should initially include a pain history and assessment of the impact of pain on the patient, a directed physical examination, a review of previous diagnostic studies, a review of previous interventions, a drug history, and an assessment of coexisting diseases or conditions.

Treatment planning should be tailored to both the individual and the presenting problem. Consideration should be given to different treatment modalities, such as formal pain rehabilitation program, the use of behavioral strategies, the use of non-invasive techniques, or the use of medications, depending upon the physical and psychosocial impairment related to the pain. An opioid trial should not be initiated in the absence of a complete assessment of the chronic pain complaint.

Passive modalities are described as the application of some form of cold, heat, or electricity to the body to assist in pain management. These modalities are referred to as "passive," as the recipient does not have to actively participate. The modality is applied while the patient is at rest.

The most common forms of heat include moist hot packs and ultrasound. Cold treatments, or cryotherapy, can be used to minimize pain as well. This can be administered in the form of cold packs and ice massage to the low back. Fluoromethane is a spray that can also be applied to the skin by the therapist, and is usually followed by a series of therapist-assisted stretches.

Electric stimulation can also be used to control pain. Some specific types include TENS (transcutaneous electric nerve stimulation) and microcurrent. In cases where TENS has been found to be helpful in controlling pain, especially chronic pain, a portable TENS unit can be obtained for home use.

Aquatic therapy can be a useful resource for patients with chronic pain conditions, or patients who are having difficulty functioning on land. The benefit of performing treatments in the pool is a reduction in weight bearing, and a safe atmosphere to work on any balance issues. " For deconditioned patients or those with global, chronic pain due to conditions such as fibromyalgia, aquatic therapy offers a faster return to functional movement and a form of maintenance exercise they can take with them after rehab.

Anesthesiologists do nerve blocks and prescribe narcotic medications. Physical medicine and rehabilitation specialists prescribe physical therapy exercises and modalities using heat and cold to relieve pain. Neurologists control pain with anti-seizure medications. Psychiatrists decrease pain with antidepressant drugs. Psychologists manage pain with psychological counseling, hypnosis and biofeedback. Rheumatologists administer steroids into painful joints.

Physical therapists will rehabilitate your body. Chiropractors manipulate your spine to control your back and neck pain by realigning your spine and taking pressure off your nerves. Surgeons operate on nerves, joints and discs to lessen the suffering of pain. In many chronic pain states a multidisciplinary approach using all or most of the mentioned pain specialists is used to manage complex pain problems such as reflex sympathetic dystrophy which will be described in a later chapter.

Which modalities actually work? Each of these modalities can help you with your pain. In many instances a multidisciplinary pain center can provide you with the most benefit. You should investigate what therapies are scientifically sound. You should have some basic knowledge about scientific studies that have been.

Suppose your neighbor tells you that you need procedure "X" to manage your pain. Her doctor does this procedure and your neighbor says that her doctor will do it on you. You should take the time to examine studies that recommend this procedure as being wonderful and revolutionary. For example injection "X" is reported in a newspaper advertisement to relieve low back pain in 80% of patients. WOW! This must be a great procedure. You do some investigating. The results are placed in the following table.

	Pain Relief (%)	No Pain Relief (%)
Group I (100 patients)	80 %	20 %

Table 1. Pain relief with new pain device.

What is missing? You need to know how many individuals with the same pain symptoms who did not have this procedure had relief of their pain. On the other hand, you could look at a group of patients with the same treatment who received another drug or substance. This is called a control group. Now compare injection "X" treatment with what is referred to as a sham treatment or a control treatment. .

A sham treatment is essentially a placebo treatment. Now examine the results comparing injection "X" with the placebo. The placebo is essentially better than injection "X". A good study will always have a comparison group. Do not be fooled by testimonials or by studies that have no comparison group. Remember that statistics can be manipulated if there is no control group.

	Pain Relief (%)	No Pain Relief (%)
Group I (100 patients)	80 %	20 %
Group II (100 patients)	81 %	19 %

Table 2. The natural course of the pain is similar to injection X.

You can see now that there is no difference in the groups that received the treatment compared to individuals who did not receive the treatment. You should not be fooled by claims of success that have no merit.

Nerve blocks are frequently used to manage pain. Local anesthetics like Novocain used in combination with steroids are deposited near the nerves or tissues that are responsible for chronic pain. These anesthetics stop pain production by numbing the nerves responsible for your pain. The steroids decrease the irritability of the pain producing nerves.

Certain techniques, such as continuous local anesthetic infusions, may warrant an escalated level of monitoring and ancillary care. Other techniques, such as the infiltration of a wound with local anesthetic or the addition of a nonsteroidal anti-inflammatory agent to a regimen of mild oral narcotics are so simple that excluding them from patient care is almost callous and inconsiderate.

Attention to the mechanisms of pain that may be present in a given situation, whether it be muscle spasm, ischemia, inflammation, edema, or nerve injury, may guide the clinician toward a more rational approach in managing that pain.

In many instances these blocks will break the pain cycle. Many patients respond to drug therapy. Mild and strong narcotics are prescribed depending on the severity of your pain. Pain patches with either a local anesthetic or a strong narcotic exist which give a patient sustained pain relief. Long acting narcotics (Oxycontin) exist which decrease the need for frequent drug dosing.

Antidepressants and anticonvulsants modulate pain transmission in the spinal cord. Muscle relaxants decrease muscle spasm that can significantly decrease your pain. Non-steroidal anti-inflammatory drugs alleviate pain by decreasing tissue inflammation. The Chinese have used acupuncture for over 2000 years. This method of pain relief consists of placing small needles into the skin and muscles over the body.

The needles stimulate larger nerves that go to the spinal cord and release endorphins and enkephalins. These substances decrease the number of pain impulses that go to the brain. Chiropractic therapy consists of manipulating the spine by a physician trained in safe spinal manipulation.

A chiropractor aligns the spine. This maneuver takes pressure off the nerves coming off the spinal cord that decreases pain conduction. Psychologists may help control pain with hypnosis or biofeedback. Hypnosis helps activate the nerves in the spinal cord that block pain signals from traveling up your spinal cord to your brain.

Biofeedback uses a machine to enable a pain patient to relax painful muscle. Physical therapists administer modalities that provide heat and cold to your muscles and ligaments. Some therapists do massage therapy that relaxes painful muscles. Electrical stimulation applied to the body decreases pain in a variety of painful conditions. The device is called a TENS (Transcutaneous Electrical Nerve Stimulator) unit. This instrument is battery powered.

A TENS unit stimulates endorphin and enkephalin production in your spinal cord. Neurosurgeons can place implantable devices in your body to control severe pain. One device is called a narcotic pump. This device gives a drop of morphine or other strong narcotic into the fluid around the spinal cord. The other surgically implanted device is called a spinal dorsal column stimulator. A wire is attached to a battery source that is placed in your body. The wire is placed parallel to your spinal cord.

This stimulation releases endorphins and enkephalins within the spinal cord. As one can see many modalities are available to patients for the control of their chronic pain. Which one is right for you? The proper treatment for your pain will depend on the severity of your pain as well as your physical and mental health status.

When considering a modality to relieve your pain, you should be aware of another important concept. Evidence-based medicine (EBM) is an attempt to more uniformly apply the standards of evidence gained from scientific medical studies to certain aspects of medical practice. Specifically, EBM seeks to assess the quality of medical evidence relevant to the risks and benefits of treatments (including lack of treatment). According to the Centre for Evidence-Based Medicine, "Evidence-based medicine is the conscientious, explicit and judicious use of current best evidence in making decisions about the care of individual patients.

EBM, however, seeks to clarify those parts of medical practice that are in principle subject to scientific methods and to apply these methods to ensure the best prediction of outcomes in medical treatment, even as debate about which outcomes are desirable continues". EBM requires clinical expertise, but also expertise in retrieving, interpreting, and applying the results of scientific studies and in communicating the risks and benefits of different courses of action to patients.

Evidence-based medicine/healthcare is looked upon as a new paradigm, replacing the traditional medical paradigm that is based on standard of care authority (which is common practice in your state). It is dependent on the use of randomized controlled trials, as well as systematic reviews (of a series of trials) and meta-analysis, although it is not restricted to these. There is also an emphasis on the dissemination of information, as well as its collection, so that the evidence can reach clinical practice. It therefore has commonality with the idea of research-based practice.

Having considered the extent to which EBM represents a departure from basing medical decisions on customary practices, there may be a change in the extent to which medical custom remains prevalent in the legal standard of care analysis. A problem ensues in the custom-based standard of care that courts have traditionally used to determine medical malpractice liability.

If you are injured from a medical procedure, should the court use the old procedure as the standard of care or the new procedure that is supported by evidence based medicine? For these reasons, current standard of care analysis is potentially inconsistent with the practice of EBM.

This concept is important because traditionally, local customs established the standard of care in medical malpractice actions. Under a custom-based standard, practicing in accordance with accepted practice generally decreases medical liability. Physicians have in the past needed only to conform to the "customs of their peers."

Often pain can be treated with physical therapy as a part of a comprehensive chronic pain treatment program through passive and active therapies. Forms of passive therapy include traction, electrical stimulation, ultrasound, hot packs, and ice packs. Active therapy includes aerobic conditioning, strengthening exercises, muscular release, and stretching. Manual therapy is an especially effective method of treating pain. Manual therapy involves restoring movement to stiff joints and reducing muscle tension in order to return a patient to full mobility.

While the mainstay of chiropractic is spinal manipulation, chiropractic care now includes a wide variety of other treatments, including manual or manipulative therapies, postural and exercise education, ergonomic training (how to walk, sit, and stand to limit back strain), nutritional consultation, and even ultrasound and laser therapies. In addition, chiropractors today often work in conjunction with primary care doctors, pain experts, and surgeons to treat patients with pain.

In 1996, the FDA gave acupuncture its first U.S. seal of approval, when it classified acupuncture needles as medical devices. In the 20 years since, study after study indicates that acupuncture can relieve pain. Pain tends to come in two varieties: acute and chronic. Acupuncture treatment can be very helpful for both.

As you can see, EBM can cause some legal problems if you are injured from a procedure in a certain medical community. If the standard of care was to do unsafe medicine that EBM demonstrated to be unsafe you need a legal consultation. For example, it used to be acceptable to put steroids in your spinal fluid for the management of back pain.

Acupuncturists insert hair-thin needles into the skin at specific points around the body. It is virtually painless. Inserting the needles into the body is thought to correct imbalances in the flow of energy in the body. Acupuncture is thought to ease pain by affecting neurotransmitters, hormone levels, or the immune system.

It is no longer the standard of care in most communities. What is your recourse if you had this procedure and developed complications? Complications could take months to years to develop in some instances. You need to realize that EBM practices may differ from customary care in your community. For this reason, you should not attempt to handle your own case. Instead, you should seek the advice of an attorney.

8. PAIN ASSESSMENT

Pain is a subjective experience for which there are no objective biological markers. There is no objective measurement of pain. Self-report is considered the most accurate and appropriate pain assessment method as family members and caregivers often underestimate a patient's pain. As researchers work toward developing better treatments for chronic pain they will need adequate ways to assess pain and its effects on life. Patients should be asked to rate their pain both to better understand its severity as well as to give a baseline assessment to determine changes in the level of pain after treatment. Pain is the most common reason why a patient visits a physician.

Pain is a complex entity and is affected by tissue injury but also by previous pain experiences, as well as by your psyche (anxiety and depression) and by any pending lawsuits. The transition from acute pain following an injury to chronic pain cannot be explained. The entity that we refer to as pain cannot be touched or felt by the treating physician. As a result, you must give your doctor an accurate assessment of your pain. Many chronic pain patients have seen a variety of physicians before seeing a pain medicine specialist. Many patients become frustrated and sometimes feel that no one believes that they truly hurt.

A patient's pain may not correlate with findings or lack of findings on a physical examination and X- rays. A patient's pain can only be adequately diagnosed after the treating physician has done a good history and physical examination. A clinician cannot feel your pain. As a result, you will be given papers to fill out with questions to answer. Questions asked will include a history of your pain, a pain diagram and occasionally a depression and/or activity assessment. Significant depression can worsen your pain.

Several different techniques are available for your doctor to use in determining your level of pain. Commonly used techniques include verbal, visual, and psychological tests. Both you and your doctor are responsible for documenting and recording trends in the intensity and frequency of your pain. This information tells each of you whether your pain has really improved or whether it has worsened.

Charting your pain levels in a diary will help your doctor see your long-range (weeks-months) pain trends, which are ultimately more important than your day-to-day pain trends. One important factor used to assess your progress is your activity. Did you return to work after taking off for a painful episode? Are you playing tennis etc.? A pain assessment provides a baseline for your doctor to assess any therapy or medications you are currently taking, and it also helps your doctor prescribe future therapy methods. Your doctor also needs to be able to determine how much disability you have in order to prescribe the appropriate types of therapy for you.

Your doctor will depend on you for accurate and reliable answers to questions about the pain you experience. Because pain involves many aspects such as sensory, emotional, and behavioral factors, it is difficult to measure the amount of pain you feel based on one single parameter. The choice of a pain-assessment test depends on the needs of both you and your doctor. A functional evaluation, such as reports of your daily activities, must be included in your assessment. If your doctor does not ask about your daily activities, voluntarily tell him your further limitations with respect to work, recreation, dressing, fixing meals, and any other daily activities. Progress continues to be made in developing pain-assessment tools.

You or your doctor should not oversimplify your pain assessment. The objective reports you are able to give, as well the observations your doctor is able to make about your behavior, are important to accurate pain management decisions. Because pain is subjective and can be observed only by you, it is important that the reports of your pain levels come from you. This will give your doctor a more accurate measurement of the type of pain you are experiencing.

For example, if you just complain of a toothache, your doctor will have almost no way of knowing how severe your pain condition is. There is no general consensus among pain medicine doctors as to the best test for the measurement of pain. An ideal test for the assessment of pain must bring together experimental as well as clinical knowledge.

One way of assessing your pain is to use a numeric scale. This is the simplest method for attempting to measure your pain. During this test, you are asked to rate your pain on a scale of 0 to 5 or to use words such as "none," "slight," "moderate," or "severe." This assessment is also a quick, simple, and reliable way to evaluate the effectiveness of any medications you are taking to manage your pain.

On the numeric scale, 0 equals no pain, 1 equals mild pain, 2 equals moderate pain, 3 equals distressing pain, 4 equals horrible pain, and 5 equals excruciating pain confining you to bed rest. This method is easily understood and may be helpful in guiding the treatment plans your doctor creates for you. Another type of verbal scale asks you to rate your pain on a scale of 1 to 10, with 1 being equivalent to pain that is barely noticeable and 10 relating to excruciating pain. A verbal numeric scale is easily understood. All you have to do is choose a number to represent your level of pain.

Another method used by some doctors is a pain diary. This is a descriptive report you keep to assess your pain. The pain diary shows a written account of your day-to-day experiences. It can be used to help diagnose the causes of your pain. The value of the pain diary is that you and your doctor can monitor your day-to-day variation of painful states and your response to therapy. You need to keep a diary of your pain patterns when you are sitting, standing, and lying down.

You should also record your sleep patterns and sexual activity. You also must note the amount of pain medication you are taking and whether it lessens your pain. Because pain can interfere with eating patterns, keep a diary of the amount of food you eat and at what time you ate. Be sure to include any types of recreational activities and whether your pain felt better or worse afterward.

Pain drawings offer a visual way to evaluate your pain. You will be asked to shade in areas on a human figure outline that correspond to the areas of your pain. The drawing will help your doctor determine where your pain is coming from and how widespread it is on your body. Over time, your pain drawings can be compared to show the changes of your pain and how you are responding to therapy.

After observing your behavior, your doctor may classify your pain behavior by using the following four-class system: Class 1 consists of patients with low physical injury but high levels of abnormal behavior patterns related to their pain. Class 2 consists of patients with lower physical injury and low behavior pattern abnormalities. Class 3 consists of patients with significant tissue injury in addition to high behavioral pattern abnormalities. Class 4 consists of patients with a high tissue injury and normal behavioral patterns.

A McGill pain questionnaire is a method for assessing pain psychologically. A McGill pain questionnaire gives a multidimensional pain score. You are given 20 word sets that describe a different dimension of your pain. You are asked to select words relevant to your pain from each of these 20 sets. For example, one set includes the words "jumping," "flashing," and "shooting." Another set includes the words "tingling," "itching," "smarting," and "stinging." You circle the word that relates closest to the pain you feel throughout the 20 word sets. The McGill pain questionnaire consists of four different parts.

The first part consists of a human figure drawing on which you are instructed to mark the location of your pain. The second part is the pain-rating index that contains 78 words divided into 20 groups. Each set contains up to six words. Five of these groups describe tension or fear. Each word is assigned a value according to its position within a subclass. The third part of this test asks additional questions about prior pain experiences, as well as the location of your pain and current usage of pain medications. The fourth part consists of a present pain intensity index.

This aspect of the test requests a pain score from 0 to 5 with word descriptors such as no pain, mild pain, discomforting pain, distressing pain, or horrible and excruciating pain. These words also are assigned different values. All the values are added to obtain a total score. All the scores are then evaluated to attempt to assess your total pain experience.

There is also a short form of this test that has been developed. This questionnaire contains fewer words and categories than the long form. This test is sensitive to evaluations of reduction in pain experiences. This test is more useful for rapid evaluation of data following procedures or surgery.

Your physician will ask many questions or give you a form to fill out which addresses the location of the pain, the intensity of the pain, the type of pain (e.g. burning, dull or sharp). Your physician needs to know what makes your pain worse and what relieves your pain. The severity of a patient's pain is the hardest entity for a physician to know because your physician is not experiencing your pain.

One way of assessing the severity of your pain is to assess your blood pressure and pulse. These are called hemodynamic parameters. They can be elevated when you are experiencing severe acute pain. These parameters are not helpful however, in chronic pain. A patient may complain of a severe toothache but have no increase in the blood pressure and heart rate. On the other hand, a patient with invasive cancer with excruciating pain will probably have significant increases in heart rate and blood pressure.

Other pain self-assessment scales are available. The horizontal visual analog scale consists of a 10 cm line anchored by two extremes of pain: no pain and extreme pain. Patients are asked to position a sliding vertical marker to indicate the level of pain they are currently experiencing; pain severity is measured as the distance in centimeters between the zero position and the marked spot.

The vertical visual analog scale is similar to the prior scale but is presented vertically, and the line is replaced by a red triangle with its summit facing downwards (no pain=0) and its base at the top (maximum pain=10). The faces pain scale consists of a line drawing of seven faces that express increasing pain (no pain=0, maximum pain=6).

Many pain physicians use Verbal Analogue Scales (VAS) to assess the severity of your pain. A scale of 0 to 10 can be used. A score of 0 indicates no pain while a score of 10 represents the worst imaginable pain. This scale is simple and is easy to be understood by the patient. This is similar to the previous scale with the exception that a patient makes a mark on a ruler with marks from 0 to 10. Your pain ratings will be kept in your patient chart and the scores will be compared with each visit. These scales serve as a gauge of your progress to treatment.

Some doctors want to have their patients keep a pain score diary on a daily basis. Your doctor may want to know the relationship between your pain and your activity such as sitting, standing and walking. Since sleep deprivation can worsen your pain, your doctor may ask you about your sleep pattern on each visit. Your doctor needs to know if you can do normal activities as well as whether or not you can work. In order for a physician to formulate your treatment plan, your physician needs to know if the pain is localized or referred. Localized pain is confined to one area such as a knee joint.

Referred pain begins in one area and travels to other areas of your body. An example is pain referred from the heart during a heart attack to the left arm. A pain medicine specialist also needs to know if your pain is superficial or deep. An example of superficial pain is that from a fingernail or from the skin as seen following sunburn. An example of deep pain is that from a structure deep within the body such as a diseased appendix or gallbladder. One treatment may only require medications while the other may require surgery. As you can see the treatment for each of these types of pain will differ. Superficial pain may be treated by analgesic creams or by pills.

Deep pain as seen in cancer patients may require needle injections or surgery to control the pain. Referred pain such as pain originating from the heart may require a surgical procedure or may require only medications. Localized pain can be treated with an injection of anesthetics that can numb the painful area. An example is an injection of a knee joint. You should begin to understand that the treatment of pain could be complex and on occasion be frustrating for both the patient and physician.

Before a physician begins pain treatments, a complete examination must be done. Strength, sensation and reflexes must be evaluated. Skin temperature should be noted as well as range of motion of the neck, back and extremities. A patient's mental status must be evaluated. Vital signs and the way a patient walks should be recorded. Swelling, skin color and hair loss should be appreciated. Loss of sensation to touch can be evaluated by rubbing a fine brush over the skin.

Strength and coordination are evaluated as part of the neurological examination. Following your examination your physician will probably want to order diagnostic studies. Plain X rays are used to diagnose bone abnormalities of the spine. A CAT scan is used to define bone abnormalities, as well in more detail than a plain X ray.

You may ask why your doctor cannot diagnose the source of your pain by looking at your laboratory or imaging studies. These studies only relate that there is an abnormality in your pathology. You need to know that if you have abnormal tests, it does not mean that you hurt.

If you have degenerative disc disease noted on X ray, you do not have to have pain. The X-ray is only a picture. For example, you may have a picture of a telephone. Is it ringing? There is no way to tell from looking at the picture that you are in pain. The same is true with respect to imaging studies and laboratory tests.

An MRI is useful for the diagnosis of soft tissue pathology such as nerve compression or muscle shrinkage, disc herniation and tumors. However, the MRI does not tell if you hurt. You can have a disc herniation, but not experience any pain. A myelogram is the injection of dye into the fluid that surrounds the spinal cord. This test can visualize a disc herniation or compression of a nerve coming off of the spinal cord.

A bone scan is the injection of dye into your vein followed by a series of pictures of your skeleton that are recorded by a scanner. This test can detect arthritis and trauma to bone as well as tumors. An EMG is the evaluation of your muscle using needle electrodes. This test can detect muscle pathology.

Nerve conduction studies evaluate abnormalities of the transmission of electrical impulses through nerves. Blood tests can detect rheumatoid arthritis and some medical diseases such as liver disease. A urinalysis may detect kidney pathology. As you can see the diagnosis and treatment of chronic pain can be difficult and challenging.

Because pain can have multiple causes, a physician must treat you as a whole and not just your area of pain. For example, you may have pain in the bottom of your feet. This pain may be the result of a vitamin deficiency. Your doctor could give you some numbing medicine (e.g. a Lidoderm patch) for your feet that may decrease your pain for a short time. However, if your vitamin deficiency is corrected, your pain may completely resolve.

The verbal rating scale is a simple, commonly used pain rating scale. To complete it, subjects select one of six descriptors that represent pain of progressive intensity: none, mild, discomforting, distressing, horrible, or excruciating. Another scale is a modified 21-point Box Scale. The scale has a row of 21 boxes labeled from 0 to 100 in increments of five. The 0 is labeled "no pain," while the 100 score is labeled "pain as bad as it could be."

Pain can be extremely difficult to assess in elderly patients. It can be difficult for elderly patients to give a numeric representation of their pain. They should be asked to verbally describe their pain as none, some or severe. Pain may be particularly difficult to identify in cognitively impaired individuals as it can manifest itself atypically as agitation, increased confusion, and decreased mobility. In many clinical settings, pain is not assessed in demented patients due to reliability concerns.

In particular, self-assessment is rarely attempted. Furthermore, when pain is evaluated in severely demented patients, the nursing staff routinely uses observational scales. These assessments include vocalizations, facial expressions, and body language.

Pain is also difficult to diagnose in infants and children. Children less than two years of age will report that they hurt but have difficulty localizing the exact area where they hurt. A child with a finger injury may just report pain but not identify the finger as the source of pain. This is because the brain has not developed enough to be able to distinguish generalized pain from localized pain. As a result infants and young children must be observed. Crying, facial expression and blood pressure and heart rate can be good indicators that pain is present.

Patients who may be unable to self-report pain intensities include: older adults with advanced dementia, infants and preverbal toddlers, critically ill/unconscious patients, persons with intellectual disabilities, and patients at the end of life.

Each of these populations may be unable to self-report pain owing to cognitive, developmental, or physiologic issues, including medically induced conditions, creating a major barrier for adequate pain assessment and achieving optimal pain control. Inability to provide a reliable report about pain leaves the patient vulnerable to under recognition and under- or overtreatment. Nurses are integral to ensuring assessment and treatment of these vulnerable populations.

Patients who may be unable to self-report: older adults with advanced dementia, infants and preverbal toddlers, critically ill/unconscious patients, persons with intellectual disabilities, and p Just like all other patients, these special populations require consistent, ongoing assessment, appropriate treatment, and evaluation of interventions to insure the best possible pain relief. Because of continued advances and new developments in strategies and tools for assessing pain in these populations, clinicians are encouraged to stay current through regular review of new research and practice recommendations for patients at the end of life.

9. DIAGNOSTIC TESTS

This chapter describes the various diagnostic tests, which may be ordered by your physician. These tests should be ordered to confirm a doctor's clinical impression. Laboratory tests check a sample of your blood, urine or body tissues. Your doctor analyzes the test samples to see if your test results fall within a normal range. The tests use a range because what is normal differs from person to person.

Some laboratory tests are precise, reliable indicators of specific health problems. Others provide more general information that simply gives doctors clues to possible health problems. Information obtained from laboratory tests may help doctors decide whether other tests or procedures are needed to make a diagnosis. The information may also help your doctor develop or revise a patient's treatment plan.

All laboratory tests are generally used along with other exams or test such as MRIs, X-rays, and EMGs etc. The doctor who is familiar with their patient's medical history and current condition is in the best position to order and to explain test results and their implications. Patients are encouraged to discuss questions or concerns about laboratory test results with the doctor. Two common tests that you should be familiar with are the complete blood count and the blood chemistry tests.

A complete blood count measures the levels of different types of blood cells. By determining if there are too many or not enough of each blood cell type, a CBC can help to detect a wide variety of illnesses or signs of infection. A blood chemistry test measures the levels of certain electrolytes, such as sodium and potassium, in your blood. A C reactive protein and erythrocyte sedimentation rate teat may be useful in the diagnosis of rheumatoid arthritis or other inflammatory disease.

Doctors order urine tests to make sure that your kidneys are functioning properly or when they suspect an infection in your kidneys or bladder. This is important if you are taking a medication like a nonsteroidal anti-inflammatory medication that can affect your kidney. A urine test can be done in the doctor's office or even at home. It's easy for toilet-trained kids to give a urine sample since they can urinate in a cup. In other cases a catheter (a narrow, soft tube) can be inserted through the urinary tract opening into the bladder to get the urine sample.

An example of pain management fraud with respect tests were detected when patients were recruited to come to the office of a pain management physician and agree to diagnostic tests. In return, patients would receive cash or prescriptions for Vicodin, Oxycontin, or Opana ER. Some patients agreed to get prescriptions for narcotics and then immediately turn them over to the pain office recruiter. The recruiters were filling the prescriptions for resale on the streets.

In a typical visit, a patient would agree to medical tests such as blood tests, breathing tests, EKGs, EEGs, ultrasounds, X-rays, and psychological testing, no matter what their medical symptoms were. An investigation revealed that for some of the tests that the clinic billed, the equipment was broken or the clinic did not even own the necessary equipment. The testing was all done before being seen by the doctor.

The doctor was initially charged in federal court with health care fraud. In a plea agreement, the doctor pled guilty to the charge of paying kickbacks. He was sentenced to 1 ½ years in jail and his medical license was suspended.

Legitimate tests for the diagnosis of back pain include: an X ray to look for bone degeneration. A bone scan can help detect certain spine conditions, such as spondylosis (spinal osteoarthritis), fractures, and infections. For a bone scan, a very small amount of radioactive material is injected into a blood vessel and is eventually absorbed by your bones. The areas with more radioactive material, called "hot spots," will show abnormalities. If there's pathology with a disc, the dye will leak out of it. A myelogram is a test to see if you have a spinal canal or spinal cord disorder. As part of a myelogram, you will also have an x-ray or CT scan to identify any abnormalities.

Tylenol (acetaminophen) can cause liver damage if you take too much (more than 4000 mg per day). Liver function tests ascertain how your liver is working and helps diagnose any liver damage or inflammation. Your doctor may order one when looking for signs of a viral infection or liver damage from other health problems.

On occasion, blood tests may be done to determine that you do not have a bleeding problem such as hemophilia. Aspirin can cause bleeding by decreasing the ability of your blood to clot. Before doing a nerve block it is prudent to know if your blood will clot in a normal time. Otherwise a needle can result in significant bleeding.

Plain X rays can be done in a physician's office. X rays can assess bone-joint arthritis. X rays can diagnose degeneration of your discs. Your bone alignment (do the bones line up with each other?) can be assessed as well. Bone fractures can also be identified. You should be aware that you are subject to radiation exposure with this diagnostic test.

If you have the possibility of having osteoporosis, your physician may order a DEXA (dual energy x-ray absorptiometry) that is a specific test for the diagnosis of osteoporosis. A Computed Tomography (CT scan) allows a physician to assess a disc in your back as well as arthritic changes affecting the bones in your neck and back.

A CT scan of your head can be useful for the diagnosis of a bleeding injury to your brain following trauma to your head. Patients receive radiation exposure with this test. Myelography or a myelogram is primarily of use when surgical therapy is planned. A dye is placed in the fluid that surrounds your spinal cord. An image is formed which tells a physician that a nerve coming off your spinal cord is compressed or not compressed by a disc herniation.

An image does identify painful areas of your body. An image demonstrates abnormal anatomy that could be an area of pain generation. Degenerative disc disease noted on an X- ray for example does not imply that you have a disease or are supposed to have pain. This entity is a normal aspect of aging. Therefore, you should not be alarmed if your doctor tells you that you have degenerative disc disease. The same is true if you are told that you have a disc herniation. Not every disc herniation causes pain and not every disc herniation requires surgery.

Ultrasound is another valuable diagnostic tool. Though ultrasound tests are typically associated with pregnancy, doctors order ultrasounds for different reasons. For example, an ultrasound test can be used to look for collections of fluid in your body, or for problems with your kidneys. An ultrasound is painless and uses high-frequency sound waves to bounce off organs and create a picture. A special jelly is applied to the skin, and a handheld device is moved over the skin. The sound waves that come back produce an image on a screen.

Computerized axial tomography is a specialized x ray. CAT scans are a kind of X-ray, and typically are ordered to examine for pathologies such as an appendicitis, internal bleeding, or abnormal organ growths. Tomography in which computer analysis of a series of cross-sectional scans made along a single axis of a bodily structure or tissue is used to construct a three-dimensional image of that structure. The technique is used in diagnostic studies of internal bodily structures, as in the detection of tumors or brain aneurysms. A scan is not painful.

A scan may require the use of a contrast material (a dye or other substance) to improve the visibility of certain tissues or blood vessels. The contrast material may be swallowed or given through an IV. CAT scans consist of a highly sensitive x-ray beam that is focused on a specific plane of your body. As this beam passes through your body, it is identified by a detector, which feeds the information that it receives into a computer. The computer then analyzes the information on the basis of tissue density.

Generally a CT is preferred where bone details necessary (long bones like your arm or leg, spine, skull), while a MRI produces much better soft tissue details (brain, spinal cord etc.). CT scans are useful for examining body cavities (thorax, abdomen, and pelvis) for calcium deposits, cysts, and abscesses.

With some diseases, either a CT scan or MRI is commonly ordered. Spinal stenosis, for example which is a bone growth around your spinal cord or around the holes in the bones of the low back and neck where the nerves from the spinal cord exit to your extremities and is usually seen in individuals over 50 years old. Stenosis can compress the nerves resulting in pain and numbness in the extremities. Because of numbness on the bottom of your feet, you may have difficulty with balance. A CT scan or MRI can identify this pathology. Magnetic Resonance Imaging (MRI) is done by utilization of a magnetic field that is applied around your body. MRIs use radio waves and magnetic fields to produce an image.

MRI's are often used to look at bones, joints, and the brain. Contrast material is sometimes given through an IV in order to get a better picture of certain structures. Nuclei within your body cells with an odd number of protons orient themselves with the magnetic field. The MRI scanner applies a certain amount of energy and the nuclei assume a new orientation with respect to the magnetic field. This energy is removed and the nuclei emit energy as they reorient in the magnetic field. The energy emitted is detected and displayed as an image. The MRI involves no radiation.

Magnetic resonance imaging provides a picture of your soft tissue that may be better than the CT scan. An MRI cannot be done if you have certain metals in your body or a heart pacemaker or a defibrillator. Magnetic resonance imaging allows visualization of the discs, spinal cord and cerebrospinal fluid. A MRI can be used with a contrast dye to identify an extruded disc, infection or tumor.

Plain X rays give physicians images in a front to back plane. A side-to-side plane and a oblique view are helpful in diagnosing your possible causes of your pain. On the other hand, a CT and the MRI image shows slices of the body as well as a three hundred and sixty degree image of a defined section of the body.

Images only show pathology. They do not show pain. Pain is a subjective experience. If you view a photograph of an old scratched and dented telephone, you have no idea if it is ringing or not. You have no idea if it works. The same is true with an X- ray image. An abnormal X ray does not mean that you hurt.

Bone scanning is done using a technetium isotope tracer injected into a vein. This tracer is distributed according to the bone blood flow. A greater blood flow to the bone from trauma such as a fracture or arthritis is compatible with greater bone absorption of the tracer. Total body radiation occurs but is low following a bone scan. The three-phase bone scan consists of the administration of a radioactive tracer followed by scanned images on three occasions. The first image is phase 1 Phase one measures blood flow on the first pass of the tracer. The second phase assesses the blood vessel system while the third phase assesses the turnover of bone, which can be seen in fractures or tumors. Bone scans are frequently used to diagnose RSD.

Electromyography (EMG) and the Nerve Conduction Velocity Tests (NCV) are two diagnostic tools that are helpful to the pain management doctor. These two tests allow the assessment of the location, the pathogenesis, and the prognosis of neuromuscular lesions. Loss of the outside wrapper (myelin) of a nerve or nerves is assessed by the nerve conduction velocity test. Abnormalities of a nerve take 3-5 days to develop. An EMG is a needle test to determine if your muscle is diseased or injured.

Abnormalities in your muscle can take five to six weeks to become evident. Muscles that are closer to your brain manifest electrophysiological abnormalities sooner than more distal muscles. Focal defects in your nerve may cause NCV slowing across the defect. A NCV measures how fast your nerve sends and impulse. Stimulation of the nerve is done at one end of your nerve and the velocity is measured at another end of your nerve. Generalized nerve pathology results in a reduced nerve conduction velocity. In other words your nerve impulses are slower than normal.

Electromyography (EMG) measures the response of muscles and nerves to electrical activity. It's used to help determine muscle conditions that might be causing muscle weakness, including muscular dystrophy and nerve disorders. A needle electrode is inserted into your muscle (the insertion might feel similar to a pinch) and the signal from the muscle is transmitted from the electrode through a wire to a receiver/amplifier, which is connected to a device that displays readout. EMGs can be uncomfortable and scary to kids, but aren't usually painful. Occasionally kids are sedated while they're done.

Distal latency is the assessment of the distal conduction velocity of your painful nerve that can be affected by the neuromuscular junction that is the location where the nerve and muscle join. Some muscle diseases may have normal NCV studies but electromyographic (EMG) abnormalities usually occur in these situations. EMG measures muscle electrical activity. A reduction in the size of the waves on an oscilloscope (a screen with waves that move across the screen) is proportional to the nerve loss to the muscle. It should be noted when a muscle is penetrated by an EMG needle, the normal muscle is quiet when it is at rest.

Muscle fiber firing at the time of needle insertion can give your doctor an indication of any muscle disease. The NCV assesses the speed at which your peripheral nerves transmit electrical signals. Your nerve is stimulated, usually with surface electrodes, which are patch-like electrodes placed on your skin over the nerve at various locations. One electrode stimulates the nerve with a very mild electrical impulse. The other electrode records the resulting electrical activity. The distance between electrodes and the time it takes for electrical impulses to travel between electrodes are used to calculate the nerve conduction velocity.

A muscle should contract when stimulated by a nerve impulse. A needle electrode is inserted through the skin into your muscle. There should be a short burst of electrical activity at this time. The electrical activity detected by this electrode is displayed on an oscilloscope, and may be heard through a speaker. After placement of the electrodes, you may be asked to contract certain muscles. The presence, size, and shape of the waveform make up an action potential. This waveform provides information about the ability of your muscle to respond to electrical stimulation. These tests are useful for investigating nerve and muscle function in diseases such as peripheral neuropathy, compression neuropathy etc.

Many standard tests can be useful in some situations but not in others. The key question in judging whether a diagnostic test is necessary is whether the results will influence the management of the patient. Billing for inappropriate tests, both standard and nonstandard appears to be much more common among chiropractors and joint chiropractic/medical practices than among other health-care providers.

Nerve conduction studies: These tests can provide valuable information about the status of nerve function in various degenerative diseases and in some cases of injury . However, "personal injury mills" often use them inappropriately "to "follow the progress" of their patients. Thermographic tests describe small temperature differences between sides of the body as images.

Chiropractors who use thermography typically claim that it can detect nerve impingements or "nerve irritation" and is useful for monitoring the effect of chiropractic adjustments on subluxations. : Diagnostic ultrasound procedures have many legitimate uses. However, ultrasonography is not appropriate for "diagnosing muscle spasm or inflammation" or for following the progress of patients treated for back pain .

Many instances have been discovered in which corrupt health-care providers bill insurance companies for nonexistent or minor injuries. The typical scam includes individuals who are paid to recruit legitimate or fake auto accident victims or worker's compensation claimants. The providers fabricate diagnoses and reports and commonly provide expensive but unnecessary services. The lawyers then initiate discussions on reimbursements based upon deceitful or exaggerated medical claims.

A patient should not have or use medical tests that are not approved or cleared by the Food and Drug Administration (FDA). They are often used to get you to buy products you don't need, and give inaccurate and/or useless results.

The need for vigilance against prescription-drug abuse is real. Overdose deaths involving opioid pain medications such as OxyContin, hydrocodone and Percocet have risen rapidly. Deaths exceeded 16,000 in 2010 for example. However, some labs encourage doctors to refer more patient specimens for drug testing by giving physicians an ownership stake or cut of test revenue.

Medical guidelines encourage doctors who treat pain to test their patients, to make sure they are neither abusing pills nor failing to take them, possibly to sell them. It is recommended that an opioid prescriber require a urinalysis test before every visit. An absence of the medications the patient is supposed to be taking is just as informative as the presence of medications that a physician has not prescribed.

Even though laboratories perform most drug tests, there are ways doctors themselves can be reimbursed, including by doing the tests right in their offices. Many pain specialists have purchased devices called mass-spectrometry machines that can count the precise number of particles of different substances in a urine sample. Other doctors become laboratory owners or benefit indirectly from arrangements made with labs.

10. QUALIFICATIONS TO PRACTICE PAIN MANAGEMENT

Did you know that the doctor doing your injection may have trained at a weekend course or may have learned pain treatment on the job? The weekend courses are cadaver courses. Do you want to be that doctor's first patient? You might be. There are no regulations on pain injectionists.

Doctors who manage pain are frequently anesthesiologists. Anesthesiologists ensure that you are safe, pain-free and comfortable during and immediately following surgery. But not everyone realizes that decades of research and work done by anesthesiologists have led to the development of newer, more effective treatments for patients who have pain unrelated to surgery. Many anesthesia techniques used to make surgery and childbirth virtually painless is now being used to relieve other types of pain. In fact, the work pioneered by anesthesiologists has led to treatments for pain control outside the operating room.

Frequently an anesthesiologist heads a team of other specialists and doctors who work together to help you manage your pain. Pain medicine doctors are experts at diagnosing why you are having pain as well as treating the pain itself. Some of the more common pain problems they manage include: arthritis, back and neck pain, cancer pain, nerve pain, migraine headaches, shingles, phantom limb pain for amputees and pain caused by AIDS. Pain medicine doctors are experts at diagnosing why you are having pain as well as treating your pain.

Like other physicians, anesthesiologists have completed four years of medical school. They spent four more years learning anesthesiology and pain medicine during residency training. Many anesthesiologists who specialize in pain medicine receive an additional year of fellowship training to become an expert in treating pain. Some also have done research, and many have special certification in pain medicine through the American Board of Anesthesiology.

This board is the only organization recognized by the American Board of Medical Specialties to offer special credentials in pain medicine. Medical specialty certification in the United States is a voluntary process. While medical licensure sets the minimum competency requirements to diagnose and treat patients, it is not specialty specific. Board certification demonstrates a physician's expertise in a particular specialty and/or subspecialty of medical practice. Pain medicine is a subspecialty of anesthesiology.

The American Board of Medical Specialties member boards (24) are responsible for setting the standards for quality practice in a particular medical specialty. Each Member Board has a board of trustees or directors, all of whom are certified in that Board's medical specialty.

Individual Member Boards evaluate physician candidates to ascertain if the candidate completed the appropriate residency requirements and if he or she has an institutional or valid license to practice medicine. If a physician meets these basic admission standards, the Member Board will evaluate the candidate using written and oral examinations. Because specialties differ so widely, the criteria that inform these tests are quite different. What makes someone a good anesthesiologist does not necessarily make him or her a competent cardiologist.

Ultimately, the measure of physician specialists is not merely that they have been certified, but that they keep current in their specialty. The American Board of Medical Specialties requires maintenance of certification that is a formal means of measuring a physician's continued competency in his or her certified specialty and/or subspecialty. To become recertified a physician must: hold a valid, unrestricted medical license, meet educational and self-assessment programs determined by the particular Board, demonstrate specialty-specific skills and knowledge, demonstrate the use of best evidence and practices compared to peers and national benchmarks.

Unfortunately, a physician needs no credentials to practice pain management other than a medical or osteopathic medicine degree and a state medical license. As a result, there are no guidelines as to who can call themselves a pain medicine "specialist". There are no local, state or national standards with respect to pain management.

The American Academy of Pain Medicine, the American Academy of Pain Management, and the American Board of Anesthesiologists administer written examinations to certify pain management doctors. These organizations provide continuing education courses annually. Some physicians do not certify through one of these organizations but classify themselves as pain physicians.

They may go to a weekend cadaver course to be able to do a certain procedure. You should ascertain that you are not the first live patient that one of these doctors practices on after finishing a weekend cadaver course. Other professionals (plumbers, nurses, teachers, policemen, etc.) must have formal training to practice their profession. Pain doctors in many instances do not! Does this frighten you? It should!! I recommend that you investigate your prospective pain physician before you receive treatments that will not benefit you or may actually harm you.

State medical boards can revoke a doctor's license if the doctor has been accused of improperly prescribing narcotic medications or other medications. For example, if a doctor has been accused of overprescribing narcotic medications to patients and if these patients have either died or have had to be admitted to hospitals, the doctor may not be allowed to practice. Patients need to know if a health-care provider has ever had his or her license suspended or revoked. A doctor may have practiced in another state, and lost his or her license there. Sometimes that individual will apply for a license in other states.

If he or she is able to obtain a license, the doctor will move to that state. A patient therefore, needs to know if the health-care provider has ever had a suspended or revoked license anywhere. Some practitioners have been suspended from practicing because they were taking drugs. However, most individuals are able to return back to their respective health-care practice after going through a rehabilitation program. A patient should not hesitate asking what the health-care provider's grades were.

Ask to see your physician's credentials. Hospitals in many instances may want anyone who will show up and has a medical degree to do potentially mutilating procedures on patients who have insurance. You should ascertain if your pain doctor has completed a fellowship (specialized training in pain medicine) or has sufficient experience through residency training to do a procedure on you.

Examine a health-care provider's curriculum vitae to see how many positions that individual has held. One may discover that the health-care provider may have been a medical director of a pain center somewhere or was head of a physical therapy or occupational therapy department. A chiropractor may have practiced at a pain center. A psychologist, for example, may have been on staff at a multidisciplinary pain center. Review the positions that the potential health-care provider may have had.

Some individuals have attended no additional courses in pain management. Some individuals have attended no additional courses for several years. However, most state medical boards now require individuals to meet continuing medical education courses to keep their licenses.

Other health professions also have this continuing education rule. A patient needs to know if a health-care provider has done a fellowship in pain medicine. This fact is important because remember that anyone can place a shingle outside of his or her office claiming a specialty in pain management.

Teaching at medical schools usually involves more expertise than nonteaching professionals. A patient should ask if a health-care provider taught at any educational facility. A patients need to know where and when they did teach. If a pain-care provider taught anatomy at a reputable university medical school, this individual should be an expert in doing nerve blocks. This individual can also be an expert in determining what anatomic site is the cause of the pain. Check the curriculum vitae or ask the health-care provider if he or she has been on the faculty of any seminars, conferences, or workshops.

Again, someone who has recognition in his or her field is usually asked to be a faculty member at a local or national seminar or local or nation conference. Some individuals are asked to help with workshops. Workshops are hands-on teaching experiences for health-care providers. For example, pain-medicine doctors can go to a workshop to learn how to do radiofrequency ablation of nerves in facet joints. These are hands-on courses with faculty who are well experienced in these procedures.

Did a health-care provider speak on reflex sympathetic dystrophy or post-herpetic neuralgia? The subject matter they spoke on usually indicates that they have some expertise in these particular fields. If a patient has a certain pain syndrome, he/she will probably want to go to an individual who has special expertise in treating this syndrome.

With these facts in mind, you must do your homework when choosing a pain medicine physician. Most university pain centers require that pain medicine physicians have a formal fellowship before they can begin to treat patients.

Because there is essentially no real state or federal requirements for an individual to be a pain-management provider, a patient are ultimately responsible for choosing the correct individual. It is also important to know if a health-care provider did publish articles, book chapters, or reviews on certain pain conditions that a patient may be experiencing. More specifically, did the health-care provider research and do an article on a patient's particular pain syndrome? Advertisements are not the place to discover new revolutionary treatments.

Remember that if this particular treatment was safe and efficacious, the local university pain center would be utilizing this procedure. If one is in doubt about the efficacy of a procedure, do not hesitate calling a university pain center to see whether anyone has heard of the procedure and if they recommend the procedure.

It is your duty to find the best-trained physician. Your insurance plan will list doctors approved by their plan. Some companies have strict criteria before admitting physicians to their plan. The American Association of health plans lists a Web site with a doctor finder at www.aahp.org. Click on to this site and follow the instructions to help locate a physician.

A patient should not be misled by false claims from sometimes unscrupulous practitioners. Unfortunately, health care is a business like any other business. This is the reason why patient need to find a health-care practitioner who is knowledgeable as well as ethical.

If a patient has been injured on the job or was injured in a motor-vehicle accident or in a fall in a store, it is helpful to know if a health-care provider usually sees patients referred by insurance companies, by attorneys, or by other doctors. If a patient has obtained a bodily injury, he/she may think that discovering this information is ridiculous.

However, many doctors have their referrals come primarily from insurance companies. If this happens, there is the chance that bias could be introduced into a patient's pain management. For example, if a patient sustained a RSD/CRPS injury in the course of a patient's employment, the employer may want to send a patient also to a doctor who they routinely use for their examinations.

Furthermore, a workmen's compensation insurance company may want a patient to see one of their doctors. Unfortunately, in some instances the company wants a patient to see a health-care provider who will find nothing wrong with patient. This is an instance where bias is introduced into pain management.

If a doctor consistently finds objective evidence to substantiate an employee's pain, that doctor may not be referred to again by the insurance company. These health-care providers are rare, but they do exist. So beware! A patient should, therefore, ask a potential health-care provider if he or she sees a significant number of patients referred by insurance companies.

Patients frequently seek treatment for chronic nonmalignant pain in primary care settings. Compared with physicians who have completed extensive specialization (eg, fellowships) in pain management, primary care physicians receive much less formal training in managing chronic pain. While chronic pain represents a complicated condition in its own right, the recent increase in opioid prescriptions further muddles treatment.

It is unknown whether patients with chronic pain seeking treatment in primary care differ from those seeking treatment in tertiary care settings. Primary care physicians care for a complicated group of patients with chronic pain that rivals the complexity of those seen in specialized tertiary care pain management facilities.1

Chronic pain management by Swiss specialist physicians with the primary hypothesis that pain clinic practitioners conform better to good practice (interdisciplinary, diagnostic/therapeutic routines, quality control, and education) than other specialists treating chronic pain was surveyed. Pain clinic practitioners were found to be more interdisciplinary and use more pain diagnostics than other specialists. Pain clinic practitioners bring particular-differing-skills to chronic pain management compared to other physicians.

A background information check can be done on every physician. Go to ama-assn.org/aps/amahg.htm. Has your physician ever been disciplined by a state medical board? Find out by going to the Web site ama-assn.org/ama/pubcategory/2645.html to find out if your doctor is a health hazard. If your doctor has been disciplined find out the reason.

A physician should have some certification from a medical specialty like anesthesiology, physical medicine etc. to do pain medicine in addition to completion of a fellowship. Ideally, the pain medicine physician should have further training in pain medicine. If your physician has no certification in any specialty you should eliminate that physician from your list of potential treating physicians.

There may be some qualified doctors who have not taken a certification test but it would be extremely difficult identifying those individuals who are truly competent. You should ask your physician if he or she has credentials in pain medicine including research publications etc. To ascertain if your physician is certified by the American Board of Medical Specialties, go to the website www.ABMS.org.

The medical board of the state of Ohio determined that pain physicians in Ohio for example come from many medical backgrounds and use different medical boards to claim board certification in the field of pain medicine. The names of Ohio physicians designating themselves as pain physicians were collected from the State Medical Board of Ohio and the American Medical Association.

The directories of the American Board of Medical Specialties (ABMS), the American Board of Pain Medicine, the American Academy of Pain Management, and the American Board of Medical Acupuncture were referenced for certification in pain medicine, pain management, or medical acupuncture. The requirements for these credentials vary widely, yet they have all been used to claim "board certification."

Board certification in medicine implies recognition by an ABMS member board as having completed the required training, met the standards, and then passed an examination that validates qualifications, and knowledge in a specific medical field. In 2002, there were 335 Ohio physicians designating themselves as pain physicians. Two-hundred-eighteen (65%) had at least one pain board certification.

Ninety-six (29%) of the Ohio pain physicians were certified in pain medicine by the American Board of Anesthesiology, the American Board of Physical Medicine and Rehabilitation, or the American Board of Psychiatry and Neurology, which are all member boards of the ABMS. One-hundred-seventeen (35%) of the self-declared Ohio pain physicians held no pain-related board certification. Anesthesiologists comprise the majority of all pain physicians and are the majority in all four pain boards.

Testimonials can be a marketing tool not only for health-care products but for almost any type of product. Most of the time, a patient can take the testimonials that appear in advertisements with a grain of salt. If patient are evaluating a medicine or a product, look for studies on the Internet or in the library.

Patients who have complex pain problems such as RSD/CRPS patients sometimes require the skills of several health-care providers to manage their pain. Pain-management techniques are now being taught in some medical schools. It is anticipated that this training will increase at least to where medical students can take an elective in pain medicine.

Hopefully someday pain medicine will become a separate specialty that is recognized as a true specialty by the American Medical Association. It is unreasonable to expect one individual to know and comprehend the entire range of knowledge associated with pain medicine without extra training in pain medicine. This is the reason why a multidisciplinary approach to pain management has evolved. This type of approach utilizes the expertise of various disciplines that are brought together in an effort to provide patient with optimum pain management care.

A patient must do his/her homework when evaluating any method for pain-relieving medicines and devices sold over the counter that range from scientific nonsense to fraud. Some companies will include testimonials from patients in their advertisements. There is no way of knowing whether these individuals actually exist.

Although guidelines discourage the use of imaging, over one-quarter of patients are referred for imaging. Guidelines recommend that initial care should focus on advice and simple analgesics, yet only 20.5% and 17.7% of patients received these treatments, respectively. Instead, the analgesics provided were typically nonsteroidal anti-inflammatory drugs (37.4%) and opioids (19.6%).

This pattern of care was the same in the periods before and after the release of the local guideline. The usual care provided by GPs for LBP does not match the care endorsed in international evidence-based guidelines and may not provide the best outcomes for patients. This situation has not improved over time. The unendorsed care may contribute to the high costs of managing LBP, and some aspects of the care provided carry a higher risk of adverse effects.

11. OPIOIDS

Physicians, patients, policy makers, pharmaceutical companies and others must work together to stem the opioid epidemic. But we often don't have complete data to understand what's happening and reduce addiction and deaths. Since 2010, more than 3,600 people have overdosed and died from opioids in Arizona. In 2015, the dead numbered 701 which is the highest of any year before, or nearly two per day, according to an analysis by the Arizona Department of Health Services.

The Centers for Disease Control and Prevention data reflects a number of state successes for monitoring programs. New York and Tennessee passed mandates for their prescription drug monitoring programs, and saw a 75 percent and 36 percent decline in doctor shopping, respectively.

The CDC calls prescription drug monitoring, "the most promising state-level interventions to improve opioid prescribing, inform clinical practice, and protect patients at risk." Prescription drug abuse is an epidemic in the United States that has been the subject of ongoing legislative control since the 1970s. The pharmaceutical dispensing of opioids increased 48 percent between 2000 and 2009 [1], and prescription drugs play a significant role in unintentional death

Narcotic drugs are prescribed for postoperative pain, cancer pain and for some chronic pain syndromes. Narcotic drugs can relieve moderate to severe pain. The term narcotic refers to agents that benumb or deaden nerves, causing loss of feeling or paralysis. Psychodelic drugs like LSD, contrary to popular belief are not narcotics. Many law enforcement officials in the United States inaccurately use the word "narcotic" to refer to any illegal drug or any unlawfully possessed drug.

Most medical professionals prefer the term opioid which refers to natural, semi-synthetic and synthetic substances that behave pharmacologically like morphine. The Opioids are a class of controlled pain-management drugs that contain natural or synthetic chemicals based on morphine, the active component of opium. These narcotics effectively mimic the pain-relieving chemicals that the body produces naturally. Opioids are the most often prescribed pain-relievers because they are so effective.

Morphine is the standard to which other opioid drugs are compared. Morphine is frequently prescribed to alleviate severe pain after surgery. Codeine can be helpful in soothing somewhat milder pain, as are oxycodone (OxyContin, an oral, controlled-release form of the drug), propoxyphene (Darvon), hydrocodone (Vicodin), hydromorphone (Dilaudid) and meperidine (Demerol), which is used less often because of its side effects. Diphenoxylate or Lomotil can also relieve severe diarrhea, and codeine can ease severe coughs.

The primary medical use of opioids is to relieve pain. Other medical uses include control of coughs and diarrhea, and the treatment of addiction to other opioids. Opioids can produce euphoria, making them prone to abuse. Opioids should only be used for moderate to severe pain that has not responded to non-narcotic drugs like aspirin or ibuprofen.

Narcotics can be used alone like oxycodone or used in combination with aspirin, ibuprofen or acetaminophen (Tylenol). Some narcotics like oxycodone or morphine are available as an extended release tablet that must be swallowed whole. Tablets, which are not extended release, may be split..

In 1914, the Federal Government passed a law that prohibited prescribing opioid drugs for recreational use. The Federal Controlled Substances Act of 1970 formulated schedules for drugs. You need to be aware of three of five schedules; I, has no current accepted medical use like heroin or marijuana, II; high abuse and dependence potential like morphine, codeine or oxycodone, and III; includes drugs with a lesser dependence and abuse liability. Hydrocodone (Vicodin) is a schedule III drug. Valium, a relaxant is a schedule IV drug and some cough medicines are schedule V drugs. Oxycodone (Oxycotin) is a schedule II drug which means that it is potentially more habit forming than hydrocodone.

There is a difference between the descriptions of narcotic drugs and opioids. Opioids are drugs like morphine, hydrocodone etc. Narcotics are extremely addictive drugs and include heroin and other drugs that can cause sedation. Opioids act by attaching to a group of proteins called opioid receptors, found in the brain, spinal cord and gastrointestinal tract. When these drugs link to certain opioid receptors in the brain and spinal cord they can block the transmission of pain messages to the brain.

For the purposes of discussion in outlining the pharmacologic activity of these compounds, the opioids will be classified as (1) agonists, (2) antagonists, and (3) mixed agonist-antagonists. All drugs bind to receptors that exist on the outer membrane of your cells. Narcotics bind to narcotic receptors on cells in the brain and spinal cord. Opioid receptors may also be recruited on tissue cells outside of your central nervous system such as your knee following an injury. An injection of morphine into your knee may alleviate your pain.

When opioids turn on a receptor, that receptor decreases pain signals usually in your spinal cord that prevents pain signals from going to your brain. As a result, your pain perception is decreased. Experimental studies involving binding of opioids to specific receptors in the brain and spinal cord have substantiated the hypothesis that these receptors exist which mediates the actions of the opioid drugs to stop pain signals to your brain. There are two basic classes of opioid receptors called mu and kappa receptors.

Other classes exist (e.g. delta) but are not important for the discussion of your pain in this chapter. These receptors also appear to be the site of action of the endogenous (pain drugs produced by your body) opioid-like substances and have been divided into three major categories, designated mu, and kappa.

It has also been proposed that at least two subtypes of each category of opioid receptors exist. Experimental evidence suggests that activation of mu receptors (found principally at sites in the brain) is associated with analgesia, respiratory depression, euphoria, and physical dependence. The kappa receptors (located within the spinal cord) are believed to mediate spinal analgesia, constriction of the pupil size and sedation. The other receptors may influence affective behavior, and although some physicians believe that activation of these receptors plays a role in opioid-induced analgesia, this remains controversial.

Since a number of different compounds, (e.g., certain antihistamines, some steroids, and anti-psychotics have phencyclidine) none of which are opioid in structure but can affect binding affinity for these sites. Agonistic (stimulating) opioids act as analgesics by binding to and activating both mu and kappa receptors in the brain and spinal cord. The opioid antagonists bind to all categories of opioid receptor sites throughout the body, but fail to activate them. These compounds are not used for pain control; rather, the utility of these drugs lies in their ability to reverse an overdose of opioids including narcotics.

The compounds that comprise the mixed agonist-antagonist group are more recent additions to the clinically important opioids. These drugs are semi-synthetic derivatives of morphine, the chemical structures of which have agonistic activity at some kappa receptors but antagonistic activity at mu receptors, e.g., pentazocine, butorphanol, and nalbuphine, or partial agonistic activity at mu receptors and antagonistic activity at kappa receptors, eg. buprenorphine. All are effective analgesics since they stimulate either mu or kappa receptors.

Chemically, the opioid agonists include a number of classes of drugs, all of which have pharmacologic effects similar to those of morphine. Morphine is the oldest known drug of this class. It remains as the prototype for the opioid group and is the standard to which all other opioid analgesic drugs are compared. Opioid drugs decrease pain but also affect all organ systems.

Your pituitary gland in your brain can be adversely affected by chronic narcotic use. For example in males opioids can decrease testosterone that can cause depression and erectile dysfunction. Drowsiness and blurred vision can occur. Changes in mood can occur. An inability to concentrate can occur.

Euphoria can be experienced in 20% of individuals taking opioid drugs. Euphoria can be the cause of addiction. Opioids can stop your respiratory drive that can cause you to stop breathing. Narcotics affect your stomach by slowing down the passage of food in combination with your brain to cause nausea and vomiting. Opioids can cause a significant decrease in your blood pressure that may cause you to fall.

Opioids decrease movement of the bowel resulting in constipation. Morphine can make gall bladder disease worse by contracting a valve where the gall bladder meets the intestine called the sphincter of Oddi. Opioid drugs can result in a release of histamine from certain cell in the body that can cause itching and a rash. As you can see opioid drugs can have side effects.

Tolerance, addiction and physical dependence can occur with opioid drugs. Tolerance occurs when it takes more of the drug to cause the same decrease in your pain. This is not addiction. Patients may find that they develop tolerance to opioid pain medications and may need to have their doses increased in order to be effective. Tolerance has not been shown to lead to drug addiction.

Physical dependence is a condition that occurs when continued use of the drug is needed to prevent a withdrawal reaction. Steady use of opioids can result in tolerance to the drugs so that higher doses must be taken to achieve the same effects. Long-term use also can lead to physical dependence—the body adapts to the presence of the drug and withdrawal symptoms occur if use is reduced abruptly.

Addiction is an intense craving for an opioid and is often associated with recreational use. Signs and symptoms of addiction include yawning, sweating, restlessness, irritability, anxiety, nasal discharge, tearing, dilated pupils, gooseflesh, tremors, loss of appetite, body aches, nausea and vomiting, fever and chills and an increase in heart rate and blood pressure. T

These symptoms last 7-10 days. Minor symptoms can begin in 8-12 hours after the last dose of the opioid. The more severe symptoms like nausea and vomiting begin 48-72 hours after the last dose of the drug. With respect to agonist drugs, morphine is the prototype. It can be administered by mouth, rectum or by injection into muscle or vein. It is prepared in a capsule, tablet or a liquid. It is available by a rectal suppository as well. This route of administration is used for those patients who cannot swallow or are having severe vomiting. Hydromorphone and oxymorphone also come in the form of rectal suppositories. The duration of action of opioids varies from drug to drug.

Sustained release morphine and oxycodone give a longer duration of action. Immediate release drugs (e.g. OXIR) give a faster onset but have a shorter duration of action. Fentanyl, which is 75 times more potent than morphine is available in a patch and sucker, forms. The fentanyl patch is used for severe constant pain. The pain relief is continuous. The sucker, which only comes in a raspberry flavor, is used for severe cancer pain in instances where the severe pain fluctuates. Fentora is another oral form of fentanyl.

With respect to the fentanyl pain patch, the amount of drug released is controlled by small holes in a membrane in the patch. A larger hole permits the release of fentanyl into your body. The patches are available in different doses. The fentanyl is released for 48-72 hours. Patients with a fever can be at a risk for an overdose as the amount of fentanyl administered to your body can increase by 25% for every 30C increase in body temperature. The advantage of the patch is that patients do not have to take frequent pills during the night. The patch should be applied to a hairless surface.

Darvon (propoxyphene which is no longer available)) and codeine are weaker opioids that are used to treat mild pain. They may be combined with acetaminophen to make each more potent. You need to be aware that smoking tobacco can decrease the potency of Darvon and hydrocodone.

Tramadol (Ultram) is an interesting drug and may be used for moderate to moderately severe pain. It has a low abuse potential. It is not a scheduled drug. It activates mu and kappa receptors. The side effects are minimal when compared to opioid drugs. Tramadol does not produce withdrawal symptoms like opioids. The advantage of tramadol over other drugs is that tramadol inhibits norepinephrine and serotonin. These two substances in the brain and spinal cord also decrease pain.

The opioid drugs do not have this effect. Tramadol can cause nausea dizziness and headaches. Tramadol does not lower the heart rate or blood pressure. Tramadol provides pain relief similar to codeine and propoxyphene. Naloxone and naltrexone are drugs that reverse the respiratory effects of opioids. Naltrexone can be given orally. The only time that these drugs are given is to treat opioid intoxication.

Butorphanol (Stadol) and pentazocine (Talwin) are called mixed agonist-antagonists drugs. These drugs show receptor selectivity and these two drugs stimulate kappa receptors. These drugs have less opioid abuse tendencies than the agonist drugs. Opioids on the other hand work on both mu and kappa receptors. Strong opioids exist which are usually reserved for cancer patients or other patients with severe pain.

Hydromorphone (Dilaudid) and levorphanol (Levo-Droman) are eight and five times more potent than morphine. Meperidine (Demerol) is an opioid that is weaker than morphine. It is used infrequently in pain management as it can cause tremors or seizures if used on a chronic basis. Methadone is a synthetic drug similar to morphine. The advantage of methadone for your pain management is that it does not cause euphoria. Methadone however, can cause a conduction problem in your heart.

Consequently, patients have died from heart problems after being prescribed methadone. Hydrocodone and oxycodone are two opioids used for moderate to moderately severe pain. These drugs are usually combined with aspirin and acetaminophen which can potentiate the analgesic efficacy of these drugs.

Another fact that you need to know is that opioid drugs can actually cause you to experience increased pain. This observation is called opioid induced pain. Many physicians are unaware of this fact. In this situation, a reduction in your dose of your medicine or stopping it can actually decrease your pain. This phenomenon can also be seen in patients who have spinal morphine drug delivery systems.

Pharmacists should be aware of the various kinds of fraudulent prescriptions which may be presented for dispensing. Legitimate prescription pads are stolen from physicians' offices and prescriptions are written for fictitious patients.

Some patients, in an effort to obtain additional amounts of legitimately prescribed drugs, alter the physician's prescription. Some drug abusers will have prescription pads from a legitimate doctor printed with a different call back number that is answered by an accomplice to verify the prescription. Some drug abusers will call in their own prescriptions and give their own telephone number as a call back confirmation. Computers are often used to create prescriptions for nonexistent doctors or to copy legitimate doctors' prescriptions.

Some patients will entice a prescriber to write prescriptions for antagonistic drugs, such as depressants and stimulants, at the same time. Drug abusers often request prescriptions for "uppers and downers" at the same time.

Prescription drug fraud, which falls under the broader heading of pharmaceutical diversion, is defined as the illegal acquisition of prescription drugs for personal use or profit. This definition excludes theft, burglary, backdoor pharmacies, and illegal importation or distribution of prescription drugs.

Prescription drug misuse is significant and rising rapidly, with some observing that it is the nation's fastest-growing drug problem. In 2010, about one in four illicit-drug users reported that their initiation into illegal drug use began with prescription drugs. Although this number is similar to that of people reporting first-time use in 2000, addiction rates are on the rise.

For example, substance abuse treatment admissions associated with prescription opiate abuse increased from 8 percent of all opiate admissions in 1999 to 33 percent in 2009. Research shows that people who misuse opioids often obtain them through a legitimate prescription to treat pain or a medical condition.

Prescription drug fraud can take many forms. The most common tactics are to forge or alter a prescription, to doctor shop, and to phone in fraudulent prescriptions posing as a doctor's office employee. Theft of prescription pads is also common.

As one can see, there are many opioids that can be used for the management of your acute chronic pain. The proper choice of your medication is dependent upon the magnitude of your pathology, the side effects of the drug prescribed, the effectiveness of the drug and your overall health.

Pill mills are prevalent in pain management. A pill mill is a doctor's office, clinic, or health care facility that routinely conspires in the prescribing and dispensing of controlled substances outside the scope of the prevailing standards of medical practice.

Pill mills give good doctors a bad name and they put people's lives at risk. Pill mills are places where bad doctors hand out prescription drugs like candy. Drug Enforcement Administration officials believe the highest concentration of pill mills are in Florida and Texas.

It is against federal law for a doctor to prescribe pain medication without a legitimate medical purpose or "outside the usual course of medical practice." If a prescription is deemed as not valid, a doctor could be charged with drug trafficking. The nationwide surge in deaths now places prescription drug overdoses as the second leading cause of accidental death behind traffic crashes and painkillers as the top narcotic contributing to death.

Until recently almost anyone could operate a pain clinic. There have been cases of a few ex-convicts who have made huge sums of money by operating pain clinics. In fact, a man convicted of drug trafficking, who could not run a liquor store in Florida, was able to run a series of seven pain pill franchises before being arrested.

Lawmakers and law enforcers have been cracking down recently on clinics, as well as doctors and pharmacies, which illegally or irresponsibly dispense prescription narcotics. Prescription pain medication is regulated by federal law, so doctors who prescribe it without a legitimate medical purpose or outside the usual course of medical practice can be charged with drug trafficking. At pill mills, the doctor, pharmacist, or other operators sell these medications to people without a valid medical reason, or in large quantities, making a significant profit for themselves in the process. People even travel from out of state to purchase medication from these mills.

Signs that a facility may actually be a pill mill include not requiring a physical exam, X-rays or medical records before being prescribed drugs, being able to pick your preferred medication, being directed to "their" specific pharmacy, and treating pain solely with pills.

12. ADDICTION

Chronic opioid therapy (defined as greater than 3 months on opioids) is a common practice for those with non-cancer pain, cancer survivors with treatment-related pain, and individuals with cancer undergoing disease-modifying therapy with a survival that can be for a year or more. Drugs are chemicals that have a profound impact on the neurochemical balance in the brain.

The risk of addiction, depression, central hypogonadism, sleep-disordered breathing, impaired wound healing, infections, cognitive impairment, falls, non-vertebral fractures, and mortality are increased in populations on long-term opioids.

Chronic pain, whether arising from bone, or any other tissue or structure, is, more often than commonly thought, the result of a mixture of pain mechanisms, and therefore there is no simple formula available to manage chronic complex pain states. One possible explanation for the severe pain described in some patients is opioid induced hyperalgesia induced by high doses of opioids.

Patients receiving chronic opioid treatment that develop paradoxical pain sensations, as well as worsening existing pain, can be diagnosed as suffering from opioid-induced hyperalgesia. As the worldwide population expands so too does the proportion of patients who experience pain that requires a strong opioid.

Opioid-induced hyperalgesia is a phenomenon associated with the long term use of opioids such as morphine, hydrocodone, oxycodone, and methadone. This entity may mimic addiction.

Identifying the development of hyperalgesia is of great clinical importance since patients receiving opioids to relieve pain may paradoxically experience more pain as a result of treatment.

As a result he/she takes more pain medication and subsequently appears to be addicted. Ketamine has been shown to be significantly beneficial in patients who require large amounts of opioid medications or exhibit some degree of opioid tolerance. Methadone is also effective in reducing high-dose opioid OIH.

The clinical use of opioids is further complicated by an increasingly deleterious profile of side effects beyond addiction, including tolerance and opioid-induced hyperalgesia (OIH), where OIH is defined as an increased sensitivity to already painful stimuli.

This paradoxical state of increased nociception results from acute and long-term exposure to opioids, and appears to develop in a substantial subset of patients using opioids. As more opioids are prescribed, especially to treat chronic nonmalignant pain, OIH becomes more of a relevant and significant issue.

In the last decade, a significant number of preclinical studies have investigated the factors that modulate OIH development as well as the cellular and molecular mechanisms underlying OIH. Several factors have been shown to influence OIH including the genetic background and sex differences of experimental animals as well as the opioid regimen.

Mu opioid receptor variants and interactions with different proteins were shown to be important. Furthermore, at the cellular level, both neurons and glia play a major role in OIH development.

People who are suffering emotionally use drugs to escape from their problems and this can lead to drug abuse and addiction. While progress is being made in treating patients with CRPS, it is important to remember that the goals of care are always to: 1) perform a comprehensive diagnostic evaluation, 2) be prompt and aggressive in treatment interventions, 3) assess and reassess the patient's clinical and psychological status, 4) be consistently supportive, and 5) strive for the maximal amount of pain relief and functional improvement.

The annual number of US deaths from prescription-opioid overdose quadrupled between 1999 and 2010 and in 2010 alone reached 16,651. Deaths from opioid overdose have now surpassed the historic death toll from another drug-related epidemic - anesthesia mortality.

Repeated, or chronic, use of opioids induces adaptive or allostatic changes that modify neuronal circuitry and create an altered normality. Patients receiving long-term opioid therapy often transitioned to chronic use after starting opioids.

Ongoing opioid analgesic use in patients suffering from chronic non-malignant pain (CNMP) has been associated with the development of opioid misuse, abuse, addiction, and overdose. Some physicians are afraid to prescribe scheduled drugs because of the possibility of causing addiction.

Chronic pain, whether arising from viscera, bone, or any other tissue or structure, is, more often than commonly thought, the result of a mixture of pain mechanisms, and therefore there is no simple formula available to manage chronic complex pain states.

It has been shown previously that the risk of true addiction in chronic pain patients was approximately 0.3%. Accurate anatomical diagnosis can be provided in only 15% of the patients utilizing traditional medical technology. The question of, "Why not relief?" should be raised in our society on a daily basis.

It is imperative to understand the true nature of pain by separating the myth of psychological pain from the reality of organic pain and manage it appropriately utilizing all available means, not only narcotics and interventional technology, but also behavioral therapy.

Prescription monitoring programs and using urine toxicology to monitor opioid use may decrease opioid abuse. CRPS patients may request opioids to control the severe pain.

Addiction is a chronic relapsing brain disease. Brain imaging shows that addiction severely alters the brain's areas critical to decision-making, learning and memory, and behavior control, which may help to explain the compulsive and destructive behaviors of addiction.

An addiction is a recurring problem by an individual to engage in some specific activity, despite harmful consequences to the individual's health, mental state or social life. An addiction can occur with drugs, gambling, overeating etc. Drugs can make one euphoric. As a result, one may request more and more drugs to maintain this euphoria.

Moreover, aversion to addiction and diversion remains a potent force that shapes prescribing profiles.1 Addiction is a hindrance in the long term treatment of complex regional pain syndrome (CRPS) because addiction in itself aggravates CRPS, causes stress in the sympathetic nervous system resulting in more severe sympathetic dysfunction.

Drug abuse or substance abuse, involves the repeated and excessive use of prescription or street drugs. In one way or another, almost all drugs over stimulate the pleasure center of the brain, flooding it with the neuro-transmitter dopamine which produces euphoria. That heightened sense of pleasure is so compelling that the brain wants that feeling back, again and again.

Addiction is frequently found in people with a wide variety of mental illnesses, including anxiety disorders, unipolar and bipolar depression, schizophrenia, and borderline and other personality disorders.

Long term pain narcotic patients should be limited to the nonaddicting pain medications (such as Stadol or Ultram) or at least to the less addicting pain medications such as Stadol or Buprenorphine (Buprenex). Methadone may be considered in severe pain that is refractive to these drugs.

Methadone can be used for the treatment of pain in addicted patients. Methadone is also an opiate that prevents users from getting high on heroin by competing with the much more potent opiates for the body's opiate receptors. Buprenophrine is another drug that is effective for the treatment of addiction and is also an analgesic.

Addiction and drug dependence occur when drugs become so important that a patient is willing to sacrifice his/her work, home and even the family. Once a patient's brain and body get used to the substances a patient is taking, a patient begins to require increasingly larger and more frequent doses, in order to achieve the same effect.

Narcotics such as Heroin may over-stimulate the pleasure centers of the brain producing euphoric effects that cause compulsive drug-seeking behaviors. The severities of withdrawal symptoms associated with narcotics include chills, shakes, muscle pain, nausea, vomiting, and headaches and cravings.

A clinician must be able to distinguish between legitimate patients with chronic pain and individuals engaged in non-therapeutic drug seeking behavior. Physicians have for years recognized the value of opioid analgesics in relieving chronic pain.

Unfortunately, drug seekers may also request opioid analgesics. They do this by feigning illnesses, and seek controlled substances from multiple doctors and by forge prescriptions. Drug seekers may be difficult to distinguish from true chronic pain sufferers.

In general, drug seekers prefer illicit drugs such as heroin and cocaine to prescription drugs. Prescription drugs however, have advantages over illicit drugs. Third-party insurers or welfare-entitlement programs may pay for prescribed drugs. Prescription pharmaceuticals are obtained in the safety of the physician's office.

Drug abuse and addiction have a devastating impact on society. Heroin use alone is responsible for the epidemic number of new cases of HIV/AIDS and hepatitis. Drug abuse is responsible for decreased job productivity and attendance, increased healthcare costs, and an escalation of domestic violence and violent crimes.

An estimated 20 percent of people in the United States have used prescription drugs for nonmedical reasons. Central nervous stimulants, depressants and opioids are prescription drugs that are frequently abused. Central nervous system depressants are used to treat anxiety, panic attacks, and sleep disorders. Examples are Nembutal (pentobarbital sodium), Valium (diazepam), and Xanax (alprazolam). Long-term use can lead to physical dependence and addiction.

Central nervous system stimulants are used to treat narcolepsy and the attention-deficit/hyperactivity disorder. Examples include Ritalin (methylphenidate) and Dexedrine (dextroamphetamine). Opioids, also known as narcotic analgesics are used to treat pain. Opioids are the most commonly abused prescription drugs. Examples include morphine, codeine, OxyContin (oxycodone), Vicodin (hydrocodone) and Demerol (meperidine).

One may obtain drugs by the following means: prescription forgery, by telephone (faking to be a physician's office), multiple doctors, and indiscriminate prescribing by physicians. Pain clinicians who prescribe chronic opioids are aware that there is an illicit market for opioid analgesics. For example OxyContin can be sold for $1.00 per milligram.

One 80 mg pill can be sold on the street for $80.00. Telephone scams occur when the drug seeker claims to be a patient of one of the other physicians in the on-call group, and asks for a prescription for an analgesic to last until they can see their regular physician. Sometimes, the drug seeker uses a telephone to impersonate a practicing physician. Prescription forgery is a common activity among drug seekers.

Drug seekers can modify a legitimate prescription to increase the dosage or quantity of an opioid. The easiest method is to increase the number of tablets on the prescription. Multiple episodes of noncompliance raise an alert of drug seeking behavior as well as multiple episodes of prescription loss. The patient with chemical dependency loses control over drug taking. The patient cannot take medications as prescribed. The patient repeatedly reports lost or stolen medications.

The physician will notice that the drug seeker frequently requests early renewals of prescriptions. A pain physician must however, be aware that aggressive complaining about the need for more drugs may indicate inadequate pain management as opposed to drug seeking behavior.

A patient should not be allowed to suffer. It should be understood that substance abusers can suffer from chronic pain which should be treated in a humane manner. Unapproved use of opioids to treat another symptom such as sleep deprivation should not be tolerated.

However, the pain management physician must objectively identify a patient's pain complaint with the appropriate medical test before prescribing an opioid. Opioid analgesics are powerful tools in the armamentarium of the pain clinician. Criminal and chemically dependent drug seekers may attempt to obtain such drugs from the physician. A pain medicine physician must therefore, use safe prescribing strategies.

A physician has no legal obligation to prescribe opioid analgesics on demand. A reasonable precaution to be taken by the pain medicine physician with an unfamiliar patient is to establish a policy of not prescribing opioid analgesics pending a complete assessment including corroboration of the patient's history.

Some patients or patient families are afraid of addiction. However, a significant number of individuals do not understand the difference between addiction and tolerance.

The American Academy of Pain Medicine, the American Pain Society, and the American Society of Addiction Medicine recognize the following definitions and recommend their use.

I. Addiction

Addiction is a primary, chronic, neurobiologic disease, with genetic, psychosocial, and environmental factors influencing its development and manifestations. It is characterized by behaviors that include one or more of the following: impaired control over drug use, compulsive use, continued use despite harm, and craving.

An entity termed pseudo-addiction exists which is not true addiction. Pseudo-addiction occurs when pain is under treated. Pseudoaddiction resolves when the pain resolves. Addictive behavior on the other hand, persists in spite of increasing the patient's pain medication.

II. Physical Dependence

Physical dependence is a state of adaptation that is manifested by a drug class specific withdrawal syndrome that can be produced by abrupt cessation, rapid dose reduction, decreasing blood level of the drug, and/or administration of an antagonist.

III. Tolerance

Tolerance is a state of adaptation in which exposure to a drug induces changes that result in a diminution of one or more of the drug's effects over time. Most specialists in pain medicine and addiction medicine agree that patients treated with prolonged opioid therapy usually do develop physical dependence and sometimes develop tolerance, but do not usually develop addictive disorders.

Addiction is a primary chronic disease and exposure to opioid medications is only one of the etiologic factors in its development. Therefore, good clinical judgment must be used in determining whether the pattern of behaviors signals the presence of addiction or reflects a different issue.

Drug overdose has become the leading cause of injury death in the United States. More than half of those deaths involve prescription drugs, specifically opioids. A key component of addressing this national epidemic is improving prescriber practices.

According to the National Institute on Drug Abuse over 2.5 million people receive treatment each year at a qualified drug rehab facility. And although the world of addiction treatment is filled with caring, expert professionals who have dedicated their lives to helping others, there are unfortunately, a number of businesses within the industry that over-promise in terms of the results offered, or flat out lie about the effectiveness of their programs.

Allegations of fraud and other criminal practices are impacting care and prompting lawmakers to consider a plan to properly license and regulate substance abuse treatment facilities. Some clinics diagnose people with addictions they don't have, so they can increase client rolls. The clinics recruit mentally ill residents from group homes to attend therapy sessions. They attract patients from the street through incentives of cash, food and cigarettes, and have them sign in for days they do not attend sessions. One clinic billed for clients who could not have attended sessions, either because they were in jail or dead.

Eight people have been indicted for allegedly participating in a scheme that submitted more than $50 million in fraudulent bills to a California state program for alcohol and drug treatment services for high school and middle school students that, in many instances, were not provided or were provided to students who did not have substance abuse problems. Kickbacks for patient referrals for addiction treatment cost payers considerable sums of money.

Fraud in health care is just like in any other industry: Fraudsters with the means and opportunity take full advantage to unjustly profit. Health care crooks inside and outside the industry include patients, payers, employers, vendors and suppliers, and providers, including pharmacists.

When addicts want to get clean, the most common path, at least for those who can afford it, is a brief chemical detox followed by a 28-day inpatient rehab. In South Florida, rehab is often followed by a much longer stint living in a halfway house (typically a low-rent apartment) with other recovering addicts. People staying in those "sober living" homes are often encouraged to get additional support from outpatient programs that offer one-on-one counseling, group therapy, and 12-step programs. Stories abound in Delray Beach of halfway house owners charging insurance companies thousands of dollars a month for simple urine tests, collecting illegal referral fees from rehab programs, and even finding ways to get addicts drugs in hopes that they will relapse.

13. ANTI INFLAMMATORY MEDICATIONS

Steroids are drugs used to reduce inflammatory pain such as joint pain. However, steroids may have significant side effects associated with their use. For example, steroids can cause weight gain, osteoporosis, avascular necrosis of your hips etc. Nonsteroidal anti-inflammatory drugs are commonly used to treat painful conditions. This may include a sprain strain injury, a headache, a toothache etc. Many individuals believe that these drugs are safe because many of them are sold over the counter. However, these drugs may have serious side effects in some individuals.

Nonsteroidal anti-inflammatory drugs inhibit prostaglandins. Prostaglandins are a related family of chemicals that are produced by the cells of your body and have several important functions. They promote inflammation, pain, and cause fevers. They are involved with the function of platelets that are necessary for the clotting of your blood, and protect the lining of your stomach from the damaging effects of acid. Prostaglandins are produced within your body's cells by the enzyme cyclooxygenase (COX). There are two of these enzymes, Cox 1 and Cox 2. However, only Cox-1 produces prostaglandins that support platelets and protect the stomach.

Nonsteroidal anti-inflammatory drugs (NSAIDs) block the Cox enzymes and reduce prostaglandins throughout your body. As a consequence, ongoing inflammation, pain, and fever are reduced. Since the prostaglandins that protect the stomach and support the platelets and blood clotting also are reduced, NSAIDs can cause ulcers in your stomach and cause bleeding. NSAIDs differ in how strongly they inhibit Cox-1 and, therefore, in their tendency to cause ulcers and promote bleeding.

NSAIDs are among the most widely used drugs, starting in infancy for pain and fever, right through to the elderly where they are standards for treating osteoarthritis and other muscle and skeletal conditions. The mechanism of action is responsible for the extensive side effects. Ulcers are the most well-known effect and hospitalization secondary to gastrointestinal bleeding from NSAIDs is common. The other well-known side effect is cardiovascular disease, and NSAIDs to increase the risks of heart attacks and strokes.

The COX-2 inhibitors like Vioxx had fewer effects on COX-1 in the gastrointestinal tract, reducing side effects, but effects on COX-2 were linked with increases in events like heart attacks and strokes. Importantly, other NSAIDs interfere with the beneficial effects of ASA (aspirin) on platelets that can give protective effects against cardiovascular disease. Another important difference between the two enzymes is their ability to cause ulcers and bleeding. Celebrex is referred to as one of the selective Cox-2 inhibitors and therefore causes less bleeding and fewer ulcers than other NSAIDs.

Aspirin is the only NSAID that is able to inhibit the clotting of blood for a prolonged period (4 to 7 days). This prolonged effect of aspirin makes it an ideal drug for preventing the blood clots that cause heart attacks and strokes.

COX-2 inhibitors do not cause your blood to not clot. This is one reason why COX-2 inhibitors are implicated in heart attacks. You should be aware that the FDA issued a public health advisory concerning use of non-steroidal anti-inflammatory drug products including those known as COX-2 selective agents. The COX-2 selective agents like Celebrex may be associated with an increased risk of serious cardiovascular events especially when they are used for long periods of time or in very high-risk settings. The drugs Vioxx and Bextra have been taken off the market because of serious side effects. Preliminary results from a long-term clinical trial suggest that long-term use of a non-selective NSAID; naproxen may also be associated with an increased cardiovascular risk compared to placebo.

Evidence in a lawsuit against Pfizer alleges that the drug company cherry-picked data on its drug Celebrex. Its claim to fame when it came on the market in 1998 was that it relieved pain without causing the gastrointestinal side effects common to other pain-relief drugs like ibuprofen.

Studies showed it didn't necessarily relieve pain any better than the other drugs on the market. The FDA does no testing of drugs that are to be approved. There an objective third party that does tests. Rather the system the FDA employs has the drug company pay for and do the studies and they only submit the studies that support the release of their drug. They are not required to submit failed ones. Celebrex is still being widely used, often by arthritis patients. Celebrex is in the same class of drugs as Vioxx and Bextra, both of which were pulled from the market because of serious heart risks.

The FDA (Federal Drug Administration) stated that patients who are at a high risk of gastrointestinal bleeding, have a history of intolerance to non-selective NSAIDs, or are not doing well on non-selective NSAIDs may be appropriate candidates for COX-2 selective agents. Non-selective

NSAIDs are widely used in both over-the-counter and prescription settings. As prescription drugs, many are approved for short-term use in the treatment of pain and menstrual discomfort, and for longer-term use to treat the signs and symptoms of osteoarthritis and rheumatoid arthritis.

NSAIDS are classified as non-opioid analgesic drugs and are aspirin like drugs. Although the pharmacologic and toxicologic properties of these compounds are similar and all possess analgesic activity, only certain drugs are indicated specifically for the relief of pain (eg. Feldene, Voltaren, Advil, Naprosyn, Celebrex etc.).

NSAIDS stop the production of prostaglandin production. Since prostaglandins are formed and released in response to cell membrane injury, these substances have become associated with pain reactions that accompany tissue injury and inflammation. Prostaglandins sensitize pain receptors (mostly C fibers) by lowering the threshold to thermal, mechanical and chemical stimuli.

The increased pain sensations induced by prostaglandins is a localized event that allows the mediators of pain such as bradykinin, histamine and substance p, to exert a greater effect on pain receptors. The receptors are stimulated to a greater extent causing more pain. All of the NSAIDS analgesics prevent the biosynthesis and release of prostaglandins by inhibition of prostaglandin cyclooxygenase, a cell membrane enzyme that is present in almost all cells. Therefore, the NSAIDS reduce the formation of prostaglandins and decrease the pain sensitivity caused by these substances. NSAIDS have analgesic, fever reducing, and anti-inflammatory effects.

Not all of the drugs are equally active, nor are all clinically useful, with respect to these effects. Dolobid (diflunisal) for example, is used exclusively as an analgesic but does not decrease a fever. With the exception of acetaminophen, aspirin, and ibuprofen, none of the other compounds are used to reduce fever.

NSAIDS are used in the treatment of various arthritic conditions such as rheumatoid arthritis, ankylosing spondylitis, osteoarthritis and acute gouty arthritis. As the particular inflammatory condition being treated is alleviated, the pain associated with the disease is also decreased. Pain associated with inflammatory diseases is effectively reduced by all of these NSAID drugs. Aspirin is the oldest NSAID.

Many patients are under the mistaken impression that these drugs not only reduce pain, but also promote healing. This information is false. Inflammation is an integral part of the healing process. One of the damaging side effects of NSAIDs is the inhibition of the healing process of soft tissues. The long term detrimental effects far outweigh the temporary positive effect of decreased pain. NSAID block inflammatory healing.

Toradol (ketolorac) has minimal antiinflammatory effects but has significant pain relieving effects. This observation suggests that antiinflammatory effects are not related to pain relieving effects. NSAIDS have a ceiling affect. This means that when you take a certain dose of an NSAID, more of the NSAID will not give you more pain relief. This affect is opposite to that of opioid analgesics. They have no ceiling effects. This means that more of an opioid will increase your pain relief.

The Bayer Company in Germany discovered aspirin in the late 1800's. Aspirin is the prototype to which other NSAIDS are compared. The side effects of the NSAIDS should be briefly discussed. Serious side effects are rare. The liver and kidneys can be affected by high doses of NSAIDS prescribed over a long duration. Patients with forms of arthritis will require NSAIDS long term for the anti-inflammatory properties of the NSAIDS.

Gastrointestinal toxicity can occur with all NSAIDS that can lead to bleeding from the stomach and may lead to hospitalization and surgery as well as blood transfusions. Localized irritation of the stomach lining constitutes the most common adverse reaction associated NSAIDS. Although epigastric distress is common at the lower doses, gastric and/or intestinal ulceration and bleeding will occur in only a small percentage of patients. At higher doses of aspirin, erosive gastritis and gastrointestinal hemorrhage is observed more often. These effects are the result of the inhibition of cyclo-oxygenase 1 (COX-1).

You need cyclo-oxygenase 1 to form protective prostaglandins that reduce acid secretion by your stomach and promote the secretion of protective intestinal mucus. Aspirin and other compounds with high anti-inflammatory activity, such as indomethacin, tend to elicit the highest incidence of gastrointestinal reactions. Other NSAIDS like naproxen are considered to produce fewer and less intense gastrointestinal reactions than aspirin.

Acetaminophen is essentially devoid of these effects. Acetaminophen has some anti-inflammatory affects. Newer NSAIDS that are specific for cyclo oxygenase 2 enzymes are safer than the rest of the NSAIDS that inhibit both cyclooxygenase 1 and 2. Celebrex is safer on your stomach. With respect to the heart and lungs all of the NSAIDS can cause swelling in your extremities as well as increase your blood pressure.

It should be noted that all NSAIDS including ibuprofen and naproxen could be linked to an increased risk of a heart attack. Because of this research, it is advisable to use the lowest effective dose of NSAID for the shortest time necessary, NSAIDS can cause clotting problems and make you prone to bleeding or bruising. This is due to the inhibition of thromboxane A, formation in thrombocytes (cells in the bloodstream associated with clotting). However, Celebrex does not cause this problem. In other words, Celebrex is the only NSAID that does not adversely affect the blood thinning effects of aspirin.

With respect to your kidneys, sodium and water retention with extremity swelling are seen with NSAID use. The higher the dose, the more prone you are for these side effects. Ask your doctor about the lowest effective dose that can be prescribed for you. If you are over sixty years of age you should be prescribed lower doses, as you may be more sensitive to NSAIDS than younger patients.

NSAIDS are excellent analgesic medications for pain in extremities, as well as for dental pain and headaches. They are furthermore, non-addicting. NSAIDS should be used with caution in elderly patients. If you are significantly sick (such as an intensive care patient, an NSAID can adversely affect your kidneys. In some instances NSAIDS can caus kidney failure.

Nonsteroidal anti-inflammatory drugs (NSAIDs) are commonly used in the elderly for the treatment of fever, pain, pain associated with inflammation in rheumatoid arthritis and osteoarthritis, neuromuscular disorders, headache, and musculoskeletal conditions. Each year in the United States, people spend 5 to 10 billion dollars to purchase prescription and over-the-counter NSAIDs. Gastrointestinal side effects such as ulcers and bleeding are the most prevalent and life-threatening problems associated with NSAIDs in elderly individuals.

Specifically in the elderly, NSAIDs have become a leading cause of hospitalization in this age group and may increase the risk of death from ulceration more than four fold. NSAIDs and the new class of cyclo-oxygenase-2 selective NSAIDs continue as drugs of choice for analgesia and anti-inflammatory effects. Physiological changes of aging worsen the side-effect profile of NSAIDs in the elderly. These side effects, when added to the increased potential for drug interactions, lead to a much greater risk for adverse outcomes when NSAIDs are used in the elderly patient.

NSAIDS should be used with caution in pregnant patients as well. These drugs are not recommended during pregnancy, especially in the third trimester. While NSAIDs as a class are not direct congenital malformation drugs, they may however, cause premature closure of the fetal ductus arteriosus and also cause a reduction in maternal amniotic fluid. As a result, pregnant patients taking NSAIDS may require ultrasound monitoring by the treating obstetrician. In addition NSAIDS may cause premature birth. Aspirin should not be used during pregnancy. Fetal bleeding could occur as a result of the inhibitory effects on the fetal platelets. Acetaminophen which does have slight anti-inflammatory properties is safe and well-tolerated during pregnancy.

Massive NSAID use in osteoarthritic patients is one of the main causes of the rapid rise in the need for hip and knee replacements. NSAIDs remain among the most commonly used drugs in the world for the treatment of osteoarthritis despite the potential for significant side effects. in view of the safety profile of NSAIDSs, physicians need to consider our results together with all known safety information when selecting the preparation and dose for individual patients. Nonsteroidal antiinflammatory medication therapy may have potentially negative effects during the proliferative phase of a healing since it was associated with decreased DNA synthesis.

14. MUSCLE RELAXANTS

Muscle Relaxers are medications which affect the skeletal muscle function. The actual term "muscle relaxer" refers to two chief groups of therapeutic drugs called spasmolytics and neuromuscular blockers. Spasmolytics, also called "central acting muscle relaxers", are often used to diminish musculoskeletal pain, as well as muscle spasms. Neuromuscular blockers have no CNS activity and work by intercepting diffusion at the neuromuscular end plate.

These particular muscle relaxers induce paralysis and are often used in surgical procedures. While both are considered muscle relaxers, the term is usually limited to spasmolytics. The most common side effect associated with muscle relaxers is drowsiness and sedation.

Muscle relaxants are effective for short-term symptomatic relief in patients with acute and chronic low back pain. However, the incidence of drowsiness, dizziness and other side effects is high. Muscle relaxants must be used with caution. Muscle relaxants are a useful adjunct in the treatment of patients with chronic and persistent pain. There are a number of categories in muscle relaxants, but one may broadly divide them into centrally acting muscle relaxants and peripherally acting muscle relaxants.

Central mechanisms of action include activity on the glycine receptors, as seen with the muscle relaxant properties of benzodiazepines, or on the GABA receptors, as seen with benzodiazepines and baclofen. Baclofen has been used to treat the spasticity of multiple sclerosis; it may also be used to treat muscle spasm associated with radiculopathy. Cyclobenzaprine differs from amitriptyline by two hydrogen ions, and it retains many of the side effects of amitriptyline (e.g., dry mouth, constipation, irregular heartbeats).

Muscle relaxants are effective for short-term symptomatic relief in patients with acute and chronic low back pain. However, the incidence of drowsiness, dizziness and other side effects is high. Muscle relaxants must be used with caution.

Muscle relaxants are a useful adjunct in the treatment of patients with chronic and persistent pain. There are a number of categories in muscle relaxants, but one may broadly divide them into (1) centrally acting muscle relaxants and (2) peripherally acting muscle relaxants. If your muscles are tense, you can have decreased oxygen in your muscle tissue that can cause you to experience pain. Muscle relaxants are drugs that decrease tension in your muscles. These drugs can be useful in pain management.

Muscle relaxants are not really a single class of drugs, but are a group of different drugs and each of these drugs can have an overall sedative effect on your body. These drugs other than dantrolene do not act directly on your muscles, but they act in your brain and are more of a total body relaxant.

Skeletal muscle relaxants are drugs that relax striated muscles (those that control your skeleton). Skeletal muscle relaxants may be used for relief of spasticity in neuromuscular diseases, such as multiple sclerosis, as well as for spinal cord injury and stroke. They may also be used for pain relief in minor strain injuries and control of the muscle symptoms of tetanus.

The muscle relaxants may be divided into only two groups, centrally acting and peripherally acting. The centrally acting group, which appears to act on the central nervous system, while only dantrolene has a direct action at the level of the nerve-muscle connection.

Dantrolene (Dantrium) has been used to prevent or treat malignant hyperthermia (severe elevation of your body temperature and muscle contractions during anesthesia) in surgery. When your muscles are tense, blood flow in your muscles can decrease. The decreased blood flow decreases your muscle oxygen level that can cause you to experience pain just as if your heart muscle has decreased oxygen following a heart attack. Decreased oxygen to your heart muscle is the reason you experience angina.

Strains, sprains, and other muscle and joint injuries can result in pain, stiffness, and muscle spasms. Muscle relaxants do not heal the injuries, but they do relax muscles and help ease discomfort. Muscle relaxants exert their effects by acting on the central nervous system. In the United States, they are available only with a physician's prescription. Several examples include; carisoprodol (Soma), cyclobenzaprine (Flexeril), and methocarbamol (Robaxin).

Most drugs come only in pill form. However, methocarbamol (Robaxin) is available in both tablet and injectable forms. Muscle relaxants are usually prescribed along with rest, exercise, physical therapy, or other treatments. One muscle relaxant, Zanaflex (tizanidine) does provide pain relief by decreasing Substance P which is one of your body's pain signal transmitters. This medication is helpful in decreasing pain associated with fibromyalgia. Although the muscle relaxant drugs may provide you with pain relief, they should never be considered a substitute for other forms of treatment like physical therapy.

Because muscle relaxants exert their effects on your central nervous system, they may potentate the effects of alcohol and other drugs. They may also add to the effects of anesthetics, including those used for dental procedures. For this reason, anyone who takes these drugs should not drive; operate machinery, or any activity that might be dangerous.

People with certain medical conditions or who are taking certain other medicines can have problems if they take muscle relaxants. Diabetics should be aware that metaxalone (Skelaxin) may cause false test results on one type of test that detects sugar in your urine. Patients with epilepsy should be cautioned that taking the muscle relaxant methocarbamol might increase the likelihood of seizures.

Common side effects of muscle relaxants are visual changes, such as double vision or blurred vision; dizziness; lightheadedness; drowsiness; and dry mouth. These problems usually go away as your body adjusts to the drug and do not require medical treatment. Methocarbamol and chlorzoxazone may cause temporary color changes in your urine. Other side effects are stomach cramps, nausea and vomiting, constipation, diarrhea, hiccups, clumsiness or unsteadiness, confusion, nervousness, restlessness, irritability, flushed or red face, headache, heartburn, weakness, trembling, and sleep problems.

More serious side effects are not common, but may occur. Anyone who experiences breathing problems, facial swelling, fainting, unusually fast or unusually slow heartbeat, fever, tightness in the chest, rash, itching, hives, burning, stinging, red, or bloodshot eyes, or unusual thoughts or dreams after taking muscle relaxants should seek medical help promptly.

Parafon Forte can cause liver pathology (injury) in some individuals. The reaction is rare, but you can develop the following symptoms: fever, rash, loss of appetite, nausea, vomiting, fatigue, pain in the upper right part of the abdomen, dark urine, or yellow skin or eyes.

Muscle relaxants may interact with some other medicines. The effects of a drug may either be lessened or potentiated. When this occurs, the effects of one or both of the drugs may change or the risk of side effects may be greater with either drug.

Anyone taking muscle relaxants should let their physician know all other medicines, including over-the-counter or nonprescription medicines that he or she is taking. Some patients for example, receive muscle relaxants from an emergency department. They may not tell their treating physician. If they develop side effects, the primary care physician would not know what is causing any new symptoms.

Most muscle relaxants are centrally acting. Central mechanisms of action include activity on the glycine receptors, as seen with the muscle relaxant properties of benzodiazepines, or on the GABA receptors, as seen with benzodiazepines and baclofen. Baclofen has been used to treat the spasticity of multiple sclerosis; it may also be used to treat muscle spasm associated with radiculopathy. This indication is not approved by the Food and Drug Administration (FDA) because the primary activity for this drug has been for myelopathies.

Metaxalone has a role, as do other muscle relaxants, such as carisoprodol and methocarbamol. Cyclobenzaprine (Flexeril) has atropine-like side effects. Cyclobenzaprine differs from amitriptyline by two hydrogen ions, and it retains many of the side effects of amitriptyline (e.g., dry mouth, constipation, irregular heartbeats

Some of these muscle relaxant drugs are antispasticity medications used to treat muscle spasms and are usually associated with disorders of your nervous system. A muscle spasm is an involuntary increase in your muscle tone that that occurs when you stretch your muscle. The cause of the spasm is not known but may be related to a decrease in your body's nervous system's ability to be able to control muscle contractions.

Drugs that decrease spasms are called antispasmodic drugs and include drugs like Valium (benzodiazepine), baclofen (Lioresal), Zanaflex (tizanidine) or dantrolene. Each of these drugs can exert their effects for a long time. Shorter acting medications will be described below.

Botulism toxin administered into your muscle can decrease pain from muscle spasms or muscle dysfunction. These toxins (7 total A-G) prevent release of a chemical called acetylcholine from the nerve ending that goes to your muscle. This action can stop muscle spasms. Botulism toxins A and B are commonly used in a medical practice.

These toxins can be used to manage pain associated with whiplash disorders, some headaches, torticolis and low back pain. Botulism toxin can relieve your pain for 3 months. It can take two weeks for the toxin to exert its effects. Botulism toxin injections can cause you to experience mild side effects. These effects may be a fever or mild joint pain.

Benzodiazepines are used for anxiety and seizure treatment, but Valium and Klonopin can both be used for muscle relaxation. These drugs exert their effects by acting in your spinal cord. These drugs are useful if you have a history of a spinal cord injury. These drugs can last for a long time once they have been introduced into your body. Valium should not be used long term. You should know Valium is a depressant and can worsen depression associated with chronic pain.

Baclofen is another powerful drug that works in your spinal cord. This drug is frequently used in patients with spinal cord injury or multiple sclerosis. Baclofen causes less sedation than benzodiazipines. However baclofen can cause some drowsiness. A sedative is a medicine used to treat restlessness.

A pump with tubing placed into your spinal cord can administer baclofen continuously throughout your spinal fluid. Dantrolene affects the muscle spasm by direct action on the muscle itself. It is used in spinal cord injuries and for the treatment of spasms associated with cerebral palsy.

Tizanidine (Zanaflex) exerts its effects on your central nervous sys-tem. It is frequently used for the treatment of muscle spasms associated with rheumatoid arthritis. This drug also decreases substance P that is a pain neurotransmitter. Because this drug can decrease your blood pressure, you should use it with caution if you have a history of hypertension.

The drugs mentioned above can have a long duration. Other drugs are available that have shorter actions. These types of drugs are used for short periods following muscle injuries. These drugs may also be used following surgery. They are not used to treat muscle spasms.

Carisoprodol (Soma) has sedative properties as well as muscle relax-ant properties. This drug should be used for muscle pain. It will not however, relieve muscle spasms. This drug furthermore, may decrease your ability to fall asleep. Methocarbamol (Robaxin) is a sedative and decreases muscle pain by its sedative action. It has no muscle relaxant effects.

Cyclobenzaprine is a drug that is chemically related in structure to amitriptyline (Elavil). This drug does not act on muscles but exerts its effects on your brain. It causes sedation. However, this drug can reduce muscle pain and tenderness. Remember that all muscle relaxant drugs may cause severe sedation. You should not drive a car or operate machinery when taking muscle relaxants.

Baclofen, when administered into your spinal fluid, may cause severe central nervous system (CNS) depression with cardiovascular collapse and respiratory failure. All of the drugs mentioned can have serious side effects. Diazepam (Valium) may be highly addictive. It is a controlled substance under federal law. Valium can be a tranquilizer (a drug that has a calming effect and is used to treat anxiety and emotional tension).

Dantrolene has a potential to cause liver damage. The incidence of hepatitis is related to the amount of drug that you have taken, but may occur even with a short period of small doses. Hepatitis has been most frequently observed between the third and twelfth months of therapy. The risk of liver injury appears to be greater in women, in patients over 35 years of age and in patients taking other medications in addition to dantrolene.

If you are taking certain muscle relaxants and experience purple colored urine, you do not have a serious illness. For example, methocarbamol and chlorzoxazone may cause harmless color changes in your urine such as orange or reddish-purple with chlorzoxazone and purple, brown, or green with methocarbamol. Your urine will return to its normal color when you stop taking the medicine. Because each of these drugs can cause sedation, they should be used with caution with other drugs including alcohol that may also cause drowsiness.

Drugs that inhibit the metabolism of Valium in your liver may increase the activity of the diazepam (Valium). These drugs include: cimetidine, oral contraceptives, disulfiram, fluoxetine, isoniazid, ketoconazole, metoprolol, propoxyphene, propranolol, and valproic acid. In females dantrolene may have an interaction with estrogens. The rate of liver damage in women over the age of 35 who were taking estrogens is higher than in other groups.

Given that no two people are alike, if you are taking any medications and begin to take nutritional supplements you should be aware that potential drug-nutrient interactions may occur and are encouraged to consult a health care professional before using any natural product. Combining certain prescription drugs and dietary supplements can lead to undesirable effects such as: diminished prescription drug effectiveness, reduced supplement effectiveness and impaired drug and/or supplement absorption.

Fibromyalgia syndrome is a common, chronic musculoskeletal disorder of unknown etiology. While available therapy is often disappointing, most patients can be helped with a combination of medication, exercise and maintenance of a regular sleep schedule. Adding nutritional supplements derived from the unicellular green alga, Chlorella pyrenoidosa, produced improvements in the clinical and functional status in patients with moderately severe symptoms of the fibromyalgia syndrome.

There is accumulating evidence that selenium plays an important role in human nutrition. A reported case report indicated that severe muscle pain disappeared after four weeks of selenium treatment.

Short-term supplementation of Montmorency powdered tart cherries surrounding a single bout of resistance exercise, appears to be an effective dietary supplement to attenuate muscle soreness, strength decrement during recovery, and markers of muscle catabolism in resistance trained individuals.3 These cherries reduced immune and inflammatory stress, better maintained redox balance, and increased performance in aerobically trained individuals as well.

It has also been reported that consumption of black currant nectar by a complex series of mechanisms, alcohol adversely affects skeletal muscle. In addition to the mechanical changes to muscle, there are important metabolic consequences, by virtue of the fact that skeletal muscle is 40% of body mass and an important contributor to whole-body protein turnover. Prior to and after a bout of rigorous exercise protein attenuates muscle damage and inflammation exercise-induced muscle damage.

On the other hand, by a complex series of mechanisms, alcohol adversely affects skeletal muscle. In addition to the mechanical changes to muscle, there are important metabolic consequences; by virtue of the fact that skeletal muscle is 40% of body mass is an important contributor to whole-body protein turnover.

Skeletal muscle disorders manifested by muscle pain, fatigue, proximal weakness, and serum creatine kinase elevation have also been reported in patients with selenium deficiency.

Watermelon is rich in L-citrulline, an effective precursor of L-arginine. There is a beneficial effect of watermelon pomace juice as a functional food for increasing arginine availability, reducing serum concentrations of cardiovascular risk factors, improving glycemic control, and ameliorating vascular dysfunction in obese animals with type-II diabetes.

An arginine and antioxidant-containing supplement increased the anaerobic threshold at both week one and week three in elderly cyclists. This study indicated a potential role of L-arginine and antioxidant supplementation in improving exercise performance in elderly cyclists. Skeletal muscle disorders manifested by muscle pain, fatigue, proximal weakness, and serum creatinine e kinase elevation have also been reported in patients with selenium deficiency.

Like any illegal drug muscle relaxants can be easily purchased in pill mills. Furthermore, the world's largest online retailer and a prominent cloud services provider, listed prescription muscle relaxant drugs for sale without a prescription, and the muscle relaxant methocarbamol. Valium may be purchased online without a prescription at many Web sites. as well.

15. NEUROPATHY

A peripheral neuropathy or PN, signifies a problem with functionality of the peripheral nerves (nerves outside the spinal cord). These nerves are responsible for transmission of signals from the central nervous system to the rest of the body. Depending upon which type of peripheral nerve is affected. PN may produce a wide variety of symptoms, with varied degrees of severity. In a lot of cases, other health conditions perpetuate PN and thus, it can be both a symptom and disease unto itself.

Neuropathy is seen with a number of different underlying medical conditions. It can also exist without the cause being possible to diagnose, when doctors called it 'idiopathic. Neuropathy is the term used to describe a problem with the nerves, usually the 'peripheral nerves' as opposed to the 'central nervous system'

Peripheral neuropathy can affect one nerve (mononeuropathy), two or more nerves in different areas (multiple mononeuropathy) or many nerves (polyneuropathy). Carpal tunnel syndrome is an example of mononeuropathy. Most people with peripheral neuropathy have polyneuropathy.

Peripheral neuropathy risk factors include: Diabetes mellitus, especially if sugar levels are poorly controlled, Alcohol abuse, Vitamin deficiencies, vitamins, Infections, and HIV Autoimmune diseases, such as rheumatoid arthritis and lupus etc., in which your immune system attacks your own tissues, Kidney, liver or thyroid disorders, Exposure to toxins, Repetitive motion injuries and a Family history of neuropathy. There are many causes of peripheral neuropathy, including diabetes, infections, auto-immune diseases, exposure to toxic chemicals, chronic alcoholism, and certain medications - especially those used to treat cancer and HIV/AIDS.

Anticonvulsant drugs have been used for the management of neuropathic (damaged nerves) pain since the 1960s. These drugs interfere with the total number of pain signals that travel to your brain. The clinical impression is that they are useful for chronic neuropathic (nerve damage) pain, especially when the pain is lancinating or burning. Pain is usually the natural consequence of tissue injury resulting in approximately forty million medical appointments per year.

In general, following most injuries, as the healing process commences, the pain and tenderness associated with your injury will resolve. Unfortunately, some individuals experience pain without an obvious injury or suffer pain that persists for months or years after their initial injury. This pain condition is neuropathic in nature and accounts for a large number of patients presenting to pain clinics with chronic pain.

Following any tissue injury (nerve, muscle, bone, etc.) your nervous system sounds an alarm to your brain to make you aware that you have been injured. Rather than your nervous system functioning properly to sound an alarm regarding tissue injury, in neuropathic pain, the peripheral or central nervous systems are malfunctioning and become the cause of the pain. In other words, after your nerve has healed it may still transmit pain signals.

An example is a car alarm. The alarm will sound if your vehicle is being tampered with. This is normal. Now imagine that your alarm sounds when no one is near your car. Somehow there is a short circuit. The same occurs within your nervous system. Neuropathic pain is a complex, pain state that usually is accompanied by nerve injury. With neuropathic pain, the nerve fibers themselves may be damaged, dysfunctional or injured. These damaged nerve fibers send incorrect signals to other pain centers. The impact of nerve injury includes a change in nerve function both at the site of injury and areas around the injury. Symptoms may include: shooting and burning pain and tingling and numbness.

In order to understand the effects of antiseizure drugs, you need to be aware that these drugs can block the ion (calcium and sodium) channels that are present throughout your nervous system. Ion channels are pore-forming proteins that help to establish and control a small electrical gradient between the inside and outside of your nerve cells.

When ions flow in and out of your neuron, this electrical gradient ceases and pain signals subsequently cease to be transmitted to your brain. Calcium and sodium channel anticonvulsant drugs block the pores or channels. When these drugs drop off of these channels, you will experience pain again.

Antiseizure drugs are frequently used in pain management. It is not known exactly how anticonvulsants work to reduce pain. They may block the flow of pain signals from your brain and spinal cord. Some anticonvulsant drugs may work better than others for certain conditions. Neuropathic pain is a form of chronic pain caused by an injury to or a disease of your peripheral or central nervous system. It does not respond well to traditional pain therapies like opioids or nonsteroidal anti-inflammatory drugs.

In neuropathic pain, it has shown that a number of pathophysiological and biochemical changes take place in the nervous system as a result of an insult to a nerve. This property of the nervous system to adapt to external stimuli plays a crucial role in the onset and maintenance of pain symptoms.

Carbamazepine (Tegretol), the first anticonvulsant studied in clinical trials, probably alleviates pain by decreasing conductance in sodium channels and inhibits ectopic nerve discharges. Results from clinical trials have been positive in the treatment of trigeminal neuralgia, painful diabetic neuropathy and postherpetic neuralgia with this medication.

Gabapentin (Neurontin) and pregabilin (Lyrica) have the most clearly demonstrated analgesic effects for the treatment of neuropathic pain, specifically for the treatment of painful diabetic neuropathy and postherpetic neuralgia. Based on the positive results of these studies and its favorable adverse effect profile, gabapentin or pregabilin should be considered the first choice of therapy for neuropathic pain. Evidence for the efficacy of phenytoin as an antinociceptive agent is, at best, weak to modest. Lamotrigine (Lamictal) on the other hand has good potential to modulate and control neuropathic pain.

There is a potential for phenobarbital, clonazepam, valproic acid, to-piramate, pregabalin and tiagabine to have antihyperalgesic and antinociceptive activities based on result in animal models of neuropathic pain, but the efficacy of these drugs in the treatment of human neuropathic pain has not yet been fully determined in clinical trials. The role of anticonvulsant drugs in the treatment of neuropathic pain is evolving and has been clearly demonstrated with gabapentin and carbamazepine.

Further advances in our under-standing of the mechanisms underlying neuropathic pain syndromes and well-designed clinical trials should further the opportunities to establish the role of anticonvulsants in the treatment of neuropathic pain.

If you have had a direct injury to one of your nerves, you may benefit from an anticonvulsant drug. The clinical impression is that these drugs are useful for the treatment of chronic neuropathic pain, especially when the pain is lancinating or burning. There are seven drugs that are useful in neuropathic (nerve injury) pain; pregabilin (Lyrica), gabapentin (Neurontin), carbamazipine (Tegretol), valproic acid (Depakote), clonazepamm (Klonopin), phenytoin (Dilantin) ,zonisamide (Zonegran)) and lamotrigine (Lamictal).

Neurontin is an effective drug for the treatment of neuropathic pain but Lyrica is becoming widely used in the management of many pain syndromes. It has fewer side effects than other anticonvulsant drugs. These drugs can be useful for the treatment of shingles, diabetic neuropathy and fibromyalgia. Reflex Sympathetic Dystrophy, diabetic neuropathy migraine headaches, sciatica, radiculitis, and pain associated with multiple sclerosis may respond to either of these drugs.

If you experience sharp shooting pain, these drugs may be helpful in decreasing your pain. If you experience side effects from either drug, other anticonvulsant medications are available. Oxcarbazepine (Trileptal), lamotrigine (Lamictal), topiramate (Topamax), and zonisamide (Zonegran) may also be effective in reducing pain caused by diabetic neuropathy and postherpetic neuralgia. Lyrica is now FDA approved in 2007 for the treatment of fibromyalgia.

Anticonvulsant drugs are effective in the treatment of chronic neuropathic pain but were not initially thought to be useful in the management of postoperative pain. However, similar to any nerve injury, surgical tissue injury is known to produce neuroplastic changes leading to spinal sensitization and the expression of nerve induced pain.

Gabapentin (Neurontin) may decrease post-surgical pain. The pharmacological effects of anticonvulsant drugs, which may be important in the modulation of these postoperative neural changes, include suppression of sodium channel, calcium channel and glutamate receptor activity at peripheral, spinal and supraspinal sites.

Your doctor may obtain a complete blood count and liver tests before prescribing some of these anticonvulsant drugs (e.g. Tegretol). Your doctor will give you a 4 to 6 week trial of the drug. It may take the medication this length of time to exert its effects. Therefore, if you have no pain relief after several days you should not stop the drug that was prescribed to you.

Because it takes your body time to adjust to one of these medications, your doctor must adhere to the phrase "begin low and proceed slow" which means that you should be prescribed a low dose and this dose may be increased gradually over days to weeks. Anticonvulsant drugs are effective in the treatment of chronic pain but may also be useful for pain management following surgery.

Similar to any nerve injury, surgical tissue injury is known to produce changes leading to spinal cord sensitization which can cause you to have pain after surgery. Gabapentin has been shown to decrease post-surgery pain. Pregabilin is effective for the treatment of diabetic neuropathy and shingles.

Pregabilin binds to calcium channels of nerves, which results in a re-duction of your pain. Some insurance plans do not pay for Lyrica because it is new and relatively expensive. However, it has been shown to be more cost effective than gabapentin. This drug can cause dizziness, blurred vision, drowsiness, weight gain and swelling of your legs. This medication may decrease your platelet count as well.

Some anticonvulsant medicines can cause a decrease in your platelets which can interfere with your ability to form a blood clot. If your platelets are too low, you will bruise easily. Gabapentin is effective for the management of oral phantom pain following a tooth extraction. Gabapentin binds to nerve calcium channels. The drug is useful in most nerve injury pain disorders. An average dose is 300 mg taken three times a day.

Tegretol is a drug that is chemically related to amitriptyline. It pre-vents repetitive discharges of your nerves. This medication works on sodium channels in your painful nerves. Inhibition of these sodium channels can decrease your pain sensations. An average dose is 200 mg every day. Side effects include dizziness, drowsiness, blurred vision and nausea. This medication can cause various forms of anemia and liver damage. As a result, your doctor will obtain a blood count and liver tests.

Tegretol has been shown to be effective for the treatment of trigeminal neuralgia (facial pain). Depakote is given in a dose of 250 mg twice a day. This medication can cause you to have liver failure. Your doctor will monitor your liver function closely. This medicine is used when the other anti convulsant medications have been tried but failed to provide pain relief. Side effects of this drug include nausea, vomiting loss of appetite and diarrhea. Tremors and sedation may also be associated with this medication.

Klonopin may be useful for the treatment of pain associated with the burning mouth syndrome. Klonipin is useful also for the treatment of lancinating pain associated with the phantom limb syndrome. The drug may also be useful for migraine headache prophylaxis and for the treatment of trigeminal neuralgia (facial pain). The usual dose is 1 mg per day. Side effects include mood disturbances and delirium. Lethargy and sedation may also be seen. This drug has a significant sedative effect. It should be initially only taken at bedtime.

Dilantin alters sodium, calcium and potassium channels in your nerves. An average dose is 300 mg three times a day. The number of side effects associated with this drug is significant. Liver damage can occur and the drug can decrease your folic acid level in your bloodstream. A decrease in your folic acid blood level may actually cause your nerves in your arms and legs to have burning sensations.

Zonegran's mechanisms of action suggest that it could be effective in controlling neuropathic pain symptoms. It also decreases sodium channel activity on the sodium channels of your nerves. Side effects can include a decrease in your blood sodium levels, kidney stones, visual difficulties and secondary angle-closure glaucoma.

A typical dose of this medication is 300 mg per day. Side effects related to this drug include agitation, anxiety, ataxia, confusion, depression, difficulty concentrating, headache, difficulty sleeping, memory problems, stomach pain as well as liver pathology. This medication may also cause weight loss. A dry mouth and flu like syndrome may also be associated with this drug.

Lamictal also exerts its effects on sodium channels. This drug decreases the release of some pain-causing chemical from the ends of your nerves. The reason why you develop chronic pain after having acute nerve injury pain remains unclear. However, it is believed that Lamictal in addition to some of the other drugs mentioned may prevent this transformation.

A typical dose will be 200 mg twice a day after starting at a low dose and going to 200 mg slowly. Adverse effects related to this drug include headaches, dizziness, blurred vision and nausea and vomiting. This medication may be of benefit for the treatment of pain associated with Reflex Sympathetic Dystrophy.

Given that no two people are alike, if you are taking any medications and begin to take nutritional supplements you should be aware that potential drug-nutrient interactions may occur and are encouraged to consult a health care professional before using any natural product. Combining certain prescription drugs and dietary supplements can lead to undesirable effects such as: diminished prescription drug effectiveness, reduced supplement effectiveness and impaired drug and/or supplement absorption.

There is evidence suggesting that omega-3 fatty acids may have neuroprotective and anticonvulsant effects and, accordingly, may have a potential use in the treatment of epilepsy. One might expect that omega-3 fatty acids may also be effective in decreasing the intensity of neuropathic pain.

Honey is the only insect-derived natural product with therapeutic, traditional, spiritual, nutritional, cosmetic, and industrial value. In addition to having excellent nutritional value, honey is a good source of physiologically active natural compounds. Honey may decrease pain associated with nerve inflammation. The ultimate biochemical impact of honey on specific neurodegenerative and neuroinflammation remains to be studied.

Neuropathic pain is one of the most common complications of diabetes mellitus. Curcumin can be considered as a new therapeutic potential for the treatment of diabetic neuropathic pain and the activation of opioid system may be involved in the antinociceptive effect of curcumin. Dietary therapy with antioxidants could be considered as a new effective strategy in the long term for CPP, and may be better accepted by patients.

PN patients are typically under the care of a physician such as their internist or family practitioner. Unfortunately for some, the treatment of peripheral neuropathy which usually includes prescription drug therapy has been unsuccessful. These patients often suffer from debilitating neuropathy pain, are desperate and are searching for relief.

Some peripheral neuropathy clinics use direct mail advertising, TV, full-page newspaper ads and the internet to gain the attention of peripheral neuropathy sufferers. The typical ad will utilize provocative pictures of feet standing on sharp tacks or pictures of feet on fire. One clinic utilized a picture of a surgical foot amputation to garner attention. One marketing tactic frequently used includes a free dinner lecture at a local restaurant to sell their peripheral neuropathy program to the desperate patient.

A typical PN scheme protocol includes expensive and sometimes painful, nerve conduction testing. These tests are used to diagnose a neuropathy and may be done at the onset of treatment and intermittently throughout the care program. The clinician may X-Ray the patient's neck, back, arms, legs and feet. These x-rays have often been found to have no value in helping the doctor reach a diagnosis.

These x-rays expose the patient to potentially unnecessary and harmful radiation. The clinic also orders a variety of elastic and hard, plastic braces for the patient's neck, back, wrists and/or ankles. In the majority of instances, these braces were found to offer little assistance to the patient's painful condition. These supports are expensive with bills totaling over thousands of dollars.

The actual treatment that the clinic renders for the peripheral neuropathy pain includes frequent (2-3 X per week) injections of an anesthetic agent, often Marcaine, into the peripheral nerves of the arms/wrists/legs/calves and/or feet. There have been instances in which patients have received over 100 treatments involving up to 5 injections per day.

In most of the scenarios identified, the patient will briefly see a medical doctor on the first visit. The medical doctor will order all the tests, braces and injections. The doctor may recommend that the patient undergo physical therapy and/or chiropractic care in the clinic as well. Typically, all of the localized anesthetic injections are given by a nurse. A chiropractor and/or physical therapist may render various treatments over the course of care, further increasing the cost. The patient rarely sees the medical doctor again.

Claims sent to the PN patient's insurance company can amount to thousands of dollars and can exhaust the patient's insurance benefits that they may need for regular health care.

The peripheral nervous system (PNS) include the nerves running from the brain and spinal cord to the rest of the body; the arms and hands, legs and feet, internal organs, joints and even the mouth, eyes, ears, nose, and skin. Peripheral neuropathy occurs when nerves are damaged or destroyed and can't send messages from the brain and spinal cord to the muscles, skin and other parts of the body.

There are many causes of peripheral neuropathy, including diabetes, infections, auto-immune diseases, exposure to toxic chemicals, chronic alcoholism, trauma and certain medications – especially those used to treat cancer and HIV/AIDS. In some cases, the cause of a person's peripheral neuropathy remains unknown. When nerves are damaged, numbness, pain or muscle weakness may occur.

The peripheral neuropathy symptoms often include: A sensation of wearing an invisible "glove" or "sock", Burning sensation or freezing pain down the nerves, Sharp, jabbing or electric-like pain,Extreme sensitivity to touch or inability to feel with hands feet. Difficulty maintaining balance or the Inability to determine the position or where your feet are located.

A review of peer reviewed scientific journals and position statements from recognized professional medical/chiropractic societies failed to identify studies that support a rationale for frequent peripheral nerve blocks for peripheral neuropathy. Patient interviews have resulted in mixed responses. Some patients have found relief with a series of injections and a maintenance schedule of injections, others have not. Complications or adverse reactions to the services are not common but could include infections and a worsening of the patient's condition.

A practitioner admitted that he submitted claims to Medicare for nerve block injections that were false and fraudulent because the nerve block injections were not medically indicated and necessary for the patients' health per Medicare coverage guidelines. Between February 2009 and December 2011, the clinic billed Medicare approximately $3,083,454, and Medicare paid the clinic approximately $879,582 for nerve block injections.

A recent trend involving collaboration between chiropractors, medical doctors and/or podiatrists has been identified in several areas of the country which involves treatment of patients who suffer from peripheral neuropathy.

The providers are typically an MD/DC clinic, a DC clinic, or a podiatric office. The providers use direct mail, TV, print advertising and the internet to garner patients. A typical protocol includes a nerve conduction study (NCS) at the onset of care. In some cases, the providers may use a mobile diagnostic provider for the testing. Interim nerve conduction studies are usually performed, followed by another at the end of care. The treatment procedure includes frequent (2-3 X per week) injections of an anesthetic agent, often Marcaine, into the peripheral nerves of the arms/legs. There have been instances in which patients have received over 100 dates of service. Providers submit claims for the number of nerves injected. In some cases, the providers were noted to up code the number of injections. e.g.) The records indicated 3 nerves injected, but 5 injection claims were submitted.

The patient also typically undergoes an electrical stimulation therapy with a HakoMed (Bioelectric) device, or other electrical stim therapy. Some clinics are using low level laser (cold laser) therapy also. In offices where there is no MD/DO/DPM, the chiropractor may use multiple PT modalities including manual massage, vibratory massage, manual therapy and ultrasound as well as manipulation.

Another easy trap that into which many patients fall is the belief of testimonials or other statements from companies that give bodacious claims with regards to neuropathy. The fact is the research and clinical trials will speak for the product if they have them. Many companies and individuals make a lot of claims without having the clinical studies to back up their statements. Do not be fooled into buying any products that does not have clinical studies behind it. Advertisers who offer testimonials and "expert" commentary instead of clinical studies probably don't have the scientific research to back their product.

A rule of thumb is to avoid treatments which taught medical cures without discussing you medical problems with your primary care physician.

16. MYOFASCIAL PAIN

The myofascial pain syndrome (MPS) is a chronic condition that affects the fascia (connective tissue that covers the muscles). It may involve either a single muscle or a muscle group. In some cases, the area where a person experiences the pain may not be where the myofascial pain generator is located.

Myofascial pain is the most common form of musculoskeletal pain. Myofascial trigger points play an important role in the clinical manifestation of myofascial pain syndrome. Elucidating the role of central sensitization in the pathophysiology of trigger points is fundamental to developing optimal strategies in the management of myofascial pain syndrome.

Myofascial pain may develop from a muscle injury or from excessive strain on a particular muscle or muscle group, ligament or tendon. Other causes include: Injury to muscle fibers, Repetitive motions or Lack of activity. A myofascial pain syndrome is a soft tissue disorder of your muscles that can cause you not only to have pain for a long time, but it can also cause you to on occasion, have some disability. Your overall activities of daily living, including work, recreation and social interaction can be significantly affected.

Myofascial pain is pain related to muscle injury or overuse resulting in taut bands and palpable areas of pain that is referred to other muscular areas of your body. The pain can be dull, sharp or burning. You may suffer from sleep deprivation depression and anxiety like fibromyalgia. Your doctor may make a diagnosis of myofascial pain if you cry out or wince and withdraw away from light palpation on an area of your body

Muscle strains and ligament sprains can cause pain in your muscles and can contribute to the onset of a myofascial pain syndrome. The pain intensity of myofascial disorders can vary from painless decreases in range of motion about your arms, legs, neck, and lower back, which are common in older individuals, to pain that is agonizing and incapacitating.

Most myofascial pain can be relieved with an appropriate diagnosis and specific treatment. Pressing on the tender spots on your body can identify myofascial trigger points. When you tender area is pressed, you will have pain in other areas of your body that are away from the area being examined. Fibromyalgia pain does not cause referred pain when tender areas are palpated.

An active trigger point is an area of extreme tenderness that usually lies within the skeletal muscle and which is associated with a local or regional pain. A latent trigger point is a dormant (inactive) area that has the potential to act like a trigger point. It may cause muscle weakness or restriction of movement.

Fascia is a strong connective tissue that runs continuously and web-like throughout the body. Fascia performs a number of functions, including enveloping and isolating the muscles of the body, providing structural support and protection. Fascia is a very important part of the body, and it has three layers, starting with the superficial fascia directly under the skin and ending with subserous fascia, deep inside the body.

The pains in the other areas of the body are referred pain patterns that demonstrate trigger points. Myofascial trigger points occur when there is trauma to your muscle or prolonged tension on your muscle from slouching over a desk or slouching over a worktable. This slouching results in disruption of your muscle cells.

When your muscle cell becomes disrupted, your cells release calcium. Calcium released inside of your muscle cell stimulates more contractions of your muscle. A prolonged contraction will exceed the available oxygen, glucose, and other nutrients that are needed for the energy to allow your muscle to continue to contract. With a sustained contraction, you run out of oxygen as well as other nutrients. This allows your muscle cell to build up a substance called lactic acid which stimulates muscle pain fibers.

Substances that cause your body to produce pain-causing substances are prostaglandins that sensitize pain fibers or substance P (a pain neuro-transmitter) that is involved in pain transmission. These pain transmitters then stimulate nerve endings around your muscle cells. These nerve endings go to other structures in your body. This is why you notice a referred pain pattern when you have a myofascial pain syndrome.

You will notice nodular, ropelike bands under your painful muscles when you have myofascial pain syndrome. The lack of oxygen in your muscle tissue will cause some of your muscle cells to die. This will cause scar tissue to form about your muscles. This scar tissue gives you the nodular feeling when you press over these painful areas.

Not all pain in your muscles is from myofascial pain. Sometimes arthritis can cause muscle pain surrounding your joints. Myopathy is a disease of muscles that can occur and cause you to have muscle pain. If you have a disc herniation, you can have referred pain to your muscles as well. Rocky Mountain spotted-Fever or Lyme disease can also cause you to have muscle pain. A myofascial trigger point in your muscle needs to be distinguished from tender areas around your ligaments as well as around your bone.

The diagnosis of your myofascial pain syndrome is made by your health-care provider's history and physical examination and expertise. No laboratory tests are useful for the diagnosis of this syndrome. If you have the myofascial pain syndrome, you will complain of localized muscle pain and tenderness as well as the referred pain. If you have myofascial trigger points around your head and neck, you may com-plain of headaches as well as problems with your vision. Remember that you can have myofascial trigger points in one muscle or many muscles.

To make a diagnosis of myofascial trigger points, you must have painful areas in a muscle that is noted by your doctor on physical examination. These painful areas must be nodular and must be reproducible. Different amounts of pressure from your examining health-care provider will give you referred pain. If you truly have myofascial pain your doctor will record whether you have a "jump sign" noted on physical examination. This means that when your doctor applies pressure on your trigger point, you jump away from the pressure. Myofascial pain may be caused by muscle injury, post-surgical scarring, poor posture, trauma or repetitive movements.

Myofascial release is simply applying pressure to those tight little knots, which, by the way, can be extremely painful. Myofascial release actually is a safe and very effective technique that involves applying sustained pressure to those tight little knots. Myofascial Release. there must be as sustained constant pressure at the fascial barrier for at least 120 seconds before the elastic component of the fascia gives enough to begin elongation of the collagen component.

Your health-care provider will usually notice a twitch about the area that has pressure applied to it. At the time of your examination, your health care provided will notice that your pain diminishes with stretching or following injection of your muscle with a local anesthetic.

Your trigger points are classified as either active or latent. Active trigger points occur following acute muscle trauma. The latent trigger point on the other hand does not cause you to have pain at rest but can cause you to have restriction of movement about a certain part of your body. Latent trigger points are from a previous muscle injury. A latent trigger point can persist for years after recovery from an injury. Latent trigger points can predispose you to have pain with overuse of your previously injured muscle. Sometimes in cold weather, your muscle will contract and cause you to have pain.

Remember, only the active trigger points cause pain. The latent trigger points cause pain when they become active. Normal muscles do not have trigger points that can be felt or have areas that can cause your pain when touched. You should feel your normal muscles. Normal muscles do not have ropelike, nodular areas or tender areas to pressure and exhibit no observable twitch when your health-care provider palpates your muscle. Furthermore, you will not have referred pain with this applied pressure.

You can have different degrees of severity of myofascial pain. Some trigger points are much more sensitive than others. An extremely sensitive trigger point can cause you to have greater referred nerve pain than a less-severe or intense trigger point. Myofascial pain is usually not symmetrical on either side of your body. However, medical conditions that cause muscle pain such as fibromyalgia are symmetrical.

Trigger points are usually activated by overuse of muscles. You can stretch your muscle beyond its normal capability, which will cause your muscle to become injured. Bleeding can occur within your muscle following injury, which may cause scar formation in your muscle. Active trigger points can develop in your muscles following excessive, repetitive, or sustained motions. For example, if you work in a warehouse and load heavy boxes all day over months, you can begin to develop active trigger points. Common areas of trigger point pain include your neck, arms, shoulders, face, back and legs.

Emotional stress can cause your muscles to stay in a contracted state. When your muscles are contracted for a length of time as previously stated, you lose oxygen and other nutrients to your muscle tissues. You must attempt to relax and do breathing exercises and range-of-motion exercises to decrease your pain. Heat and cold my help decrease your pain. Myofascial pain can vary in pain severity from hour by hour or from day by day. If you do not exercise and do aerobic activity and are under a lot of stress, you have susceptibility to develop active trigger points.

Viral illnesses can cause muscle pain as well. If you have a virus, do not put cold packs on your muscles. A virus will activate chemicals in your body that activate pain signals. That is why you ache all over your body when you have the flu.

Myofascial pain may outlast any precipitating traumatic musculoskeletal event. The pain duration is of myofascial pain is longer in duration than the muscle strain duration. The duration depends on your overall muscular prior to an injury. If you are a professional football player for example, you can have a muscle strain and never develop trigger points. If you are not physically fit, a minor muscle strain can result in myofascial pain.

Eventually your active trigger points will become latent. If you rest your muscle and use a splint or an elastic bandage, your active trigger point may revert to become a latent trigger point. Occasionally you may do an activity that will activate your latent trigger point. This not unusual and you should expect this occurrence on occasion. Many of your muscles around your active trigger point can decrease their function, causing your muscles to become weak. If enough of your muscles lose a significant portion of their function, you can develop weakness of an entire extremity.

Myofascial pain is caused by pressure over your muscles. When you are lying in bed, you may have some pressure on your body in the area of the trigger points from your mattress. This pressure from your bed can cause you to have pain. On the other hand, be aware that sleep disturbances can cause your muscles to contract and become stiff and can worsen your myofascial pain syndrome.

There are no blood tests that will show abnormalities that can be attributed to a myofascial pain syndrome. X-rays, MRI images, and CAT scans have not demonstrated any changes that can be associated with myofascial trigger points either active or latent. There have been no reported electromyography (EMG) changes when you have a myofascial pain syndrome.

The highest incidence of the onset of trigger points occurs between ages 31 and 50. When you are over 50, maximum activity could cause you to suffer from myofascial pain. As you continue to age and reduce your activity as a result of pain, your range of motion as a result of latent trigger points will become manifest. Many health-care providers are aware of myofascial trigger points.

Chiropractors treat myofascial trigger points, as do physical therapists, acupuncturists, anesthesiologists, dentists, pediatricians, rheumatologists, and specialists in physical medicine and rehabilitation all treat myofascial pain syndrome. The manner in which each of these health-care providers treats myofascial pain will vary from each of the health-care provider specialties.

If your pain is not relieved with conservative measures another method that can decrease your pain is a botulism toxin injection into your painful muscles. This drug is a gram-negative bacterium. In small doses it can relax or even paralyze small muscle fibers. The relief from the injection of the Botox can last up to three months. The problem with the Botox injection is that some individuals develop what appears to be fever and generalized joint pain associated with the bacteria that gets into their bloodstream. These side effects should however, subside over several days.

Given that no two people are alike, if you are taking any medications and begin to take nutritional supplements you should be aware that potential drug-nutrient interactions may occur and are encouraged to consult a health care professional before using any natural product. Combining certain prescription drugs and dietary supplements can lead to undesirable effects such as: diminished prescription drug effectiveness, reduced supplement effectiveness and impaired drug and/or supplement absorption.

Prevention of myofascial trigger points should be considered. This may be accomplished by doing stretching exercises both before and immediately after engaging in strenuous exercise. This concept may also be used if you are not physically fit and want to work in your garden for example. Do stretching exercises both before and after gardening. This may prevent the onset of myofascial pain.

A newer treatment for myofascial pain is Airrosti. The name Airrosti stands for Applied Integration for the Rapid Recovery of Soft Tissue Injuries. There is not enough evidence to determine whether Airrosti is safe or effective, much less whether it's the best treatment method out there.

Dry needling, also known as myofascial trigger point dry needling, is the use of either solid filiform needles (also referred to as acupuncture needles) or hollow-core hypodermic needles for therapy of muscle pain, including pain related to the myofascial pain syndrome.

Dry needling is a neurophysiological evidence-based treatment technique that requires effective manual assessment of the neuromuscular system. Physical therapists are well trained to utilize dry needling in conjunction with manual physical therapy interventions. Research supports that dry needling improves pain control, reduces muscle tension, normalizes biochemical and electrical dysfunction of motor end plates, and facilitates an accelerated return to active rehabilitation.

Many physical therapists and chiropractors have asserted that they are not practicing acupuncture when dry needling. The American Medical Association adopted a policy in 2016 that said physical therapists and other non-physicians practicing dry needling should at a minimum have standards that are similar to the ones for training, certification, and continuing education that exist for acupuncture. It would constitute fraud if a practitioner billed for dry needling treatments if he/she had no training in this modality. Some therapists bill Medicare for myofascial pain treatments that were never done on a patient.

Nearly $1.2 million in payments from Medicare, mostly for "physical therapy" was not provided by licensed physical therapists or not provided at all. Despite Medicare's best efforts to control costs, what Medicare has paid for outpatient PT services since the installation of the therapy cap has steadily risen since 2006.

A physical therapy clinic located at 27 Lois Street in Norwalk and was a part owner of Achieve Rehab and Fitness, a gym located at the same address in Norwalk. The indictment alleges that Faux engaged in a scheme to defraud Medicare and Anthem Blue Cross Blue Shield by referring some of her patients for personal training sessions at Achieve Rehab and Fitness and then billing the sessions as if they were physical therapy procedures. The indictment also alleges that Faux created and altered patient records when Medicare audited her practice in August 2009.

A massage by a massage therapist in another location was all billed to the patient's insurance company insurance as physical therapy. It is illegal to bill for such services as physical therapy. The codes all health care providers use to bill insurance companies are called CPT codes. Physical Therapists are allowed to bill only a few of these codes for things like evaluations, exercise and manual therapy.

These "therapy" codes can only be billed by a physical therapist, a licensed physical therapy assistant (not a technician) or a doctor. Some insurance does allow a chiropractor to bill for the codes but they also have to be the person providing the care. It can't be delegated by the chiropractor to a technician or trainer. If you were treated by a trainer or massage therapist it would be illegal for it to be billed as physical therapy. There is an epidemic of practices in Arizona that are billing for physical therapy services fraudulently.

Patients are provided most of their care by a trainer in some physical therapy practices. These types of practices are making money illegally. These people are hired by physical therapy practices because they are cheaper than hiring a licensed Physical Therapist. One individual was reported to law enforcement that he fraudulently represented to patients and insurance companies that he was a licensed physical therapist. He submitted more than $300,000 in fraudulent claims, most of which were for services provided to persons who had been injured in motor vehicle accidents. Evidence was determined that this individual allegedly engaged in daily and systemic overbilling, up coding, and billing for services not provided. Bills were submitted to Medicare or Medicaid for physical therapy services that were not provided and for services not medically necessary. Prescriptions had been written to patients in one scam for unnecessary physical therapy services.

Physical therapy can help patients with myofascial pain as well as other pain syndromes. Most insurance policies cover physical therapy services when provided by a licensed physical therapist. Physical therapists who are members of the American Physical Therapy Association (APTA) pledge to comply with the Association's Code of Ethics and Guide for Professional Conduct. APTA members maintain and promote high standards in the provision of physical therapy services.

17. TOPICAL ANALGESICS

The fastest-growing categories of compounded drugs are topical creams and gels, often used for pain. Pain relievers can be applied directly to your skin. These topical pain relievers are a noninvasive and convenient method for delivering pain-relieving medications. This is especially important and beneficial if you are not able to take medications by mouth. Topical pain relievers include complementary and alternative medications as well as conventional medications. Topical forms of analgesics, or pain relievers, have been used through-out human history.

The use of ointments for medicinal purposes is mentioned in the Bible. The purpose of a topical analgesic is to transmit a medication through your skin into your body. The amount of drug that actually gets through your skin is determined by the amount of pressure applied as you rub it over your skin, the area of your skin covered by the drug, the thickness of your skin and the way in which the drug is dissolved, and the use of dressings over your skin. Analgesics are available in ointments, creams, and gels. They also may be placed in patches that may be applied to your skin.

The advantage of topical analgesics is that they can be placed on your skin over the site of your pain. When compared to oral medications, you will have a lower blood level of the drug and will have fewer side effects and fewer drug interactions. There are different types of topical pain relievers. Ointments are semisolid preparations that melt at body temperature and spread easily. Ointments are not routinely used in the practice of pain medicine unless the ointment is specially compounded by a pharmacy.

Ointments are defined in three categories based on your skin penetration. One type of ointment does not penetrate beyond the external layer of your skin called the epidermis. Ointments of this class can be used for the treatment of sunburn. A second type of ointment penetrates to the internal layer of your skin called the dermis. The third type of ointment actually goes through your skin to the nerves and ligaments and in some instances into your bloodstream. The latter two types of ointments are frequently used in pain management.

Substances applied on your skin can evaporate. You do not want your analgesic drug evaporating from your skin. Your pharmacist will add substances such as glycerin to the ointment to keep this evaporation from happening. Ointments can be prepared by your pharmacist or purchased over the counter or by prescription. Some ointment preparations will contain absorption enhancers. Absorption enhancers make it easier for the drug to be absorbed through your skin. Azone and DMSO can both enhance the absorption of ointments through your skin. Ointments should be packaged in tubes.

Creams are opaque, thick, liquid substances that consist of medications dissolved in a cream base that usually vanishes through the skin. They are less of a liquid consistency than ointments. Gels are a drug-delivery system that usually contain penetration enhancers and are usually used for administering anti-inflammatory medications. The anti-inflammatory medication must be absorbed through your skin to provide you with pain relief. Gels are useful treatment methods if you have arthritic and/or muscle pain. Gels usually are thicker than creams or ointments and are usually clear, unlike creams and ointments.

The concentration of medication in gels is usually no greater than 2 percent. For example, lidocaine, which is a numbing medicine for the control of pain, is dispensed as a 2 percent gel. However, the cream is available in a 5 percent concentration. This is because medications are usually absorbed through the skin better if used in gel form. Gels usually have clarity and sparkle. They maintain their thickness even with an elevated body temperature. Some gels have been developed that may be given nasally. Some drugs are absorbed well through your nose than through your skin. Gels are usually dispensed in tubes or squeeze bottles.

Another delivery system for analgesics is a transdermal patch, which contains medication that is transmitted directly through your skin. A patch containing a medication is placed on your skin and remains there for a specified time so that the drug within the patch can be delivered through your skin to your bloodstream. Local anesthetics such as lidocaine, capsaicin cream, and fentanyl (a potent opioid medication), are some of the medicines that can be delivered through your skin using a transdermal drug delivery system.

Patches should be applied only to areas on your skin that have no blisters or open areas such as a cut. The patches are made of adhesive materials. You should not use the patch if you are allergic to some adhesives. The amount of drug that is absorbed from the patch is directly related to the length of the application of the patch, as well as the area of your skin to which it is applied. The advantage of the patch is that it gives you a continuous flow of analgesic medications.

When you take a pill, after it leaves your stomach or intestine and enters into your bloodstream, you receive a high concentration of the drug initially. As the drug is distributed to other tissues in your body, your blood level concentration of the drug decreases. Once your body breaks down the drug, you will no longer have an analgesic effect of that particular drug. However, when using a patch, you will have a continuous release of the drug from the patch into your bloodstream. You will have constant pain relief without the peaks and valleys of the drug concentration in your bloodstream associated with oral medications.

Natural compounds such as herbs or leaves and roots also can be used to treat your pain topically. Aloe Vera can be used to decrease your pain if you have sunburn. The use of this natural topical product for the treatment of various medical conditions was discovered in 1935. This drug is effective for the treatment of skin inflammation as well as minor burns. Capsaicin is a drug that has been extensively studied in both the clinical and laboratory settings.

Capsaicin is the active component of chili or red peppers. Capsaicin can be placed on your skin over your joints if you have joint pain (osteoarthritis). The capsaicin first stimulates the small pain-transmitting fibers (C fibers) by depleting these fibers of the neurotransmitter substance called P. After the substance P has been depleted, you will have a block of the pain fibers that cause burning pain sensations.

Observations in Hispanic individuals demonstrate that they did not have mouth or stomach pain after ingesting red peppers. The reason is the depletion of the pain-transmitting chemical (substance P) in the nerve endings in these areas following continual exposure to red peppers. Sub-stance P is also present in your joints throughout your body. For this reason, capsaicin can be an effective pain reliever for the treatment of pain associated with osteoarthritis and rheumatoid arthritis.

It may take a week for you to feel the pain-relieving effects of capsaicin. As substance P is being depleted from your nerve endings, you nerve endings still manufacture substance P. As a result, it will take several days to deplete enough of the substance P to provide you with pain relief. Once you discontinue use of this cream, your nerves will replenish substance P and your pain may return.

If you have a neuropathy, (e.g. burning foot pain) related to your diabetes you could have significant pain relief with topical capsaicin. Some pain-medicine physicians have used topical capsaicin to relieve the pain associated with shingles. You may have a brief burning sensation following the use of capsaicin.

You should be warned to avoid contact with your eyes and genital areas. It is recommended that you use rubber gloves when applying the capsaicin cream. You should use the capsaicin cream no more than three times a day. Various concentrations of capsaicin exist. Begin with a small concentration that contains 0.025 percent capsaicin. You may eventually increase your capsaicin dose to 0.075 percent capsaicin.

Menthol is an oil that is one component of peppermint oil. This oil in a cream base can significantly decrease your pain. When you place a menthol preparation on your skin, the menthol will feel cold to your nerve endings. While you feel the cold, your pain-stimulating nerves will be depressed. Following the initial cool sensation, you will feel a period of warmth. Menthol products can be used for the treatment of pain associated with arthritis, muscle pain, and tendonitis. Application of a menthol-containing cream may be of benefit to you if you suffer from tension headaches. It can be rubbed around the neck muscles just below the skull. It can be an extremely effective method for the treatment of your headaches.

Allergic reactions with menthol have been reported. It is recommended that you test a small amount of menthol on your skin before applying it extensively to assure yourself that you are not allergic it. You should not use the menthol preparation more than three times a day. Do not use a heating pad or a cold pack over the area of your skin where the menthol substance was placed. Some natural herbs and vegetable juices can be used as topical analgesics as well. One example is onion juice.

It is reported by some doctors that spreading the juice of a sliced on-ion over one of your painful areas could reduce your pain. A tincture can be made by putting 100 grams of minced onions in 30 grams of ethanol for a 70 percent solution. There are no hazards or side effects associated with the topical administration of an onion. However, frequent contact with the onion over time could possibly lead to an allergic reaction. The bark of a poplar tree also can be used for relieving your pain. The bark can be used for control of your pain over your joints or nerves or if you have rheumatoid arthritis. You should not use the bark if you are allergic to aspirin.

When externally applied to painful areas of your skin using the poplar bark and leaves, you should use no more than five grams of the drug per day. Either when using these topical natural products, you must follow the directions for the use of these medicines that are contained on the outside of the package or from an insert that may be placed in a box that holds a tube of any of these substances. You should remember that although these are natural products, they could have side effects like any other medication.

Another topical medication used to prevent pain is EMLA cream. This cream is dispensed only by prescription. It is used as a numbing agent more than it is used for reducing pain. This is a cream consisting of lidocaine and prilocaine, which are both numbing agents. This local anesthetic combination is packaged in tubes. An EMLA cellulose disc can be applied over your painful area. The purpose of EMLA is to provide pain relief over the painful area of your skin. It is used in children to reduce the pain of starting intravenous lines. Some pain-management doctors advocate its use to decrease the pain associated with reflex sympathetic dystrophy or the pain associated with shingles. This cream should be placed on an intact skin area.

The EMLA should be applied under a bandage for at least 60 minutes to provide relief over the painful area of your skin. This cream is not recommended if you have an allergy to lidocaine or prilocaine. If you have the blood disorder called methemoglobinemia, you should not use this cream. You should not exceed the recommended dose prescribed by your physician.

The problem with this cream as opposed to the Lidoderm patches is that it does provide pain relief for your skin but it can also numb your skin. This could be a problem if your skin becomes numb. This means that you have a block of all sensation in the skin treated with this cream. You should avoid causing any trauma to the area, including scratching your skin or rubbing or exposing your skin to extreme hot or cold temperatures until you have complete return of sensation to your skin. It is recommended that you not use this medication if you are taking heart medication. The local anesthetics in this cream can interact with some heart medicines.

Another analgesic cream that is available over the counter is a combi-nation of methyl salicylate and menthol. This is a cream that is effective for the temporary relief of arthritis and pain in your muscles. You should not use this medicine if your skin is sensitive to the oil of wintergreen. You should apply this cream around the sore areas on your body. You should not apply this cream more than three times a day. Do not place this cream over areas of the skin that are broken

Steroid creams are sometimes used for the treatment of joint pain. Topical steroids are anti-inflammatory agents. Pramoxine hydrochloride is a topical anesthetic agent that sometimes is combined with steroids to attempt to manage pain. This cream provides a temporary relief from pain. You should not use this cream if you are allergic to any of the substances in the cream such as the steroid or the pramoxine. If you develop a rash or blistering, you must stop using the cream. You should not use this cream more than three times a day. Furthermore, do not use this steroid preparation for more than five days. Do not reuse this cream until you have discussed the situation with your doctor.

Nonsteroidal anti-inflammatory agents (NSAIDS) may be compounded into creams by your pharmacist. These creams should not be used more than three times a day. Side effects with the nonsteroidal anti-inflammatory creams are the same as with the NSAIDs taken by mouth. However, the side effects of the topical NSAIDS are less than the oral NSAIDS. The side effects of any NSAID can include stomach upset and allergic reactions. If the dose is high enough, it could affect both your liver and kidneys. These NSAIDs can be very effective for the management of your pain when applied over your skin.

The use of a ketoprofen gel and a diclofenac gel, both NSAIDs, were compared at painful sites in a four-week study. The ketoprofen gel gave positive results for the treatment of knee pain and was shown to be better at relieving pain than the diclofenac gel. If you have joint pain, you may want to discuss these facts with your pain-medicine doctor or orthopedic doctor. Aspirin creams also may provide you with some pain relief when applied over your painful joints or muscles. Amitriptyline and ketamine are prescription drugs that may be mixed together to provide pain relief.

Ketamine is a potent analgesic that requires a prescription. Ketamine is a medication that can cause you to hallucinate if the dose is too high. A high dose of Ketamine is similar to LSD in its pharmacological effects. Elavil, an antidepressant can be applied topically to provide you with pain relief. A study in animals has used both of these agents together to treat pain in the laboratory setting. Amitriptyline, which is an antidepressant, has recently been shown to have pain-relieving properties when applied topically. Amitriptyline cream may be advantageous if you do not want to take amitriptyline pills by mouth.

An amitriptyline cream will not help you if you are suffering from significant depression, but can be helpful in decreasing your pain. Some patients complain of being tired while taking amitriptyline. However, amitriptyline can contribute to pain relief in fibromyalgia and the topical application may be a way of avoiding significant side effects that can be associated with oral use. There is ongoing research in this area. You may want to keep informed of the research on both of these drugs through the National Library of Medicine website at www.nlm.nih.gov.

The transdermal fentanyl patch system has become popular since it was introduced in the 1980s. This strong opioid medication was used initially for cancer pain management and then for noncancerous, chronic pain management. Fentanyl is able penetrate your skin easily. Fentanyl is 75 times more potent than morphine. It produces less histamine release from cells in your bloodstream and causes less itching than morphine. The fentanyl patch is primarily used for chronic or cancer-related pain.

A fentanyl patch can be used for most moderate to severe pain syndromes. In the fentanyl patch, the medication exists as a gel in a drug reservoir. Between this reservoir and your skin is a release membrane that has various-size holes that regulate the amount of fentanyl that is delivered to your skin. The larger the size of the holes will allow more fentanyl to be distributed to your skin and eventually through your skin which gives you a higher dose of the drug. The adhesiveness around the patch keeps it in place.

When the fentanyl patch is placed on your skin the fentanyl diffuses through the holes in the release membrane to the surface of your skin. It then goes to the outer layer of your skin and is deposited in a storage area. From the storage area, it is gradually absorbed into your blood-stream. This is the reason that it takes at least an hour before the fentanyl has begun to enter your bloodstream.

You will probably not notice any pain-relieving effects from this drug delivery system for about six hours. The patch is usually removed every three days. After the patch is removed, you will still have some drug that remains in the storage area under your skin. If you remove the patch and do not replace it, you will still receive fentanyl for hours after the patch has been removed.

Fentanyl patches come in different concentrations. The concentrations correlate with the area of the skin to which they are applied. The effectiveness of the patch is not affected by placing it on your chest, your back, or your upper arm. An increase in temperature will cause the medication to be rapidly delivered from the patch to your bloodstream.

Your skin's thickness also can affect the amount of fentanyl that is absorbed through your skin. The thicker your skin, the slower the rate of delivery of the fentanyl will be. The patch should not be applied over broken skin because the blood level of fentanyl can be significantly raised. There is no barrier to slow the absorption of the fentanyl. The fentanyl patch can cause a decrease in breathing and even death if you receive a significantly high dose of the fentanyl.

Occasionally, you may require medication for breakthrough pain if you do something to aggravate your chronic pain syndrome. For example, if you are using the patch for chronic pain and you go into your garden and do lifting, pushing, or digging, you may cause the onset of temporary pain on top of your chronic pain. At that time, an oral medication can be taken for treatment of your breakthrough pain. Another popular patch that is readily available by prescription from your pain-management doctor is the lidocaine-containing patch called Lidoderm.

The Lidoderm transdermal drug-delivery system exerts a significant amount of its pain-relieving effects by releasing a small amount of lidocaine into your bloodstream. Lidocaine is a local anesthetic. The patch does not cause numbness over your skin but does give you some degree of pain relief below the patch. There also is an effect on the nerves under your skin that are transmitting pain. This patch is used for the treatment of shingles. The Lidoderm patch contains 5 percent lidocaine. The lidocaine essentially does not reach your bloodstream like fentanyl.

The lidocaine penetrates your skin just enough to reach the nerve endings that are transmitting your pain. As a result, there are minimal side effects from the use of this patch other than from the adhesive layer of the patch. The amount of the lidocaine that is absorbed from the Lidoderm is related to the length of application over your skin. The patch should be used for 12 hours over your painful area and then removed for 12 hours. If an irritation or a burning sensation occurs around the adhesive aspect of the patch, you should discontinue use of the patch. None of the patches mentioned in this chapter should ever be reused.

If you suffer from back or muscle strain, or joint pain from osteoarthritis, these topical treatments might provide an alternative to swallowing acetaminophen (Tylenol), aspirin, ibuprofen (Advil), or naproxen (Aleve).

You must be aware that the Lidoderm patch does contain methyl paraben, which is found in many suntan lotions. Do not use the Lidoderm patch if you have allergies to any suntan lotions that contain this chemical. You should not use the Lidoderm patch if you are using a heart drug to control your heartbeat. Even though the amount of lidocaine that you can absorb is small, it can interfere with some heart medicines. If you are using heart medications, discuss any potential drug interactions with you doctor. If you become lightheaded following application of the patch, you must stop using the patch immediately.

Clonidine is another transdermal medication (Catepress). This patch is applied weekly to one area of your skin. The clonidine patch inhibits the release of norepinephrine, which is a pain transmitter. The clonidine patch also is used for the treatment of hypertension. If you have neuropathic (nerve injury) pain or reflex sympathetic dystrophy, the clonidine patch may provide you with significant pain relief. It also can be successfully used if you have pain following shingles.

The application of the clonidine patch can be most useful for pain associated with a nerve injury or inflammation of a nerve. The clonidine patch will not completely relieve your pain if you have reflex sympathetic dystrophy or post-shingles pain, but it can significantly decrease the burning component of your pain. The patch comes in different doses. The usual dose is the 0.1-milligram patch that is applied weekly.

Given that no two people are alike, if you are taking any medications and begin to take nutritional supplements you should be aware that potential drug-nutrient interactions may occur and are encouraged to consult a health care professional before using any natural product. Combining certain prescription drugs and dietary supplements can lead to undesirable effects such as: diminished prescription drug effectiveness, reduced supplement effectiveness and impaired drug and/or supplement absorption.

The plant polyphenol, resveratrol, naturally occurring in a number of fruits and other food products, has been extensively studied over the last two decades for its beneficial properties. Recently, its possible topical use in ameliorating skin conditions has also been proposed. The topical use of resveratrol can provide a good defense against induced skin damaged pain.1

Experiments have shown that soybean-germ oil (SGO) possesses a remarkable protective activity against UVB-induced skin inflammation. These results suggest that SGO might have interesting therapeutic and cosmetic applications in the management of some painful skin diseases initiated, sustained, or exacerbated by an over production of free radicals.2

The effect of dietary supplements based on Resveratrol, Lycopene, Vitamin C and Anthocyanins in reducing skin toxicity pain due to external beam radiotherapy in patients affected by breast cancer has been reported as well

Some compounding pharmacies are preparing compounded pain creams and ointments that contain a combination of multiple potent medications. Many include drugs that can cause central nervous system depression or cardiac effects such as ketamine, baclofen, cyclobenzaprine, lidocaine, tricyclic antidepressants, gabapentin, clonidine, and nifedipine. Most of these drugs have not been US Food and Drug Administration (FDA)-approved for topical use.

Southern California doctors were bribed to prescribe a pain-relief concoction as part of a $25 million workers' compensation scam. Prosecutors contend that Kareem Ahmed hired pharmacists to produce a pain-relief cream, gave kickbacks to doctors and chiropractors to prescribe it to workers' compensation patients, and conspired to submit phony claims.

Prosecutors alleged insurance fraud and conspiracy in a 44-count indictment, with crimes occurring from Oct. 1, 2009, through Jan. 31, 2013. Kickbacks to individuals were as high as $8 million over multiple years, the indictment said. It's a robocall, and it tells you that you have been selected to receive free pain relief cream. All you have to do is follow the prompts and arrange for delivery.

Sometimes a patient will receive a robocall to promote a topical pain cream. "In an attempt to stop the growing use and abuse of prescription narcotic pain pills, America's national health-care providers are now authorized to provide a new experimental pain relief compound to anyone suffering from physical pain or discomfort," the robocall says."This compound cream is directly applied to the pain-related areas," it continues. "It is non-narcotic and extremely effective. This new pain relief compound is provided to you by your insurance carrier with no out-of-pocket expense to you, and your pain relief cream can be shipped immediately."

The Food and Drug Administration (FDA) is warning five firms, Triangle Compounding Pharmacy, University Pharmacy, Custom Scripts Pharmacy, Hal's Compounding Pharmacy, and New England Compounding Center, to stop compounding and distributing standardized versions of topical anesthetic creams, which are marketed for general distribution rather than responding to the unique medical needs of individual patients. Firms that do not resolve violations in FDA warning letters risk enforcement such as injunctions against continuing violations and seizure of illegal products.

The FDA is concerned about the serious public health risks related to compounded topical anesthetic creams. Exposure to high concentrations of local anesthetics, like those in compounded topical anesthetic creams, can cause grave reactions including seizures and irregular heartbeats. Two deaths have been connected to compounded topical anesthetic creams made by Triangle Compounding Pharmacy and University Pharmacy, two of the five pharmacies receiving warning letters. Similar topical anesthetic creams are compounded by the other firms, and today's action serves as a general warning to firms that produce standardized versions of these creams.

Some of the prescriptions may not have been medically necessary or even dispensed at all, notes the report, which also details recent fraud cases brought by U.S. attorneys in several states. use among Medicare beneficiaries and federal employees in workers' compensation insurance plans has recently soared.

In Florida, federal prosecutors unsealed an indictment against a doctor who allegedly was given kickbacks including a BMW for sending prescriptions to a particular pharmacy, which then billed Tricare, Medicare and other government health programs for compounded creams. Prices ranged from about $900 to $21,000 for a one-month supply

Compounded pain creams are made with ingredients that may include not only pain relievers such as ketamine but also local anesthetics, blood pressure agents, muscle relaxants, nonsteroidal anti-inflammatory drugs, and antidepressants. The pharmacy may convert the ingredients into a cream from their original form as a liquid, tablet, capsule, or bulk dry powder.

Compound creams are not approved by the Food and Drug Administration and are intended for limited use, typically for people who can't take oral medication. CPCs often prescribed by pain clinics but also promoted or sold by other specialties, chiropractors, physiatrists and pharmacists.

Although individual ingredients are approved by the US Food and Drug Administration, the pain creams themselves, similar to all other compounded drugs, are not. Still, compounding pharmacies are allowed to operate, and are reimbursed by third-party payers, because they offer patients customized versions of drugs that meet their needs in ways a drug approved by the US Food and Drug Administration cannot (think adding a flavor to a child's cough syrup).

The pain creams, marketed to weekend athletes and the elderly alike, come with risks similar to any other drug. The Institute for Safe Medication Practices warns that many of the creams include ingredients that can cause "central nervous system depression or cardiac affects that result in slow breathing, a low heart rate or irregular beat, and drowsiness or loss of consciousness.

Two pharmacies paid kickbacks to prescribing physicians in the form of "research fees." For researching pain creams. Another Florida pharmacy disguised $70,000 in kickbacks as speaker's fees for an Indiana physician. Marketing firms that steered Tricare beneficiaries to compounding pharmacies received kickbacks as well, prosecutors said.

The United States alleges that four physicians had an incentive to refer prescriptions to their pharmacy, as steering costly prescriptions to the pharmacy Topical Specialists resulted in lucrative revenue streams for the doctors. The United States contends that these four physicians wrote hundreds of prescriptions for pain and scar creams. After speaking with patients, the government contends that these prescriptions were often not used by patients, despite the tremendous cost to the government.

While the pharmacies billed the federal government tens of thousands of dollars for these creams, the cost to actually compound them was often 4-5% of the submitted cost. Records reviewed by the government showed that the pharmacy was making up to 90% profit for each cream submitted to the Tricare health insurance program. This profit was then disbursed to the doctors who wrote the prescriptions.

In some cases, the four physicians recruited other doctors to write prescriptions – and shared their revenue with them. The government alleges that in some cases, the doctors who wrote prescriptions to Topical Specialists and WELL Health received up to 40% of the reimbursement. All four physicians received hundreds of thousands of dollars in reimbursements.

Topical cream manufacturers have fallen under scrutiny of the law for incentivizing prescribers to utilize these products. In Southern California, the Orange County grand jury has indicted 15 people involved with defrauding over $100 million from insurance companies. "We believe there were thousands of prescriptions being written and thousands being filled by multiple pharmacies in Orange County," and there were "huge markups billed to insurance companies," Workers' compensation insurers were billed in "the $1,500 to $3,000 range" for creams that had a wholesale cost of about $70.

The FDA keeps watch over topical medication scams.

18. ANTIDEPRESSANTS

Antidepressant drugs can decrease your pain intensity from an unbearable to a more bearable pain, although they will not completely resolve your pain. Antidepressant drugs are chemicals that go to your nerve connection areas in your brain and spinal cord. Neurons are not physically connected. Signals are transmitted by chemicals that go from one nerve ending to another. These drugs are chemicals that can attenuate the total number of pain signals that go to your brain.

As a result you experience less pain. Side effects such as dizziness and sedation caused by high doses of amitriptyline (Elavil) cause doctors to increase doses of antidepressants very gradually over several weeks. Initially only low doses of antidepressants like Elavil are needed. However, the dose needed to control pain may need to increase over time.

The analgesic properties of anti-depressant drugs were at one time felt to be related to the alleviation of depression, which can often accompany persistent chronic pain. However, several anti-depressants have been found to reduce pain symptoms in patients not experiencing depression. These agents are now believed to have primary analgesic abilities, which are most likely related to their effects on certain chemicals within your body. Cymbalta is one example. The efficacy of both serotonin and norepinephrine selective anti-depressants would suggest that effects on pain pathways which involve increases of either of these transmitters might contribute to analgesia.

Other suggested mechanisms of analgesia involve the antihistamine properties of some agents, increased endorphin secretion, and an increased density of cortical calcium channels. Antidepressant drugs can increase two chemicals in your brain and spinal cord that can decrease the number of pain signals that go to these structures. These chemicals are called serotonin and norepinephrine that were previously mentioned in this paragraph.

A tricyclic antidepressant drug used commonly for pain is amitriptyline (Elavil). This agent can cause constipation and dry mouth, and some patients complain of dizziness when they stand quickly (orthostatic hypotension). Sedation and tremors may also occur. Weight gain and sexual dysfunction have been also been reported. Some people even complain of a craving for chocolate. An overdose of tricyclic antidepressants or related drugs may cause you to experience a dangerous and even fatal abnormality of your heart rhythm.

Elavil taken in combination with opioids can cause more constipation than either of the drugs used alone. No antidepressant drug should be stopped abruptly without the advice of a doctor. When stopped suddenly, anxiety, vivid dreams, nausea, vomiting, and dizziness may result. Because of the frequent side effects associated with tricyclic antidepressants.

A newer class of antidepressant drugs called selective serotonin reuptake inhibitors (SSRIs) with fewer side effects is starting to take the place of Elavil. You do need to know however, that Elavil may have an effect on acid production in your stomach. Some of these drugs can actually decrease acid production and be of some benefit in patients who suffer from ulcers, reflux, or gastritis.

The newest antidepressant that is effective for some forms of pain is a combination serotonin and norepinephrine inhibitor called Cymbalta (duloxetine). This drug is effective in decreasing pain associated with diabetes called diabetic neuropathy. Cymbalta however, can make you sleepy and impair your thinking in some situations.

Another class of antidepressants is monoamine oxidase inhibitors (MAOIs). This class of antidepressant drugs is used for significant depression and is not usually used for pain management. MAOI'S drugs have a high incidence of side effects and overdoses can be lethal. These drugs increase the appetite of some patients. This class of drug increases the concentration of epinephrine, norepinephrine, and dopamine in your central nervous system, and when combined with foods such as cheese and wine high in tyramine may cause severe hypertension. For this reason, MAOIs should not be used by people with preexisting hypertension.

Side effects of MAOIs include constipation, nausea, vomiting, dry mouth, drowsiness, and dizziness. Sexual dysfunction may occur. If a MAOI is taken with meperidine (Demerol), a significant and potentially lethal elevation in body temperature can occur. MAOIs can also be associated with liver damage. Blood tests that assess liver function should be monitored routinely when anyone is taking any of these medications. Examples of MAOIs include Marplan and Parnate. The only time that a pain-management doctor usually sees a patient taking these drugs is when another doctor who was treating the patient for severe depression refers a patient.

You should be aware of some of the drugs in the selective serotonin reuptake inhibitors (SSRIs) class. The first drug of this class was fluoxetine (Prozac), introduced in 1987. Overall, this class of drugs causes fewer side effects than the tricyclic antidepressants or the MAOIs. The SSRIs exert their pain modulating and antidepressant effect by increasing serotonin levels in the central nervous system. This neurochemical is extremely valuable in reducing pain. Other SSRIs include piroxitine (Paxil), sertraline (Zoloft), and fluvoxamine (Luvox).

A SSRI, venlafaxine (Effexor), has been studied for its pain-modulating effects in chronic pain situations. This medication been shown to be effective in the control of pain in many painful disorders. The selective serotonin reuptake inhibitor class of drugs can cause nausea and diarrhea. Jitteriness and lack of sleep have also been reported as side effects in a small number of patients. Other individuals complain of sedation after taking this medication. If sedation is a problem, the medication should be taken only in the evening. The drug can be used as a nonaddicting sleep aid. A decreased libido is occasionally associated with this class of drugs.

Some reports exist that Prozac may lead a depressed patient to commit suicide. The drug itself does not cause suicide tendencies. Severely depressed patients can frequently have strong suicidal ideations and probably should be hospitalized while antidepressant medications were started. An individual who is sincere about committing suicide should be placed immediately under the care of a psychiatrist.

Be aware that SSRIs can decrease the efficacy of the opioid analgesics hydrocodone or oxycodone if taken in combinations with these agents. Both opioids are broken down in the liver to morphine, a chemical reaction that can be slowed by the SSRIs. As a result, less morphine is produced for pain relief.

A relatively new selective serotonin reuptake inhibitor, escitalopram oxlate (Lexapro), is now available to patients that do not affect liver metabolism. This medication does not interfere with the transformation of oxycodone and hydrocodone to morphine. Consequently, its use with these drugs will not decrease the efficacy of the opioid prescribed. This drug should be prescribed if you are taking hydrocodone (Lortab or oxycodone (Percocet). Patients must be told that the selective serotonin reuptake inhibitors can cause generalized muscle pain in a small number of patients. Muscle pain is not associated with tricyclic antidepressant use.

Trazodone (Desyrel) is essentially in its own antidepressant class and is known as an "atypical antidepressant" medicine. Like the other classes of antidepressants, this drug exerts its effect by increasing serotonin in your brain and spinal cord. It is not as potent as the tricyclic antidepressants but it does cause drowsiness and may be used to enhance sleep. Side effects include dizziness and dry mouth.

Priapism, a painful, persistent erection, is one of the most serious side effects of this drug in males and may precipitate a visit to an emergency room for treatment. The incidence of priapism associated with this medication in males is 1 in 10,000. The drug should be stopped immediately if there is any change in erectile function.

Studies have demonstrated that antidepressants can lessen the pain of the following syndromes in many patients: phantom pain, acute herpes zoster, post-herpetic neuralgia, cancer pain, cluster headaches, migraine headaches, reflex sympathetic dystrophy, and tension-type headaches. Is one class of antidepressant more effective than another? The drug of choice depends on the incidence of side effects as well as the effectiveness of the drug. This is one reason why your physician may try several different antidepressant drugs to attempt to determine which one works the best for you.

The occurrence of serious adverse effects resulting from antidepressant administration is low. These complications would be rare at the generally lower dosages utilized in the treatment of pain. While cardiac side effects are uncommon, tricyclic antidepressants are contraindicated in those individuals with heart failure or serious cardiac conduction abnormalities. Orthostatic hypotension (decrease in blood pressure following standing) is the most frequent cardiovascular adverse effect, and the elderly are particularly at risk. The sedating effect often observed with anti-depressant use can be beneficial as patients with pain often demonstrate diminished daytime functioning from inadequate sleep.

You may anticipate occasional side effects such as dry mouth, blurred vision, and urinary retention is more likely with amitriptyline use than with other TCAs. These effects are also less likely at the lower dosages used for analgesia. Nortriptyline and desipramine have been found to induce fewer side effects and are less sedating.

While antidepressant drugs have been demonstrated as useful adjuncts in the treatment of pain, their analgesic mechanism remains unclear. Initial dosing should be low and then slowly increased to minimize side effects. In other words start low and go slow with respect to drug dosing. When taken at night, the sedating properties of these agents can be beneficial in those pain patients experiencing difficulty with sleep. Today, antidepressants are the ninth-most popular type of prescription medicine, with annual sales topping $20 billion worldwide; according to health data firm IMS Health.

Depression affects the brain, so drugs that work in the brain may offer hope. Common antidepressants may help ease your symptoms, but there are many other options as well. Each drug used to treat depression works by balancing certain chemicals in your brain called neurotransmitters. SSRIs are common drugs for depression. In fact, they are the most commonly prescribed class of antidepressants. An imbalance of serotonin may play a role in depression.

These drugs fight depression symptoms by decreasing serotonin reuptake in the brain. SNRIs help improve serotonin and norepinephrine levels in the brain. This may reduce depression symptoms. TCAs are often prescribed when SSRIs or other antidepressants don't work. MAOIs are older drugs that treat depression. They work by stopping the breakdown of norepinephrine, dopamine, and serotonin. T

Paroxetine, which was marketed under the names Paxil and Seroxat, was introduced in 2001, following the publication of a trial carried out by the company itself that claimed the drug was "generally well tolerated" by children and adolescents suffering from depression. The drug was prescribed to more than 2 million American children the following year.

An independent re-analysis of the drug efficacy study trial was recently conducted by investigators from The British Medical Journal. Their research concluded that paroxetine was no more effective than a placebo and caused suicidal thoughts in 12 of 93 children who took the drug. The new study also revealed that the company ignored data related to the increased risk of suicide and noted that the original study known as Study 329 was written by a hired medical writer while one of the pharmaceutical companies senior scientists involved in the trial was being investigated by U.S. authorities.

Critical thinkers have difficulty placing faith in any depression treatment because science tells them that these treatments often work no better than placebos or nothing at all, and if one lacks faith in a depression treatment, it is not likely to be effective. According to the first comprehensive scientific review to include all available studies, including negative data that have long been withheld from public scrutiny by the pharmaceutical industry, four popular antidepressants being used to treat thousands of depressed American children are unsafe, ineffective or both.

In an article previously published in Newsweek explained the story of the cover up of the ineffectiveness of antidepressants. Americans are wondering how to contain health care costs. One of the best ways is for government programs not to pay for drug-based treatment options that cannot show effectiveness.

Much has been written about the benefits of modern anti-depressants of which Prozac is a popular antidepressant. A 2002 study analyzed FDA data on the 6 most widely prescribed antidepressants. It found that placebos had about 80% as much affect as the drugs themselves, suggesting that the pharmacological effects of antidepressants are clinically negligible. A large dose had no more effect than a smaller one.

A widely read 2010 JAMA article reported that most people taking anti-depressant drugs do no better than if they had received a sugar pill. It is clear that antidepressants are vastly over-prescribed and that the many behavioral and psychological interventions for depression are under used and under researched. The placebo effect is one psychological intervention strongly supported by evidence.

A Harvard Medical School psychologist, Irving Kirsch, who has been studying placebo effects for three decades, recently came up with the documented conclusion that pharmaceutical anti-depressants don't work. Antidepressants in particular have a well-established history of causing violent side effects, including suicide and homicide.

A pharmaceutical company was ordered to pay a record $3 billion in damages for wrongly promoting the dangerous drug between 1997 and 2004. The company paid doctors to attend events promoting Paxil and provided them with other perks, such as hunting trips and spa sessions.

Twenty-two years after the US marketing of Prozac, which changed the marketing, prescribing and widespread consumption of psychoactive drugs a meta-analysis of six large studies published in the Journal of the Medical Association (JAMA) confirms that industry's blockbuster drugs, SSRI antidepressants were unable to outperform placebos for moderate symptoms of depression. Just like the older, much cheaper tricyclic antidepressants, SSRIs show a clinical value only for severely depressed–i.e., clinically dysfunctional patients. Even cautious reporters of The New York Times could no longer avoid reporting the obvious–despite efforts to deflect from the scientific verdict:

The findings could help settle a longstanding debate about antidepressants. While the study does not imply that the drugs are worthless for anyone with moderate to serious depression many such people do seem to benefit it does provide one likely explanation for the sharp disagreement among experts about the drugs' overall effectiveness.

Taken together, previous studies have painted a confusing picture. On one hand, industry-supported trials have generally found that the drugs sharply reduce symptoms. On the other, many studies that were not initially published, or were buried, showed no significant benefits compared with placebos.

Antidepressants can cause some people to become hostile and aggressive. Both hostility and aggression are mentioned in some package inserts for antidepressants sold in the United States, but fall under the category of side effects that are qualified with the words may have no association with the drug or "It is important to emphasize that although the events reported occurred during treatment with [antidepressant, they were not necessarily caused by it."

The maker of Zoloft was sued in an unusual case alleging the popular antidepressant has no more benefit than a dummy pill and that patients who took it should be reimbursed for their costs. Drug maker GlaxoSmithKline (GSK) has agreed to pay $3 billion US in criminal and civil fines and plead guilty to misdemeanor criminal charges related to the sale and marketing of its antidepressants Paxil and Wellbutrin and the diabetes drug Avandia in the largest health-care fraud settlement in U.S. history.

The British pharmaceutical giant has admitted to misbranding the antidepressants Paxil and Wellbutrin and marketing them for uses not approved by the U.S. Food and Drug Administration (FDA), including the treatment of children for depression and the treatment of ailments such as obesity, anxiety, addiction and ADHD. In some cases, the company did so despite warnings about possible safety risks from the FDA, such as an increased risk of suicide for children under 18 taking antidepressants.

Lexapro has proven widely effective in the treatment of depression and anxiety disorders and has grown immensely in popularity over the last several years. Numerous lawsuits have been filed against Forest Laboratories, the makers of Lexapro, for the birth defects and dangerous medical conditions that have been linked with the usage of this drug.

New documents uncovered by ABC News suggested that GlaxoSmithKline, the maker of the popular antidepressant Paxil, failed to disclose important information about the possibility of an increased risk of suicidal behavior in some children taking the drug, as well as serious withdrawal symptoms when some patients stop taking Paxil.

Researchers have documented an alarming link between the use of antidepressants and the development of serious heart disease. The link was discovered by following 63,449 women as part of the Nurses' Health Study. The results show a specific relationship between antidepressant use and sudden cardiac death. In this cohort of women without baseline coronary heart disease, depressive symptoms were associated with fatal coronary heart disease, and a measure of clinical depression including antidepressant use was specifically associated with sudden cardiac death."

This antidepressant news followed another recent and rather stunning finding, that antidepressants cause significant bone loss. The commonly used SSRI antidepressants double the risk for fractures in anyone over the age of 50 who uses them regularly. The mechanism involved is that too much serotonin2 from the drugs directly interferes with the formation of new bone.

On top of this disturbing news, it has become quite clear that the majority of negative studies about popular antidepressants such as Prozac, Zoloft, Paxil, and Effexor were never published, according to a study in the New England Journal of Medicine, as reported in the New York Times. Thirty-seven studies the FDA considered positive were published, whereas only three negative studies were published. Thirty-three studies the FDA considered negative or questionable were either not published or published with a twist to look positive when they were not. This made antidepressant studies appear 96% positive in the literature, when in fact the studies were only 51% positive.

In the Western medical model of treating symptoms as they arise, without identifying the cause, women on antidepressants losing bone mass will simply be put on the bisphosphonate drugs. This is another drug con job, as these drugs actually disturb the health of bone and at best keep old bone in place while blunting the formation of new and healthy bone.

Two dimensional pictures can appear to show more bone density with their use, which is nothing but smoke and mirrors, as the bone is actually swollen and malformed (like a swollen ankle). The FDA has warned that these drugs can cause serious bone pain. Bone drugs are actually linked to rotting jaw bone, increased risk of fracture with long-term use, and a poor bone-healing response if you happen to fracture a bone while taking them.

Bone drugs also increases a person's risk for atrial fibrillation, which can also cause sudden cardiac death. A report in the Archives of Internal Medicine offers conclusive proof that users of Fosamax are at an

86% increased risk for developing heart-related damage in the form of atrial fibrillation. The FDA, looking at the same data, has stonewalled the issue, allowing Big Pharma to go on injuring without proper notification of risks for the public.

Adding to the list of suspect cardiovascular drugs are the widely prescribed statins. These drugs are now proven to disturb how your cells make energy, meaning they are directly making aging worse. Also, energy is required to make your brain function normally and have a good and positive mood. It is amazing that a society is so brainwashed by their pill-pushing physicians that 20 billion dollars' worth of fatigue-producing and nerve-deteriorating drugs will be gullibly swallowed this year. The side effects of statins are so bad, especially in older people, that a new study demonstrates their risks in people 70 or over far outweigh their benefits even if the person has heart disease.

This is a real double-edged sword. Statins cause depression by directly interfering with normal nerve transmission, a problem that gets worse with extended use and higher doses, the primary way these drugs are used. The anti-energy effects of statins can weaken the heart muscle, setting the stage for cardiomyopathy and congestive heart failure. Partly, this is because statins directly interfere with the production of Q10, an important nutrient your heart must have to work properly so as to make energy. Partly, it is because statins are directly toxic to muscle and injure muscle in more than 15% of users, and your heart is a muscle.

Thus, men and especially women can find themselves on a potentially devastating cocktail of drugs, any of which increase the risk for heart failure and taken together are really likely to boost risk. The drugs are so bad for health that they create the symptoms that imply the need for more drugs! It is a vicious cycle that is hard to break. In fact, when combinations of cardiovascular and diabetes drugs are used to aggressively treat type II diabetic patients the results are abysmal, resulting in an increase in deaths.

This problem is not theoretical. At a previous meeting of the American Heart Association researchers presented data showing an unexpected increase in congestive heart failure in patients 65 and over. During the past several decades, paralleling the expanded use of such drugs as statins, bone drugs, and anti-depressants, the rate of heart failure amongst Americans had risen to extra 450,000 cases per year. This statistic cannot be explained by an increased population of older Americans. People are being injured and killed and virtually nobody is doing anything about it.

Drug injuries are still on the rise as well. The newer drugs people are taking are still likely to injure patients. Doctors at one time were being paid on the side at by large pharmaceutical companies to prescribe drugs to patients. This activity has decreased because of the watchful eye of the Federal Drug Administration. Sadly, patients themselves must investigate the risks and benefits of the medications which have been prescribed to them.

19. ALTERNATIVE TREATMENTS

The term "alternative medicine" encompasses a wide array of health care practices, products, and therapies that are distinct from practices, products, and therapies used in conventional medicine. Examples of alternative medicine include homeopathic, traditional Chinese, and Ayurvedic medicine. Alternative medicine may be very effective in decreasing your pain. Many conventional medicine pain practices include alternative medicine clinicians as part of their multidisciplinary treatment. For example practices include alternative medicine clinicians as part of their multidisciplinary treatment. For example, acupuncture may be offered in some pain practices. "Conventional medicine" is practiced by medical doctors (M.D.) or doctors of osteopathy (D.O.).

Conventional medicine includes methods practiced by allied health-care professionals such as physical therapists, occupational therapists, psychologists, and registered nurses. Other terms for conventional medicine include allopathic medicine, mainstream medicine, and orthodox medicine. There are two main categories of frauds in alternative medicine. One category consists of illegitimate therapies that are emulations of poisonous orthodox medicine, such as the use of radiation. The other category of alternative medicine frauds is much more disturbing. This latter category is heavily influenced by dark religions.

Complementary and alternative medicine is referred to as unconventional or non-conventional medicine. The following is a definition for alternative medicine specialties by the National Center for Complementary and Alternative Medicine. "Complementary and alternative medicines are practices and products that are not currently considered to be part of conventional medicine." Complementary and alternative medicine practices change and update continually.

In general, health fraud drug products are articles of unproven effectiveness that claim to treat disease or improve health. In addition to wasting billions of consumers' dollars each year, health scams can lead patients to delay proper treatment and cause serious—and even fatal—injuries. FDA is very concerned about these fraud products, and removing these products from the market remains one of the Agency's top priorities.

The National Institute of Health (NIH) is reviewing alternative therapies and is confirming efficacy and safety in some areas. Complementary and alternative medicines, unlike many conventional medicine therapies, are designed to help you develop control over your health. If you are going to use any of these methods, you are encouraged to learn the side effects of some of these medicines as well as learn about drug interactions with conventional medications.

These interactions can be lethal. Do not be afraid to tell your physician what complementary medicines you are taking. Remember that when you are using alternative medicines that these medicines are not strictly controlled with respect to dosage and the amount of drug in a pill, capsule, or tea.

All plants have different amounts of substances in them. A true dose of an alternative medication in a pill is unknown in many instances. You should look carefully at the label before taking one of these substances and not take more than the label recommends. The overall drug interactions of herbal substances have not been established because they are not required to be studied by the FDA.

Conventional medical professionals are beginning to recognize the benefits of alternative medicine. As an example, the National Institute of Health Office of Alternative Medicine was established in 1992. In addition, there has been a significant increase in professional interest in the area of alternative medicine. Medical schools are beginning to offer elective courses on alternative medical therapies. The attitudes of medical school faculty toward the use of complementary medicine practices are important because the attitude of these individuals can influence their students.

Some health plans have now announced their intention to incorporate payment for some alternative medicine practices into their insurance coverage. Some managed care corporations have revealed their intentions to include alternative medicine practices for payment. Some state governments are considering legislation pertaining to the practice of alternative medicine by health-care professionals.

If you are going to use a natural substance or therapy, you are responsible for your own care. You must not self-diagnose yourself. You must discuss your symptoms of pain with your physician before taking any nutritional supplement. Grapefruit juice taken for weight loss for example may decrease the absorption of some medications from your stomach. As a result, you may not be getting the medicine that you need.

There are risks and benefits that you should be aware of when using alternative medications and therapies to manage your pain. In addition, the alternative medications you take could react with the prescription medications your doctor has given you and cause you even more problems. For example, high doses of vitamin E can decrease your blood's ability to form a blood clot.

If you are taking a blood thinner like Plavix in addition to vitamin E, you could develop a serious bleeding problem. If in doubt, consult the Physician's Drug Reference for herbal medicines. This will advise you about safe doses and any precautions and drug interactions that you may need to be aware of.

There was a study published in the New England Journal of Medicine in 1993 that was a survey of individuals in order to get their opinion of alternative medicine practices. More than 30 percent of those surveyed at that time chose alternative medicine over conventional medicine methods to prevent and treat disease.

In 1994, Congress passed the Dietary Supplement Health and Education Act. In passing this act, Congress recognized that many individuals believed that dietary supplements offered health benefits. The bill gave dietary supplement manufacturers freedom to produce more products and to provide information about their products' health benefits. The Food and Drug Administration (FDA), on the other hand, is responsible for overseeing any claims by the dietary supplement The FDA monitors manufacturers to the truthfulness of their claims.

The Federal Trade Commission regulates the advertising of all of the dietary supplements. You should be aware that the quality control standards for natural substances are a problem within this industry. Some of the manufacturers of these products will not have the amount of substance in the natural medication as stated on the container label.

You need to know that when you are using alternative medicines that these medicines are not strictly controlled with respect to dosage and the amount of drug in a pill, capsule, or tea. All plants have different amounts of chemicals in them. A true dose of a medication is unknown in many instances. You should look carefully at the label before taking one of these sub-stances and not take more than the label recommends.

The overall drug interactions of herbal substances have not been established because they are not required to be studied by the FDA. You must do your own research to determine whether the natural substance that you are taking has an accurate dosage as stated on the container label for the product.

Alternative medicine is now recognized as a legitimate medical practice. Many physicians have had personal experience with alternative medicines and felt that they were effective. Before treatment by an alternative medicine specialist, inquire to ascertain that they are properly trained. In other words, inquire as to whether or not that they have had training in alternative medicine science.

For example if you want acupuncture, you should inquire if there are state requirements for the practice of acupuncture. Someone that is not trained could cause you harm. The NIH does award grants for the study of research in complementary as well as alternative medicines. Clinical trials are being done throughout the United States with respect to complementary and alternative medicines. You may want to participate in one of these trials.

Study trials with respect to herbal medicines are an important part of the medical research process. The results from clinical trials can define better ways to treat your painful conditions. A clinical trial is a research study in which a therapy is tested on individuals like you to ensure that the medicine being tested is safe and effective. Always remember that clinical trials have risks. Before participating in a clinical trial, discuss this trial with your primary care physician. To find out about ongoing clinical trials for example, studies on arthritis and neurological disorders go to www.nccam.nih.gov.

You also may want to access the National Library of Medicine online (www.pubmed.com). Complementary medicine on PubMed is available that contains citations to articles on recently published research. You may want to see a homeopathic or naturopathic specialist. Homeopathic specialists prescribe dilutions of natural substances from plants, minerals, and animals. Homeopathy has been around for more than 200 years.

About 500 million people around the world receive homeopathic treatment. The World Health Organization has recommended that homeopathy is a system of traditional medicine that should be integrated with conventional medicine, which is considered the traditional approach to medicine.

It is important to know that the U.S. Food and Drug Administration recognizes homeopathic remedies as official drugs and regulates their manufacture. This is unlike the herbs used for medicinal use. Conventional physicians in Europe use homeopathy qualities of medicine frequently. In Britain, homeopathy is a part of the national health system.

The basic principles of homeopathy are that a disease can be destroyed and removed by a type of medicine that is able to produce the disease in humans. In other words, a substance that in large doses would produce symptoms of a disease can be used in very minute doses to cure it. In conventional medicine, this is called the theory of antibiotics.

Homeopathic practitioners adhere to the fact that the more a substance is diluted, the more potent it is. In conventional medicine, it is believed that a higher dose of the medicine will lead to a greater effect. The purpose of diluting out substances in homeopathic medicine is to avoid side effects. Homeopathic practitioners adhere to the fact that illness is different for every person. Homeopathic treatments are unique for each patient.

Homeopathic medicine emphasizes that patients are individuals and have individual signs and symptoms of an illness and should be treated only on an individual basis. The entire individual is treated, which includes the physical, psychological and spiritual portions of each person. Naturopathic medicine treats disease by using your body's natural ability to heal itself. Naturopathic practitioners invoke healing processes by using a variety of treatment options based on your particular needs. In naturopathic medicine, disease symptoms are a sign of your body's attempt to heal itself.

The steroid can be given over approximately two weeks. Sometimes your doctor will inject your painful joint with a steroid. Colchicine is the medication that has been used extensively over the past two decades for the treatment of gout. It is most effective during the first 24 hours of an acute attack. Colchicine can cause you to have vomiting and nausea. If you have liver problems, you should not take colchicine.

Allopurinol is another drug that can decrease your uric acid levels. Allopurinol is usually used in people who produce excessive uric acid. Allopurinol should not be used during an acute gouty arthritis episode because Allopurinol can prolong the attack. Some rheumatologists prescribe probenecid because it has fewer side effects than Allopurinol. Some patients may need narcotics for management of their pain.

Dietary supplements are recommended in complimentary medicine. Dietary supplements also have unseen harms. For example, kava can cause severe and occasionally fatal liver damage; blue cohosh can cause heart failure; nutmeg can cause hallucinations; comfrey can cause hepatitis; monkshood can cause heart arrhythmias; wormwood can cause seizures; stevia leaves can decrease fertility, concentrated green tea extracts can damage the liver, bitter orange can cause heart damage, and

Aristolochia, found in Chinese herbs, can cause kidney failure and bladder cancer.

If you have developed tophi (nodules under your skin) that are painful, you may need to have these uric acid crystals removed surgically. If you have had significant destruction of one of your joints, an orthopedic surgeon may need to surgically correct any malformation that may be related to uric acid deposition in your joints and the resultant joint naturally. Naturopathic medicine gets its data from Chinese, Native American, and Greek cultures.

Reflexology is another method used in nonconventional medicine practice to decrease your pain. Reflexology relieves muscle stress and relaxes your muscles through the application of pressure on specific areas of your feet. Reflexology has been used for thousands of years in mideastern coun-tries. In the early twentieth century, a doctor mapped the foot areas that related to areas of the body that affected different medical conditions.

This doctor divided the body into 10 zones and he labeled parts of the foot that he believed controlled each zone. Gentle pressure on an area of the foot would generate not only pain relief but healing in general in the defined zone. These areas of pressure in your feet are called reflex points.

The philosophy of reflexology is that your body contains an energy field. When your energy field is blocked, you develop pain and/or illness. Stimulation of your foot and the nerves that end in your feet can unblock the energy flow and increase energy to various parts of your body and promote healing as well as decrease your pain. It also is believed that stimulation of your feet can release the natural painkillers in your body called endorphins. Reflexology treatment sessions can last from 30 to 60 minutes. Usually you will receive a four-week treatment program.

Reflexology can be used for the management of your back pain. Re-flexologists believe that nerve endings in the feet have inner connection throughout the spinal cord and brain to reach all areas of the body. The problem with reflexology is that it has not been scientifically studied and still remains an unproven treatment regimen for the management of your pain.

A therapeutic massage can significantly help you control your pain, especially if you have muscle spasms. Massage therapy can decrease your stress as well as decrease your headaches and pain associated with whiplash injuries.

Massage therapy promotes generalized body relaxation. Massage is the application of touch to your muscles or ligaments that does not cause you to move or change position of a joint. Massage therapy can decrease your lower back pain as well as your neck pain. It also has been effective to reduce pain associated with sciatica. Massage therapy can decrease the pain associated with tension headaches.

There are different types of massage therapy. The Swedish massage is the most common form of massage therapy in the United States. Swedish massage works on the superficial layers of the skin as well as the superficial muscles of your body. Swedish massage promotes relaxation and improves circulation in your superficial muscles. Another type of massage is deep-tissue massage. This is more direct pressure on the deeper muscle layers of your body.

Deep-tissue massage is highly effective for the treatment of lower back pain. Sports massage combines Swedish massage with deep-tissue massage. This type of massage therapy can decrease your pain following a vigorous athletic workout. It may not be a good idea to use therapeutic massage if you have certain forms of cancer, heart disease, or some infectious diseases.

Another method to help you control your pain is aromatherapy. Women have a better perception of smell than men. Therefore, women are more likely to use aromatherapy because they have better results from this method than men.

For hundreds of years, oils extracted from plants have been used to relieve pain. During your first session with an aromatherapy specialist, the specialist will select the oil that is appropriate for relieving your pain. You may have a treatment for up to nine minutes.

Aromatherapy stimulates pleasure centers in your brain from nerves in the nose that senses smell. Aromatherapy can be used to improve your quality of life and provide you with some relaxation. It has been used for pain management during childbirth. It can be used if you have arthritis, back pain, neck pain, and other chronic pain syndromes.

Aromatherapy is reportedly effective for the treatment of muscle pain as well as pain that originates from a nerve injury. You must not use any of the aromatherapy oils if you are allergic to the herbs from which the oils were derived. If you have trouble breathing, you should not use aroma-therapy. Some aromatherapy can cause drowsiness.

Sage, rosemary, and juniper oils may increase uterine contractions if you are pregnant. You should not use these oils during pregnancy. Essential oils such as clove, cinnamon, and thyme can have anti-inflammatory proper-ties and are useful in decreasing your joint pain if you have arthritis. Aroma-therapy can be used in the following preparations: nose drops, air sprays, steam tents, candles, and drops in your bath.

Acupuncture is another popular method that can be used for pain management. Acupuncture can decrease both your pain as well as your stress. Acupuncture originated in China more than 2,000 years ago. Acupuncture is based on the belief that your health is determined by a balanced flow of vital life energy referred to as chi.

There are 12 major energy pathways in your body called meridians. Each meridian is linked to a specific internal organ. There are more than 1,000 acupoints within the meridians of your body. Stimulation of these meridians enhances the flow of your vital life energy.

Needles are inserted just under your skin to stimulate these meridians and provide you with pain relief. It is believed that acupuncture releases the body's own chemicals that relieve pain, called endorphins and enkephlins. These two chemicals are your body's natural pain-killing chemicals. Acupuncture can decrease the production as well as the distribution of substances that cause pain nerve impulses to go to the brain. Acupuncture, therefore, can decrease your need for conventional pain pills. Acupuncture has been demonstrated to decrease muscle-tension headaches.

In 1997, the National Institutes of Health endorsed acupuncture for postoperative pain, dental pain, tennis elbow, and carpal tunnel syndrome. The World Health Organization has reported that acupuncture can be useful for the treatment of migraine headaches, trigeminal neuralgia, sciatica, and arthritis.

Acupuncture also can be used to treat fibromyalgia, neck pain, and back pain. In some states there is no licensing required to be an acupuncturist, whereas other states limit the practice to medical doctors and chiroprac-tors. In some states acupuncturists are considered primary health-care professionals and may see you without your doctor's referral.

Some states require that an acupuncturist graduate from an approved school and pass a state licensing examination. To find physicians that practice acupuncture, you can go to the website www.medicalacupuncture.org. Furthermore, the American Association of Oriental Medicine has a website, www.aaom.org, which is a national trade organization of acupuncturists who have met acceptable standards of competency. This organization can provide you with the names and locations of competent members of this organization in your community.

Naturopaths recommend healing of the person and not the disease. Naturopathic medicinal treatments will include doses of natural substances that are much higher than those used by practitioners of homeopathic medicine. To best choose a natural product to decrease your pain, you should know which chemicals in the body produce pain. With this knowledge, you can pick the analgesic best suited to relieve your pain. If you have joint pain, for instance, you will want to use an alternative medicine that has anti-inflammatory properties.

If you are injured or have inflammation, your body makes a variety of chemicals that transmit pain impulses to a pain-processing center in your brain. These chemicals include the prostaglandins, cytokines, substance P, glutamic acid, and nitric oxide. Nitric oxide is a gas that is a pain chemical transmitter in your nervous system. Some remedies will be mentioned in this chapter. For in depth information, it is recommended that you consult a naturopathic book.

Given that no two people are alike, if you are taking any medications and begin to take nutritional supplements you should be aware that potential drug-nutrient interactions may occur and are encouraged to consult a health care professional before using any natural product. Combining certain prescription drugs and dietary supplements can lead to undesirable effects such as: diminished prescription drug effectiveness, reduced supplement effectiveness and impaired drug and/or supplement absorption.

The spice, turmeric has anti-inflammatory and antioxidant effects and has been shown to inhibit prostaglandin formation. This drug should not be used if you have gallbladder disease. Furthermore, do not use this medicine if you have hypertension. No significant serious health risks or side effects with use of this substance have been reported to date. The average dose is 3 grams of turmeric per day. This dose can be divided up into 1-gram doses and be taken 3 times per day with meals. For example, you may take 1 milligram with each meal for a total dose of 3 grams.

Ginseng has anti-inflammatory effects and is used in homeopathic medicine for the treatment of rheumatoid arthritis. Do not use ginseng with caffeine. Exercise caution if you use ginseng along with any antidiabetic medicine or insulin. You should not use ginseng with MAOI inhibitors, which are used to decrease your blood pressure.

Do not use ginseng in combination with diuretics. Side effects include sleep deprivation, nosebleeds, headaches, nervousness, and vomiting. The average daily dose of this root is 1 to 2 grams. Do not take more than 2 grams per day. The 2 grams can be divided up and taken 3 times a day.

Resveratrol is an antioxidant and a COX-2 inhibitor that some believe prevents heart disease and cancer. It is largely found in the skin of red grapes. Therefore, many people obtain resveratrol by drinking red wine. This substance can prevent clot formation, whereas the conventional COX-2 inhibitors do not prevent clot formation. The usual dose is no more than 600 mg per day. There are no known side effects or drug interactions for resveratrol itself. Fish oils contain the omega-3 fatty acids and can decrease prostaglandins.

Fish oils are used for the treatment of rheumatoid arthritis. You also may use fish oils for the control of joint pain. The most common side effect that you may experience with fish oil supplementation is mild stomach upset. The fish oils can decrease your blood's ability to clot. If you are taking blood-thinning drugs, you should not take fish oils, because it will give you an increased risk of bleeding. You may take up to 10 grams of fish oil per day.

N-acetylcysteine is an amino acid produced by your body that will decrease prostaglandin formation. It can help prevent some diseases and boost your immune system. You should not take this drug if you are taking carbamazepine (Tegretol). Side effects include headaches, nausea, vomiting, and an upset stomach. The recommended dose is 200 milligrams 3 times a day.

Cayenne is an anti-inflammatory medication that is helpful for the treatment of muscle pain and arthritis. This drug may be helpful for inhibit-ing the release of substance P (a pain signal transmitter) as well. Cayenne side effects include diarrhea and intestinal colic. It can decrease your body's ability to form a normal blood clot. It also can reduce the effects of aspirin, so you should be aware of this fact if you are taking aspirin as a blood thinner. High doses of cayenne over a prolonged time can cause kidney and liver damage. You should not use this drug for more than two days in a row. After two weeks you may use it again for two days. The daily dose of cayenne should not exceed 10 grams.

Ipriflavone can be used as a prostaglandin inhibitor. Women also use it to decrease the incidence of osteoporosis. This medicine can actually stop bone loss. It can decrease the risk of fractures in bone pain in females. This drug, like the other drugs that are prostaglandin inhibitors, can increase the blood-thinning activity of other drugs that you may be taking, such as Coumadin. It also can increase the effects of some asthma drugs such as theophylline, so avoid taking ipriflavone if you are using such medications.

Procyanidolic oligomers are natural substances extracted from grape seeds. They are useful for their antioxidant effects. They can decrease arthritis pain. There are no significant side effects associated with this drug. The daily dose of this drug ranges from 150 to 300 milligrams per day. However, another important effect of this medicine is that it can decrease the effects of nitric oxide.

Nitric oxide is sometimes released from cells in your bloodstream. Nitric acid essentially exists in a gas form in your body and this gas stimulates pain fibers to transmit pain impulses to your brain. Nitric oxide inhibitors include the fish oils. Cytokines are chemicals produced in your bloodstream that also enhance pain impulses. They contribute to the formation of substances that can destroy your joint linings if you have rheumatoid arthritis. Fish oils can reduce these substances in your body. These are just some examples of natural substances that can help you control your chronic pain.

Increased recognition of the limits of conventional medicine has helped drive the growing interest in complementary and alternative medicine which is now being commonly used in patients with chronic diseases, including individuals with Crohn's disease and ulcerative colitis.1

Alternative and complementary therapeutic approaches, such as the use of a wide array of herbal, nutritional, and physical manipulations, are becoming popular for relieving symptoms of osteoarthritis (OA). There is evidence of possible beneficial effects of alternative medicines in the management of OA. Treatments without scientific merit have included ion-exchange machines, lymphatic drainage massage, electrical or magnetic stimulation, Rife machines, hyperbaric oxygen chambers, and intravenous immunoglobulins. Genuine alternatives are comparable methods that have met science-based criteria for safety and Effectiveness. Experimental alternatives are unproven but have a plausible rationale and are undergoing responsible investigation. The most noteworthy is use of a 10%-fat diet for treating coronary heart disease.

When someone feels better after having used a product or procedure, it is natural to credit whatever was done. This is unwise, however, because most ailments resolve by themselves and those that persist can have variable symptoms. Even serious conditions can have sufficient day-to-day variation to enable useless methods to gain large followings. Another drawback of individual success stories is that they don't indicate how many failures might occur for each success. People who are not aware of these facts tend to give undeserved credit to "alternative" methods.

The FDA has issued a number of warning letters against companies that promoted alternative medicine products. In 2009, the FDA advised consumers not to use certain Zicam cold remedies; FDA also warned consumers against loss of smell associated with certain intranasal cold remedies containing zinc. Further research is needed

20. CHIROPRACTIC

Daniel David Palmer discovered the power of spinal manipulation by allegedly healing a deaf man by repositioning a vertebra in his spine. Shortly after, he healed someone with heart trouble through the same technique. Convinced he discovered a new medical technique, he opened the Palmer School of Chiropractic in 1897.

Palmer claimed that 95% of all diseases were caused by displaced vertebrae, a belief many chiropractors today still hold. To explain this, he invented new terms like "subluxation" (a displacement of the spine). Chiropractors believe bones can get subtly out of line and cause muscle spasms or nerve irritation. This causes the pain. Realigning the bones by manipulations called adjustments supposedly helps relieve it.

Further, most chiropractors claim their adjustments do more than just relieve pain; they allow the body to function better. If nerves aren't being pinched, all messages they transmit, from digestion to muscle relaxation to hormonal activation, can proceed more normally.

Chiropractic researchers have documented that fraud, abuse and quackery are more prevalent in chiropractic than in other health care professions. A study of California disciplinary statistics during 1997–2000 reported 4.5 disciplinary actions per 1000 chiropractors per year, compared to 2.27 for medical doctors, and the incident rate for fraud was 9 times greater among chiropractors (1.99 per 1000 chiropractors per year) than among medical doctors.

Chiropractic therapy was established as a profession in 1895. It is now the second-largest primary health-care field in the world. You may be scared of the dangers and side effects of pills and procedures that may lead you to seek out chiropractic therapy. Chiropractic therapy as a profession emphasizes your body's natural health abilities. Many people associate chiropractic therapy with only back and neck pain. However, chiropractic therapy has been shown to be safe for the treatment of headaches, carpal tunnel syndrome, and pain in your arms and legs.

Low back pain may have many causes. In most cases of injury or strain it takes time for your back to heal. Back pain lasts just as long if you go to a chiropractor, if you go to a physical therapist or if you seek no treatment at all. Chiropractic manipulation and conventional medical care are about equally effective for relieving acute low back pain. Chiropractic treatment is based on the concept that restricted movement in the spine may lead to pain and reduced function.

Spinal adjustment is just one form of therapy chiropractors use to treat restricted spinal mobility. During an adjustment, chiropractors use their hands to apply a controlled, sudden force to a joint. Chiropractors may also use massage and stretching to relax muscles that are shortened or in spasm. Many use additional treatments as well, such as ultrasound, electrical muscle stimulation and exercises.

Chiropractic medicine can improve your body function and enhance your body's healing powers. Some chiropractors emphasize a healthful lifestyle, a healthful diet, and stress reduction. They will educate you with respect to your lifestyle at each visit. Many times you doctor will refer you to a chiropractor or physical therapist if you have neck and back pain. In many instances your doctor will refer you to a chiropractor, who often works together with a physical therapist working at their clinic. Both of these professions can help you with your chronic pain.

The definition of chiropractic therapy is the correction of problems that exist in your spinal column. This enables your body to function at its peak level without medications, surgical procedures, or steroid injections. In 1999, more than 25 million Americans were treated by chiropractors. Not only do chiropractors take care of back injuries, they also can help you with your neck, hip, leg, ankle, foot, arm, and hand pain. Most back and neck pains are the result of mechanical disorders in your spine.

The problem with chiropractic medicine is that it has been maligned for a long time in the United States. However, it is now widely accepted. In Canada, which is under a national health-care system, chiropractic care is included among treatment methods that are reimbursed by the national system. If you have a back injury caused by a twist or turn, you may want to go to a chiropractor. If you have a back injury and need strengthening exercises, your doctor may refer you to a physical therapist.

Chiropractic medicine focuses attention on the relationship between the structure of your spine and how it affects your nervous system. If your spine is not in alignment due to slouching or poor posture, this can cause some of your nerves to be compressed by your spine. Your chiropractor will adjust your spine to remove any spinal abnormalities to reduce pressure off of the nerves in your arms and legs.

When your spine is not aligned correctly, it can cause you to experience tension in your muscles that will in turn affect your nervous system (spinal cord and the nerves emerging from your spinal cord). Compression on your spine and the nerves that come off of your spinal cord can cause you significant health problems and pain. In many instances an adjustment of your spine can remedy these problems.

Following your initial care, your chiropractor may re-evaluate your progress from time to time. After your spine has been misaligned for any length of time, your body may have a tendency to resume that misalignment again. Therefore, periodic visits with your chiropractor are recommended.

Traction is another method that is frequently used by chiropractors and physical therapists and can be an effective treatment for back pain. Traction involves mechanical forces that separate adjacent body parts away from each other. If you have problems with a disc in your neck or back, traction can separate the bones in your back and increase your blood flow to your injured disc, which can speed up the healing process.

If traction worsens of your pain, you should inform your health-care provider so that the traction can be immediately discontinued. Because of the differences in muscle mass between men and women, the amount of traction applied will differ between men and women. If you have a ruptured disc in your neck or back, traction can help heal this painful entity.

Chiropractors treat other entities besides back pain. For example, if you have a carpal tunnel syndrome, chiropractic manipulation can sometimes correct this condition. On occasion, you may not need surgery after chiropractic treatment.

Given that no two people are alike, if you are taking any medications and begin to take nutritional supplements you should be aware that potential drug-nutrient interactions may occur and are encouraged to consult a health care professional before using any natural product. Combining certain prescription drugs and dietary supplements can lead to undesirable effects such as: diminished prescription drug effectiveness, reduced supplement effectiveness and impaired drug and/or supplement absorption.

Chiropractic and nutritional treatment contribute to the amelioration and perhaps reversal of osteoarthritis (OA). It is further proposed that the chiropractic manipulative thrust, is in effect, treating dysfunctional bio-mechanics of joints, affecting positive cartilaginous change. The pathophysiology and multi-factorial causes of OA are reviewed. New interpretations of the literature surrounding OA are discussed which offer arguments for OA's treatment and reversal through chiropractic manipulation and nutritional support.

Some chiropractors recommend DRX 9000 machine treatments. The DRX 9000 is a fancy traction table billed by those who treat back pain (mainly chiropractors and in an area of a group of DO's) as a spinal "decompression" unit. I initially became suspicious and concerned about the device when I had several back pain patients that were previously treated at the DO's facility. They all said that their treatment consisted of daily treatments for 6 weeks of spinal decompression in the DRX 9000, water massage and blowing up a balloon.

The latter is a whole other subject to post about. The point here is the daily treatment for 6 weeks. Regardless if they had simple mechanical LBP, HNP, stenosis, etc, everyone received the same treatment. The worst part is, in many cases, their insurance companies did not pay for this plan of care.

A Wichita, Kan., chiropractor pleaded guilty to one count of health care fraud, two counts of aggravated identity theft and one count of tax evasion. In his plea, he admitted that from March 2011 to October 2013 he executed a health care fraud scheme through his businesses. He submitted false claims to Medicare, Blue Cross/Blue Shield of Kansas and Coventry Health Care of Kansas, Inc., and the Federal Employees Health Benefits Program.

Chiropractors have a limited scope of practice. They are not allowed to perform injections, dispense drugs or supervise ARNPs and physicians. A chiropractor developed what he called an "integrated practice," hiring physicians, advanced registered nurse practitioners and physical therapists and ostensibly having them perform procedures he was not qualified to perform. He misrepresented to the Kansas Board of Healing Arts that medical doctors had an ownership in his clinic. He used the names of physicians he employed to submit false claims for services.

This chiropractor fraudulently billed for nerve conduction tests, nerve block injections, subcutaneous infiltrate proceedings, fine needle aspirations and ultrasound procedures.

A chiropractic scheme perpetuated involved paying individuals to stage accidents, and then report to the clinics with a list of symptoms that they were coached to provide. Various accusations were made in court documents including: having patients sign bills for numerous dates of service when treatment was not rendered, up coding exams and billing for more services than provided. The clinic submitted almost $40,000 in fraudulent insurance claims to 6 separate insurance companies. An owner of a local collision repair shop was paid to provide patients (motor vehicle accidents) for a referral fee.

More than 36,000 chiropractors were paid nearly $500 million by the federal government in 2012, making chiropractors one of the largest groups of Medicare providers. And one chiropractor in Brooklyn topped the list, receiving more than $1 million that year alone. Overall, chiropractors provided 21 million taxpayer-funded treatments for 2.5 million beneficiaries, the Medicare data show. But just 600 chiropractors accounted for more than 10% of the Medicare payments.

Many patients report being told that because they have pain, an x-ray is warranted. While pain is one of the criteria that can constitute the need for an x-ray, it is not, in and of itself, enough. An x-ray should only be taken if your history leads the physician to believe that you may have serious spinal pathology, or if the patient has already undergone 4-6 weeks of conservative care without satisfactory improvement.

Another way that x-rays can be detrimental has to do with how they are used rather than any exposure to radiation. Many physicians like to sit down and show each patient their study, including the x-ray images. And while this seems like a commendable thing for a physician to do, there are studies indicate that showing a patient their x-rays can decrease their rate of progress .

Some chiropractic and pain physicians will take this one step further. They will show a patient all of the areas of degeneration and tell them that the degeneration is causing the pain. However, leading studies refute this idea and show that mild to moderate degeneration does not cause pain. Even though this information has been available for some time, many physicians continue to blame low back pain on degeneration when the fact is that there are many people out there with no back pain that have degeneration. In addition, as you age, you are more likely to have degeneration; therefore, the majority of the time, the x-ray ends up illustrating what was already known and does not change the treatment.

Over the past few years non-surgical spinal decompression devices have become the latest trend within the Chiropractic field. Insurance companies do not cover this procedure therefore patients need to pay for this treatment out of pocket with no guarantees. Many doctors only bill the insurance company if the patient has insurance and no ability to pay. This is accomplished by using fraudulent codes in order to obtain payment. Non-surgical spinal decompression devices can very well cause further injuries.

Chiropractic often involves many expensive but quick treatments and marketing and sales tactics that many people consider to be aggressive and distasteful, if not downright unethical, especially pre-paid treatment packages, and the emphasis of many other services and products. A 2016 federal US audit concluded that more than 80% Medicare payments to chiropractors were for medically unnecessary procedures, and 100% of treatments were unnecessary after the first thirty.

Two chiropractors were indicted by a federal grand jury in Georgia on charges of health care fraud. .S. Attorney for the Northern District of Georgia, said during that time, the chiropractors billed Blue Cross/Blue Shield of Georgia for approximately $633,990 based on vertebral axial decompression, a mechanical procedure performed on patients.

The insurance company considered the procedure to be not medically necessary. The chiropractors instructed employees at the Back Pain Institute of Columbus to alter the patient files to hide the use of VAX-D from Blue Cross, and to bill the insurer for other medically covered procedures.

A Camden County chiropractor is facing up to five years in prison after admitting that he defrauded insurance companies of more than $6,400 reimbursed for treatments he never provided to patients, authorities said. The investigation also implicated Camden police officers accused of illegally obtaining accident reports and delivering them to American Spinal Care for use to solicit business, authorities said.

New Jersey Manufacturers Insurance Co. said that it has filed suit to try to recoup hundreds of thousands of dollars paid in allegedly bogus medical claims. The civil suit, filed last week in Superior Court in Trenton, names 55 claimants as defendants for allegedly faking injuries and 11 health care companies and three doctors as "defendants in interest" because they collected money on the claims.

The insurer alleges that claimants, primarily from the Irvington area, had pretended to be accident victims between November 2000 and August 2004 and received diagnostic tests and medical treatment. The accidents "either never occurred or were staged," The claims indicated little or no damage to the vehicles, but multiple passengers complained of injuries requiring medical treatment. Many of the defendants sought care at the same chiropractic centers and were represented by the same lawyers, the insurer said in the news release.

A Deputy District Attorney said a chiropractor provided weekly chiropractic treatments for her husband and two children for several years, then turned in claim forms that said the services were provided by another employee. The claimant's insurance policy does not cover treatments done by a family member.

A chiropractor in Tampa, Florida Investigators said a chiropractor would pay patients up to $1,000 each to come to his clinic for "treatment". He would then bill each individual's insurance company for nonexistent treatments." He was subsequently charged with three counts of patient brokering.

Chiropractic therapy can be beneficial for the management of some chronic pain. However a potential patient should seek the services of a reputable and honest chiropractor.

21. PHYSICAL THERAPY

Physical therapy is an important modality that can be used to help manage your pain. A therapist will rehabilitate you following an injury. Your strength and range of motion will be evaluated and treated. Your doctor will refer you to a physical therapist if he or she feels that this modality can be of some benefit to you. Physical therapists are highly trained individuals who will obtain a medical history from you and perform an examination on you.

Your physical therapist will decide which treatment is best for you based on your overall health after an evaluation. Your physical therapist will emphasize to you that you yourself are a major component in your rehabilitation and in the management of your chronic pain. Your physical therapist also will train you to avoid future re-injury and/or a recurrence of your pain problems.

Not only is a physical therapy evaluation a planned treatment course for your pain, you also will receive an education on future injury prevention. If you were injured in your workplace, your physical therapist will tell you how to avoid further injury in that environment. You also may be placed in a work-hardening program to enable you to become maximally conditioned for your occupation. This program duplicates your regular work duties and helps increase your muscle strength and endurance so that you can return safely back to work, hopefully without further injury.

Your physical therapist will emphasize flexibility exercises for you and show you how to do them. You have to learn to be able to move your joints without stiffness and pain. Furthermore, your physical therapist will work with you on your endurance and strength. Most importantly, your pain will be addressed. In many instances, a reduction in stiffness in combination with increases in strength and endurance will significantly reduce your pain.

Your physical therapist will also tell you how to deal with your ongoing pain and emphasize to you that you should try to minimize drug therapy. Your therapist will attempt to get you back to normal daily activity as soon as possible in a safe manner. You do not want to return to activity too soon following the onset of sudden pain because you could re-injure yourself or cause yourself a worse injury. When you see your physical therapist on your first visit, you should expect the therapist to obtain a detailed medical history from you. To provide you adequate treatment, your therapist will want to know your complete medical history as well as your pain history.

For example, if you have a history of angina, your therapist will not overly stress you during exercise-related treatments because this may cause an increase in your heart rate and cause you to have chest pain. If you have had surgery or have been involved in a motor vehicle accident, it is important that you tell your therapist while he or she is taking your history. Your therapist will need to become familiar with your pain history as well as your current pain complaints in order to formulate a treatment plan specific for you.

The history that you tell your therapist will give the therapist important information about your pain syndrome, your prognosis, and the appropriate time that you will need to be under the physical therapist's treatments. Your therapist also will assess your behavioral response to your pain associated with your injury if you were injured in an accident or at work. If you have arthritis, your therapist will evaluate your pain input and behavior response to the arthritic pain. For example, your therapist will note if you grimace when you move your joints.

You should inform your therapist about any previous treatments that you have had for the control of your pain, including injection therapies with steroids. Your therapist may additionally want to ask questions about your social history and family history if they may be relevant to your condition. If you have back pain or neck pain, for example, a family history of rheumatoid arthritis is important for the therapist to know. If a family member has this disease, you run the risk of having this disease, which can influence what modality, you need in physical therapy.

You should not be reluctant to give your therapist your age. Many conditions occur within certain age ranges. Osteoarthritis and osteoporosis are known to occur in an older population. Your therapist must know your occupation. If your job involves heavy physical labor, for example, you may be prone to overstress of your back muscles. Tell your therapist when the pain gets worse during the day or notify your therapist if you have increased pain with certain activities. With this information, your therapist can direct an appropriate therapy program for you.

If you have had a similar pain syndrome before your most current pain syndrome, again tell your therapist. If the intensity, duration, and frequency of your pain are increasing during therapy, your therapist may want to send you back to your doctor. This is an indication that you are becoming worse with respect to what is causing your pain and not from the physical therapy.

Try to remember where your pain was when you first noticed it and keep a diary of your pain. For example, if your pain was originally in your back and then later it moved to your leg may indicate a disc rupture. If your pain has moved or spread since you first noticed it, be sure to tell your therapist. Tell the therapist what exact movements worsen your pain. Even pain with bowel movements can be an important history fact. A disc rupture can be associated with back pain during the act of defecation.

If your pain is worse in the morning and becomes progressively better during the day, this may be an indication that you have arthritis. Your therapist will need to know this information in order to prescribe the proper treatment for you. Providing a good medical history to your therapist will make it much easier for the therapist to prescribe the proper method of treatment for you.

You should write down pertinent information about yourself prior to your first physical therapy visit. Your therapist will need to know if your pain is in your bones, muscles, nerves, or all of them together. If the pain is in your bones, the pain is usually confined to that particular area. If your pain is in a nerve, the pain will usually go down your arm or leg from where the therapist is pressing on your spine or neck. If your pain is in your muscles, your physical therapist will note increased contractility of the painful muscles. Your therapist will examine the range of motion of your joints, including the range of motion of your neck and lower back.

If you have a history of dizziness or fainting, tell your therapist before you begin an exercise program. You should expect your physical therapist to look you over when you are disrobed. Your physical therapist will record how well you move and will also examine your posture. Your willingness to cooperate with your physical therapist also will be noted. Your therapist will evaluate how you walk. Your muscle size will be observed for unevenness between the right and left sides of your body from your neck down to your feet.

The color of your skin will be noted by your therapist. Sometimes if you have arthritis, there may be redness about your joints. Your hair pattern in your arms and legs will be evaluated. If you have decreased blood flow, there may be a loss of hair on your skin. Movements of your joints, neck, and lower back will be done to see how flexible you are. Any movements that are painful will be recorded and then will be addressed during your therapy session. Your therapist will decide whether heat or cold could help you with your range of motion or decrease your muscle spasms, which in turn will help decrease your pain. Your physical therapist's examination will emphasize the joints of your body as well as your muscles.

The examination by your therapist may be more thorough than the examination by your doctor with respect to joint movement. On examination, your therapist will try to determine what movements worsen your pain. Your physical therapist will examine you for paralysis or a loss of your reflexes in your arms and legs. Any shrinkage of the muscle in your arms and legs will be addressed. For example, if you have decreased muscle size in your thigh, your therapist will target this area to increase strength and muscle mass.

Your therapist will, furthermore, examine you for any loss of sensation in your arms and legs. For example, if you have a loss of sensation in your right shoulder, your therapist will be careful not to apply heat on this area for any significant length of time. If you have limited range of motion about your arm or leg, your therapist will work with you to increase your range of motion. A heating pad could cause a burn on your skin if you are unable to detect the sensation of heat about your shoulder.

After your therapist has examined you, the therapist may call your doctor to recommend any further laboratory tests or x-rays. After the history and physical examination has been completed, your physical therapist will determine what is causing your pain problem and will design a treatment program for you based on these findings. You will be treated as a complete individual, and not as just a pain symptom. If your assessment was not done thoroughly, your treatment regimen may not help you with respect to your pain syndrome.

If you are experiencing significant pain during your therapy, immediately notify your therapist and discontinue the treatment. One goal of physical therapy is to identify the cause of your pain with an attempt to treat the cause of your pain syndrome. In addition to rehabilitating you following your injury or illness, your physical therapist will attempt to correct any mechanical flaws in your body that could lead to further injury, such as your posture.

Your therapist may do a muscle and joint stabilization program to increase your strength and flexibility. You, on the other hand, must always feel that you are a main component in your rehabilitation. If your therapist gives you exercises to do at home you follow the instructions on how to do them and do them on the prescribed schedule. Your physical therapist will treat you with exercise and strengthening techniques, but also may complement your therapy with whirlpool baths, paraffin baths, or other methods such as using electrical current.

Heat packs can provide you with surface heating, which may reduce the pain in some surface muscles in your back, arms, or legs. Ultrasound is a deep application of heat. This method can relax your deep muscles. Elastic exercise bands and medicine balls may be used to increase your arm and leg strength. The elastic bands can be used to increase your strength, and medicine balls can be used to increase your range of motion and your flexibility as well as your strength. Some physical therapists use traction for the management of your pain.

Electricity can be used to treat your pain syndrome as well. Over the years, many claims have been made for the therapeutic application of electrical current for the treatment of some pain syndromes. Electrical current is applied to your body by placement of electrodes, which are patches with adhesive that stick to your body. The current is directed over the painful areas of your body. Electrical current can vibrate the molecules of your tissues similar to ultrasound therapy. The vibration produced by friction between the molecules of your tissues will increase your tissue temperature. As a result, heat is produced. As electrical current passes through your tissue, some nerves are excited while others are not.

It has been shown that electricity can stimulate tissue growth and repair such as bone and is sometimes used by orthopedic surgeons to stimulate bone growth following bone surgery. Sometimes stimulators can be placed following orthopedic surgery to enhance bone growth. Theoretically, the electrical current should speed up your healing time. A popular electrical current emitting device that is used frequently in pain medicine by conventional physicians, chiropractic physicians, and physical therapists is the transcutaneous electrical nerve stimulator (TENS).

A TENS unit applies electrical current to your body through electrodes that are adhered to your body. The TENS unit is used for pain control. The power source is battery operated. TENS unit therapy became popular in the late 1960s and early 1970s. The use of a TENS unit for the treatment of your chronic pain syndrome if you have neck, back, arm, and leg pain is well documented.

A TENS unit has an amplitude knob that lets your control your pain relief. These TENS units are about the size of a pager. The TENS unit patches can be placed over your muscles or nerves for the management of pain both in your muscles as well as the nerves in your arms and legs. You can use a TENS unit for the control of your pain long term without any significant side effects. Some people have allergic reactions to the adhesive in the patches.

A TENS unit can reduce your pain as well as your stress. However, you should still strive for proper body mechanics and posture. You must remember that a TENS unit is only treating your symptoms. You are incharge of the cause of your pain. If your pain is related to poor body posture, strive to correct this problem.

Iontophoresis is another use of an electrical current to drive medications through your skin. Different medications can be applied through your skin to decrease your pain. Not only is electrical current used for pain relief, it can also speed up your tissue healing. Phonophoresis is another device that uses energy to drive medications into your body.

Traction on your neck or back can increase blood flow to the injured area of your neck or back. However, if the traction does significantly increase your pain, you must immediately notify your physical therapist. Your therapist may instruct you in stretching exercises to be done at home. You must be diligent in doing these exercises provided for you. If certain exercises that you are doing do not provide you with pain relief, ask your physical therapist to recommend some other exercises or range-of-motion methods that you can do at home or at work.

Physical therapists can help you decrease your muscle tension. Your therapist also can educate you on how to decrease muscle tension yourself. Most muscle tension is related to the stress of everyday life. While flying on an airplane for example, you may experience stress when the plane bounces around in turbulent weather. You may experience stress in your job if you have to make a presentation in front of a group. The muscles in your body naturally tense up when you are stressed.

When you experience stress, your body has a protective mechanism that increases your muscle tightness. This is an early part of the fight-or-flight response to stressful situations. This response can be helpful for your protection if you are threatened. However, when your muscles stay contracted the blood flow to your muscles decreases. This cuts off the oxygen supply to your muscles that in turn cause you to experience muscle pain.

Without oxygen, your muscles begin to hurt. Over a long time, you can develop a chronic pain syndrome as a result of your posture. Prolonged slouching over several years can make some of your muscles contract while the opposite muscles can become longer. This could cause chronic muscle pain. For example, if you slouch over a computer you can put pressure on the discs in your neck and back that act as absorbers. Slouching can cause these discs to rupture.

You must attempt to balance the muscles in your body. This will decrease your pain associated with increases in your stress levels. When you are standing, sitting, or driving, remember that your head weighs approximately 10 pounds. If you do not keep your head aligned with your body your head will pull muscles, tendons and joints out of alignment. You must therefore, attempt to keep your head in line with your neck as much as possible. Your physical therapist will instruct you in proper posture techniques.

You should also pay attention to your neck position when you are using a telephone. If you band your neck to one side while talking on the telephone, ask your therapist if a headset could be of benefit. If you feel that your neck is stuck or "catches" in a certain position when doing exercises, that cause may be related to a small joint in your neck called a facet joint. The bones in your neck and back stack on top of each other like blocks. Sometimes these joints can get out of position, especially if you slouch over a desk all day. Your physical therapist may be able to help you with this misalignment of your neck.

Remember if you slouch or have bad posture, your back or neck can become out of alignment. Your muscles then can pull to one side and stretch on the opposite side of your back. If you slouch over a chair for a long period of time, your spine is going to adapt to these positions. If you sit hunched over a desk all day, your ability to stand or sit upright will be compromised. Slouching puts more pressure and stress on the discs of your back than any other posture. When you are sitting for any length of time, you should stand for 10 minutes each hour to take the pressure off the discs in your lower back. Your therapist will show you some stretching exercises to do while you are at work.

The so-called "Rock Doc" who pleaded guilty to defrauding Medicare of $2.6 million through bogus physical therapy services has been sentenced to 6 years in prison. In addition to the billing fraud, this practitioner also admitted to illegally prescribing controlled substances and receiving kickbacks for referring patients for physical therapy which was never done and has been ordered to repay Medicare about $1.65 million. The sentencing, which occurred, was reported in the Wall Street Journal and Miami Herald, among other outlets.

This health care provider was the subject of a 2010 WSJ front-page article that tracked nearly $1.2 million in payments from Medicare, mostly for "physical therapy" that was not provided by licensed physical therapists or not provided at all as mentioned. The family physician earned his nickname thanks in part to his high-profile lifestyle and punk appearance, complete with spiked blond hair.

Another case alleges that a physical therapist was the owner and operator of a physical therapy clinic. Patients would seek treatment at the clinic for minor injuries, generally sustained in car accidents. This clinic employed , a physical therapist; , a physical therapy assistant; and an office manager. The indictment alleged that all off these employees conspired together to falsify patient treatment charts to reflect therapy that was either never given, or was performed by unlicensed personnel, including the clinic owner herself. The owner caused these fraudulent physical therapy claims to be submitted by mail to private insurance companies for payment. Various insurance companies paid more than $400,000 in bodily injury claims to the clinic and its "patients" during a two-year period, based on these fraudulent submissions.

In the next example, nothing about the clinic mentions at the money that is said to have flown there. But in 2012, according to federal data, $4.1 million from Medicare coursed through the billing office in a modest white house. In all, the practice treated around 1,950 Medicare patients that year. On average, it was paid by Medicare for 94 separate procedures for each one. That works out to about 183,000 treatments a year, 500 a day, 21 an hour. What makes those figures more remarkable, and raises eyebrows among medical experts, is that judging by Medicare billing records, one person did it all.

But physical therapy, it turns out, is a big recipient of national Medicare dollars and physical therapy in Brooklyn is among the biggest of all. Of the 10 physical therapists nationwide who were paid the most by Medicare in 2012, half listed Brooklyn addresses, according to an analysis of Medicare billing data by The New York Times. Two others listed addresses on Long Island, one in Queens, and one each in California and Texas.

According to court documents in another case, a physical therapy assistant was paid beginning in June 2009 to falsify medical documentation, a home health agency owned by his alleged co-conspirators. This individual, a physical therapy assistant, pleaded guilty to creating evaluations, therapy revisit notes, and other medical documentation memorializing purported physical therapy for patients he did not see or treat.

According to court documents, an alleged co-conspirator instructed this individual on how to falsify medical documentation. This individual also signed therapy revisit notes as a physical therapy assistant for patients he did not see or treat and admitted to knowing that the documents he falsified and the documents he signed would be used to support false claims to Medicare for home health services.

Another case involved a partner in a gym, which provided exercise, strength, conditioning and performance coaching services to students, faculty and staff at certain independent high schools in New Jersey. These conspirators developed a scheme to enrich themselves by billing their personal training sessions as physical therapy services covered by health insurance even though no one at the gym was a physical therapist.

The co-conspirators would ask clients for their health insurance information and then lie to the insurance companies, indicating that the gym provided physical therapy. Some clients came to the gym with a doctor's prescription for physical therapy, and the gym would treat those individuals under the prescription and then bill the insurers. For other clients who had never seen a doctor. The physical therapy assistant made up his own diagnosis and then billed insurers as if he had provided physical therapy.

Another employee admitted that she hired an uncertified occupational therapy assistant, who fabricated and signed notes for occupational therapy patient visits that the assistant purported to perform. This employee the uncertified assistant for creating these fictitious patient visit notes and countersigned them. She also filled out patient discharge paperwork. She provided no services to the patients whose files she created and countersigned. She was paid for each patient file that she created and knew that neither she nor the uncertified occupational therapy assistant were providing occupational therapy services to the beneficiaries as stated in the falsified files.

In Los Angeles authorities said court documents show clients who visited a rehabilitation facility and other related facilities sometimes received services like massage or acupuncture, which are not covered by Medicare, and were billed from practitioners not licensed to perform physical therapy, but received no covered services. In exchange for patient referrals, kickbacks were paid by "principals" at the facilities equal to about 55 percent of the reimbursement received from Medicare, the U.S. Attorney's office said.

In Florida an indictment was made against a couple which stated that falsified patient records, and submitted fraudulent claims for services never provided, submitted claims by a therapist who wasn't enrolled as a

Medicaid provider and submitted false claims for individual therapy that was actually performed in a group setting.

This couple purportedly provided services to indigent or disabled patients and billed Medicaid for those services. They purportedly offered services to elderly people in assisted living homes and billed Medicare. The couple agreed to forfeit $319,415, which is the total amount they collectively received from Medicare and Medicaid.

Some of the largest perpetrators of Medicare fraud are nursing homes. When engaging in Medicare fraud, nursing homes provide patients with services that they do not need, and bill Medicare for the reimbursements. In one particularly egregious case, a nursing home within in a national chain billed Medicare for physical therapy, occupational therapy, and speech therapy for a single patient all in the same day. Meanwhile, the patient, who was 92-years-old and very ill, died the next day.

The rise of for-profit nursing homes is proving tragic for some of the nation's most vulnerable people, resulting in a spike in waste, fraud and abuse charges brought by federal authorities, according to a new report. Seventy percent of nursing homes were operated on a for-profit basis in 2010, according to an audit by the Medicare Payment Advisory Commission, which counsels Congress. For-profit nursing homes perform better financially: Their profit margins from treating Medicare patients were 21 percent in 2010 compared to 10 percent for non-profit nursing home companies, the commission reported.

Cases filed against the for-profit nursing homes by law enforcement and by families of patients who died allege that for-profit nursing home companies pressure facility managers to minimize the number of employees and keep down their hours to save costs. At the same time, these firms pushed for patients to receive services they did not need, according to the allegations.

A Texas federal jury on Monday found that the CEO and two other top executives of a chain of physical therapy clinics focused on treating federal government employees committed health care fraud and money laundering, but acquitted a chiropractor who was allegedly in on the scheme. The jury deliberated for about 14 hours following a 16-day trial before finding the CEO, chief financial officer and vice president of the five-state chain of these clinics guilty of all counts related to their alleged scheme to defraud the government under the Federal Employees Compensation Act, according to court records and the U.S. Department of Justice.

Prosecutors alleged the executives directed chiropractors at four of their clinics to submit $9.6 million worth of false and fraudulent claims under FECA for services that weren't provided to patients.

22. NECK PAIN

The pathology that affects your lower back also affects your neck. In other words, muscles, nerves, ligaments, discs and facet joints may cause neck pain. At any given time, neck pain affects 10 percent of the general population in the United States. Neck pain is a frequent reason why patients seek medical attention. Neck pain can range from mild discomfort to severe and throbbing and is experienced by everyone at some point in his or her life. Most of your neck pain is self-limited and does not usually require medical attention. However, if you have serious cervical spine problems such as that seen rheumatoid arthritis, notify your doctor if you have the sudden onset of significant neck pain that does not go away within two or three days.

Neck pain is caused by conditions that compress nerves or irritate the outer part of discs that are cushions between the bones in your neck. Ligaments in the front and in the back of your bones in your neck can cause pain because they have many pain fibers within these ligaments. These ligaments are called the anterior and posterior longitudinal ligaments.

The vertebrae in your neck stack on top of each other and are separated by discs. They form joints called facet joints where each vertebra joins. The outer capsule of each joint has a rich supply of pain fibers. The outer capsule holds the top and bottom of the facet joint together not unlike a clamshell. If this capsule is pulled or stretched by an injury, the joint can become loose and make the joint unstable. This instability can cause neck pain.

If your neck becomes misaligned, you can also develop significant neck pain. Over time, the bones and joints in your neck can wear out as well. This is called degenerative disc or joint disease or in medical terms is called osteoarthritis. The disc between your bones can rupture. Your facet joints in your neck can deteriorate and cause you to develop chronic neck pain. Your neck muscles can become tense as well and cause you additional neck pain.

Neck pain in general does not occur as often as low back pain. Therefore, the overall cost of neck pain to society is much less than that of lower back pain. There is fewer work days lost and less medications prescribed in patients with neck pain when compared to lower back pain. Your head weighs between 10 and 12 pounds. The bones in your neck are relatively small in comparison to your head. Your neck muscles are necessary to hold your head in a proper position. Your neck muscles must be strong to hold your head up. Try holding a bowling ball vertically for as long as you can. You will notice that your arm muscles get tired easily. The same analogy is true with respect to your neck muscles tiring from holding your head up.

The bones in your neck that are called vertebral bodies contain many pain fibers. If you fracture one of the bones in your neck, you can have severe pain. The tissue wrapper (periosteum) around your neck vertebra can be injured. The fracture of a bone in your neck can cause abnormal stress to the ligaments, muscles, and joints around the fracture as well as injury to your periosteum (an outer wrapper around the vertebral body).

Osteoporosis is a weakening of your bones from a loss of your bone density and calcium. This disease can cause small, tiny fractures in the bones of your neck and in turn can be a cause of your pain. Osteoporosis can be a source of severe neck pain.

Discs are cushions between the bones in your neck. These discs act as shock absorbers in between your bones. The cushions are important because without them your neck bones would stack on top of each other. Remember the periosteum and the pain fibers contained in the periosteum. Without these cushions, you would have terrible neck pain.

In the very center of your disc in your neck is a thick fluid like substance called a nucleus pulposus. This fluid ball is surrounded by an outer tough fiber called an annulus. Annulus is Latin for "outer ring." When the annulus bulges, pain fibers on the outer aspect of this structure can cause pain signals to be propagated. A fluid nucleus pulposus acts as a ball bearing that enables you to bend your head forward and backward or from side to side. It also is a ball bearing when you rotate your neck.

The ligaments around your disc prevent your neck from having excessive motion. Otherwise, your bones would sit on a fluid-filled ball and flop around like a Slinky toy. You can imagine that your neck would not be very stable without ligaments. Your annulus at its outer layer has many pain fibers. Neck degeneration flattens your discs. When the disc loses height, it pushes your annulus outward. This action stimulates pain fiber activity. This is why you hurt constantly as your disc degenerate.

Magnetic resonance imaging (MRI) and computerized tomography scanning (CT) can help your doctor identify any bone or disc abnormalities that may be a source of your neck pain. Be aware, however, that an abnormal imaging study does not necessarily mean that you will have neck pain. It is possible that you can have a ruptured disc in your neck and you may not experience any neck pain.

There is a normal C-shaped curve in your neck (figure 1). Your neck bones form a C curve with the C part of the curve located in the middle of your neck. The C curve is called a lordosis. The curve is sharper at the lower level of your neck. The curve in your neck determines your posture. If you have a neck injury, the muscles in your neck may pull your neck in a straight line and the curve is obliterated. If you have an X-ray following an injury, your doctor may note that your neck is straight as opposed to being curved. If your neck muscles are in spasm your neck may be straight.

A whiplash injury which will be described in this chapter can cause your neck muscles to develop spasm. This will cause your neck to straighten. If you look at your X ray, you will not see your normal C curve in your neck. Normally your neck is not straight. It should have a curve. Remember that the muscles of your neck stabilize your neck. Following an injury, your neck muscles may be stretched and compressed.

Trauma can cause your neck muscles to contract without relaxing which is called a muscle spasm. Muscle spasms compress the arteries that bring oxygen to your neck muscles and nerves. If your blood flow is decreased, acid (lactic acid is formed in your muscle tissue). Tissue oxygen deprivation causes pain. This is similar to heart pain when you have a heart attack. Muscle relaxant medications, massage therapy or injections into your neck muscles can relax your muscles and restore blood flow. This will decrease your pain.

The outer ring of your disc, called the annulus, will contain the nucleus pulposus within its structure. Think of this anatomy as a jelly doughnut. The jelly in the doughnut is held in place by the outer doughnut ring. Be aware that a basic law of physics states that the nucleus pulposus, which is a liquid, cannot be compressed. Therefore, any pressure applied to your disc at any point can cause the nucleus pulposus to spread outward and even rupture through the outer annular ring. When this happens, you suffer what is called a disc herniation or rupture. This pathology may require surgery on occasion.

A whiplash injury can be extremely painful. To understand the concept of a whiplash injury, consider that your head is as if it is a bowling ball attached to a flexible whip called your neck. At the time of an accident, your bowling ball flies away from the traumatic event but fortunately or unfortunately, it is still connected to your neck. This connection causes your neck and head to snap like a whip that can cause an injury not only to your neck but also to your brain.

Whiplash is a relatively common injury that occurs to a patient's neck following a sudden acceleration–deceleration force, most commonly from motor vehicle accidents. Whiplash is the common name for neck sprains. Whiplash associated disorders describe a more severe and chronic condition. It was known for many years that accidents involving rear-end collisions caused more neck pain than side-impact or frontal-impact collisions. This was noted in 1882 with railway accidents.

The cervical spine is subjected to a compressive force from weight of the head during a rear-impact collision. The problem occurs when the body starts to move forward and the head remains. Subsequently, the head begins its movement backward and the weight of the head compresses down on the cervical spine.

The exact injury mechanism that causes whiplash injuries is unknown but may be caused by stretching the anterior longitudinal ligament. While cervical myofascial injury is the most common problem with whiplash-associated disorders, the cervical facet joints are routinely injured in these accidents. Whiplash-associated disorders may result from rear end or side-impact motor vehicle collisions, but can also occur during diving and other accidents.

Symptoms of this disorder include neck pain, neck swelling, tenderness along the back of your neck, muscle spasms, difficulty moving your neck and headaches. Whiplash-associated disorders predispose one to premature degenerative changes. A history of psychiatric disease was more common in patients with chronic symptoms. The dominating psychiatric diagnosis both before and after the accident was depression. Psychiatric morbidity may be a patient-related risk factor for chronic pain symptoms after a whiplash injury.

Four grades of Whiplash-Associated Disorder have been defined by the Quebec Task Force on whiplash-associated disorders: Grade 1: complaints of neck pain, stiffness or tenderness only but no physical signs are noted by the examining physician, Grade 2: neck complaints and the examining physician finds decreased range of motion and point tenderness in the neck, Grade 3: decreased range of motion plus neurological signs such as decreased deep tendon reflexes, weakness, insomnia and sensory deficits and Grade 4: neck complaints and fracture or dislocation, or injury to the spinal cord.

Most whiplash injuries resolve with conservative treatment. Chiropractic and/or physical therapy are very effective modalities. If these modalities fail, trigger point injections or facet joint injections may be of benefit. A facet rhizotomy may be done if the pain persists. If none of these modalities resolve the pain, a consultation with a surgeon is indicated.

You are probably aware that if you sustained an injury to your head and if your neck bends to far toward one of the sides of your body, the holes (called foramina) for the nerves going to your arms on the side where the head bends will be narrowed. This can cause you to have a nerve injury because the closed hole can compress one of your nerves coming off of your spinal cord. On the opposite side, the holes where the nerves emerge from your spinal cord will be opened.

When your head is thrown to the side, as frequently happens when you suffer a whiplash injury, the side on which the head is thrown to can compress the facet joints on that side of your neck. On the opposite side the facet joints are opened. Either of these maneuvers can cause you to have a facet joint injury or can cause you to suffer significant pain.

If you have arthritis, osteophytes can irritate or compress one or more of your nerves. Osteophytes are abnormal bone growths. Osteophytes themselves are not painful. However, when they brush over your nerves or ligaments, they can cause you to have neck pain. Osteophytes, if they occur, are usually pointed. If one of your nerves brushes up against one of these osteophytes, or if the osteophytes compress your or irritate one of your nerves which can cause you to experience mild to moderate pain.

Steroid injections in and around your nerves can decrease the swelling of the nerve and decrease your pain. Sometimes your doctor may give you steroids by mouth. The problem with oral steroids is that they can cause you to have a significant weight gain. The injection places a tiny amount of steroids at the area of your pain.

Oral steroids have to go to your stomach and pass out of your gastrointestinal system to reach your bloodstream. The total amount of the steroid that will reach your swollen nerves will vary. This is why pain medicine doctors advocate the use of special needles to place steroids at the level of your nerve swelling. The amount of drug placed at your nerve is more reliable than that given by mouth.

The muscles in the base of your skull can compress a nerve that comes off of your spinal cord and travels to the top of your head. This is called the occipital nerve. If a tight muscle compresses this nerve, you can develop a headache called an occipital headache. If you put some heat over the muscle that is compressing this nerve, it can relax the muscle and relieve your headache. Occipital headaches can be treated by a neurologist. Sometimes an injection of a steroid at the occipital nerve can decrease your headache. An epidural steroid injection may also be helpful. Cryoanalgesia (freezing your nerve) may also be of benefit. Botulism toxin (Botox) may also be of benefit as well.

The picture of the model looks at your neck from a posterior (rear) view. In addition to similar structures in your low back, you also have a spinal cord that can be a source of pain. A syringomyelia or defect in your spinal cord can be a source of your neck pain. A syringomyelia is an abnormal fluid space within the spinal cord that is sometimes associated with a tumor or trauma of the spinal cord, or a Chiari malformation. If the abnormal fluid channel or "syrinx" enlarges enough, it can cause pressure on the nearby nerve fibers in the spinal cord resulting in numbness in the arms and or legs. In such cases, consideration can be given to operating on the syrinx in order to drain it.

Nerves that come off your spinal cord travel to the top of your head. Some of these nerves form the Greater and Lesser Occipital Nerves. If these nerves are compressed from trauma, muscle spasm or degenerative disc disease or facet joint degeneration, you may develop pain that begins in the base of your skull and then travels to the top of your skull.

The treatment of this pain consists of anticonvulsant drugs, anti-depressant drugs or injections with steroids and local anesthetics. The nerves can be deadened by freezing them (cryoanalgesia) or with phenol. If the pain persists, a peripheral nerve stimulator can be implanted that may decrease your pain.

If you do develop degenerative disc disease in your neck, you will have decreased range of motion about your neck. The decreased range of motion around your neck is an early indication that you are developing degeneration of the discs and joints in your neck. You will have trouble turning your head and attempting to look behind you. Looking up or down also can be difficult as well as painful. Attention to your neck posture and doing daily range-of-motion exercises for your neck can reduce the progression of degenerative disc disease involving your neck.

If you have severe contractions of a muscle in your neck, you may have severe pain. This prolonged contraction of a neck muscle is called torticollis. This usually occurs on one side of your neck. Your head is usually twisted to one side with your chin pointing to the opposite side. Torticollis usually results from disease or an injury to your brain or spinal cord. Injuries to the muscles of your neck can also be a cause of torticollis as well. Sometimes an injection of botulism can relieve your pain.

You should be aware of your posture. You should use a telephone headset if you have a job that requires considerable telephone time. Avoidance of improper neck posture while using a telephone can contribute to your neck pain. You should avoid the use of large pillows. A flat pillow can keep your neck in a proper position while you sleep. Be aware that women can suffer neck injuries in beauty parlors and hair salons when they go and have a shampoo. Occasionally the beautician will place the client in a chair and bend the client's neck backwards under a faucet to do a shampoo.

You could have a stroke if your arteries are clogged with fat and calcium and if you extend your neck backward for a long length of time. Furthermore, when you bend your head backward into a sink to have your hair washed, the angle of the compression of the neck sometimes causes a disc in your neck to rupture. Some people also pass out when their head is bent backward because of compression of arteries that go to their brain. It is important to let your doctor know if you have experienced any of these problems after going to a hair salon.

If you have significant pathology you should avoid hyper extending your neck. You should be aware of your posture. You should use a telephone headset if you have a job that requires considerable telephone time. Avoidance of improper neck posture while using a telephone can contribute to your neck pain. You should avoid the use of large pillows. A flat pillow can keep your neck in a proper position while you sleep.

Treatment depends on how severe the symptoms are and may include: NSAIDs to reduce pain, A neck brace for added support, Steroid injections, Physical therapy, or Stretching Neck exercises. Most neck pain is caused by activities that involve repeated or prolonged movements of the neck. Nonsurgical treatment works well on this type of pain. Most cases of neck pain caused by activities get better in 4 to 6 weeks. The most common cause of shoulder pain and neck pain is injury to the soft tissues, including the muscles, tendons, and ligaments within these structures. This can occur from whiplash or other injury to these areas. Degenerative arthritis of the spine in the neck (cervical spine) can pinch nerves that can cause both neck pain and shoulder pain. Degenerative disc disease in the neck (cervical spondylosis) can cause local neck pain or radiating pain from disc herniation, causing pinching of nerves (cervical radiculopathy)

The evaluation and treatment program you have described is typical of the scare tactics and misinformation used by some chiropractors who exploit their patients by treating imaginary subluxations and harmless spinal curvatures. I am angered when I hear of chiropractors using such methods. And I am saddened that persons seeking health advice and relief from pain become victims of unethical practitioners who attempt to brainwash every member of the family into becoming a lifelong chiropractic patient. I wish everyone could read your letter and use it as a guide in avoiding this type of chiropractor.

A "new patient evaluation" that requires an x-ray exam of every portion of the spine is the first clue of what is to follow. A "report of findings" requiring the presence of the husband or wife or a parent, the use of videos and mandatory "health classes" to explain the chiropractic subluxation, and a proposed long-term treatment program are signals to cancel further appointments. Chiropractors who use this type of salesmanship always find "subluxations" and/or abnormal spinal curves an recommend months of chiropractic adjustments and years of "preventive maintenance."

It's not unusual to have an abnormal neck or back curve, which is usually harmless or insignificant. Such curves cannot be corrected by manipulation. Patients are often told that they are in a "Phase 1" stage of spinal degeneration and that they need spinal adjustments to halt the progress of a curvature and to prevent spinal degeneration from progressing to "Stage 3 or Stage 4." This is pure nonsense.

No matter what your spine looks like, it has nothing to do with sinus infection or menstrual irregularity. Neck pain and tension headache can sometimes benefit from appropriate spinal manipulation that stretches muscles and loosens joints. But such treatment should not be painful, and it should be done only as-needed by a chiropractor who does not use any of the tactics you described.

Surgery should be contemplated within the context of expected functional outcome and not purely for the purpose of pain relief. The concept of "cure" with respect to surgical treatment by itself is generally a misnomer. All operative interventions must be based upon positive correlation of clinical findings, clinical course and diagnostic tests. A comprehensive assimilation of these factors must lead to a specific diagnosis with positive identification of pathologic conditions.

Motion evaluation of specific joints may be indicated. Range of motion should not be checked in acute trauma cases until fracture and instability have been ruled out on clinical examination, with or without radiographic evaluation; iii. Palpation of spinous processes, facets, and muscles noting myofascial tightness, tenderness, and trigger points iv. Motor and sensory examination of the upper muscle groups with specific nerve root focus, as well as sensation to light touch, pin prick, temperature, position and vibration

More than 2 cm difference in the circumferential measurements of the two upper extremities may indicate chronic muscle wasting; and v. Deep tendon reflexes. Asymmetry may indicate pathology. Inverted reflexes (e.g. arm flexion or triceps tap) may indicate nerve root or spinal cord pathology at the tested level. Pathologic reflexes include wrist, clonus, grasp reflex, and Hoffman's sign.

The Quebec Classification is used to categorize soft tissue and more severe cervical injuries. Grade I, Neck complaints of pain, stiffness, or tenderness only, without physical signs. Lesion not serious enough to cause muscle spasm include whiplash injury, minor cervical sprains or strains as well as Grade II, neck complaints with musculoskeletal signs, such as limited range of motion. It includes muscle spasm related to soft tissue injury, whiplash, cervical sprain, and cervicalgia with headaches, sprained cervical facet joints and ligaments. Grade II,I Neck complaints, such as limited range of motion, combined with neurologic signs and includes whiplash, cervicobrachialgia, herniated disc, cervicalgia with headaches, Grade IV, neck complaints with fracture or dislocation.

Radiographic imaging of the cervical spine is generally accepted, well-established and widely used diagnostic procedure. Basic views are the anterioposterior (AP), lateral, right and left oblique, and odontoids.

A Complete Blood Count (CBC) with differential can detect infection, blood dyscrasias, and medication side effects; b. Erythrocyte sedimentation rate, rheumatoid factor, Anti-Nuclear Antigen (ANA), Human Leukocyte Antigen(HLA), and C-reactive protein can be used to detect evidence of a rheumatologic, infection, or connective tissue disorder; c. Serum calcium, phosphorous, uric acid, alkaline phosphatase, and acid phosphatase can detect metabolic bone disease; and d. Liver and kidney function may be performed for prolonged antiinflammatory use or other medications requiring monitoring.

An MRI is useful in suspected nerve root compression, in myelopathy to evaluate the spinal cord and/or masses, infections such as epidural abscesses or disc space infection, bone marrow involvement by metastatic disease, and/or suspected disc herniation or cord contusion following severe neck injury.

Diagnostic cervical injections are generally accepted, well-established procedures. These injections may be useful for localizing the source of pain, and may have added therapeutic value when combined with injection of therapeutic medication(s).

Medial Branch Blocks are primarily diagnostic, used to confirm the diagnosis of cervical facet pain. When used for diagnosis, two injections at different times with different duration of local anesthetic are recommended. B) Intra-Articular Facet injections are principally diagnostic yet some patients may obtain therapeutic response. If the patient demonstrates definite short-term but not long-term response, confirmatory medial branch blocks and possible medial branch neurotomy should be considered.

Acupuncture: is the insertion and removal of filiform needles to stimulate acupoints (acupuncture points). Needles may be inserted, manipulated and retained for a period of time. Acupuncture can be used to reduce pain, reduce inflammation, increase blood flow, increase range of motion, decrease the side effect of medication-induced nausea, promote relaxation in an anxious patient, and reduce muscle spasm. Indications include joint pain, joint stiffness, soft tissue pain and inflammation, paresthesia, post-surgical pain relief, muscle spasm, and scar tissue pain.

Therapeutic spinal injections are generally accepted well established procedures. They may be used after initial conservative treatment, such as physical and occupational therapy, medication, manual therapy, exercise, acupuncture etc., has been undertaken. Therapeutic injections should be used only after pathology has been demonstrated.

For all cervical injections (excluding trigger point and occipital nerve blocks) fluoroscopic, arthrographic and/or CT guidance during procedures is required to document technique and needle placement, and should be performed by a physician experienced in the procedure.
Cervical epidural steroid injections

Epidural steroid injections (ESIs) are injections of corticosteroid into the epidural space. The purpose of the ESI is to reduce pain and inflammation, restoring range of motion and thereby facilitating progress in more active treatment programs.

Facet injections may be considered in those patients whose history and examination are suggestive of a facet pain generator. The therapeutic value of facet injections provides short-term pain relief for patients to progress through a functionally directed rehabilitation program. A procedure designed to denervate the facet joint by ablating the periarticular facet nerve branches is percutaneous radiofrequency. Trigger point injection consists of dry needling or injection of local anesthetic with or without corticosteroid into highly localized, extremely sensitive bands of skeletal muscle fibers that produce local and referred pain when activated.

Disk disease is not a simple black-and-white diagnosis. Up to 40 percent of adults without back pain have herniated disks that show up on MRIs, so a positive MRI may or may not identify the cause of pain. There is a place for surgery in preventing permanent nerve damage, but too many operations are being done—often with poor results. Intensive rehabilitation may be preferable to surgery for many patients.

One of the most popular forms of treatment currently being offered by chiropractors is a form of motorized computer-controlled traction called "decompression therapy." In reality, the cost is usually several thousand dollars, and insurance doesn't pay for anything except perhaps the original exam. VAX-D is an expensive high-tech form of mechanical traction that can provide relief in some cases of back pain but is widely promoted with unsubstantiated claims that it can correct degenerated and herniated discs without surgery. The equipment is expensive, the protocol is for treatment five times a week for four weeks, and the charge is at least $250 a session.

While surface electromyography (not to be confused with needle electromyography) testing might be helpful in evaluating the function of muscles, and thermography might be helpful in detecting the symptoms of such things as reflex sympathetic dystrophy (an autonomic disturbance affecting blood flow to the skin), it is an oxymoron to suggest that either of these tests can locate a chiropractic subluxation that has never been proven to exist. Thermography and surface electromyography are considered to be experimental and investigational with no established validity as diagnostic techniques.

Needless to say, computerized instruments used to locate subluxations that "cannot be detected any other way" can be an effective gimmick for selling chiropractic adjustments to asymptomatic patients who have imaginary vertebral subluxations.

Chiropractic patients have paid thousands of dollars in advance for a course of treatment lasting several months after succumbing to a high-pressure sales pitch involving scare tactics. These patients have usually opted to discontinue treatment because symptoms have either worsened or disappeared. Most have signed a contract, however, that does not allow a refund, even if the treatment regimen was not completed.

Some have used a chiropractic "health care credit card" to borrow the advance payment from a loan company, leaving the patient legally bound to repay the loan.

It's never a good idea to pay for chiropractic services in advance. Treatment should be discontinued if symptoms have worsened after one week of treatment or have not improved after two to four weeks of treatment. In many cases of neck or back pain, symptoms will often resolve after a few weeks, eliminating the need for further treatment. Patients who have signed a contract for discounted long-term treatment that involves correction of vertebral subluxations, however, may be told that subluxation-detection instruments indicate that they still have subluxations that need to be corrected to prevent a recurrence of symptoms.

Treatment may then be continued as a preventive-maintenance measure, even in the absence of symptoms all in keeping with subluxation theory which proposes that correction of vertebral subluxations will "restore and maintain health." Such unnecessary treatment is a needless expense, and it poses a risk that outweighs benefit, especially in the case of neck manipulation which is potentially dangerous. Insurance companies spend millions of dollars each year investigating and prosecuting fake injury claims. While a fair number of fraudulent claims slip through, companies catch and deny many more. Some of the most serious cases of fraud wind up in criminal courts.

Sometimes a chiropractor may be involved in injury fraud. On April 5, 2010 an incident occurred involving a city route bus in Florida. The bus company received ten allegedly fraudulent personal injury claims. On April 5, 2010, the route "C" bus was traveling north on Broad Street when the bus's exterior side view mirror made contact with an abandoned newsstand. Digital video surveillance on the bus shows that no passengers on the bus were disturbed or made sudden movements as a result of this contact.

The damage to the bus consisted of a broken passenger side mirror and a crack in the fifth window on the passenger side of the bus. Philadelphia police did not respond to the accident and no one that was on the bus at the time of the occurrence reported injuries to the operator.

Despite the initial absence of reports of any injuries, the bus company subsequently received notices of personal injury claims from attorneys from seven different area law firms who were representing the ten defendants. All of the claims included demands of money from the bus company for medical bills and pain and suffering. The medical bills included emergency room visits and trips to different chiropractic clinics. The settlement requests sought compensation ranging from $5,000 to $225,000.

As a result of reviewing the accident report, a witness list filled out by the bus operator at the time of the incident and the surveillance video from the bus, detectives determined that only six of the ten individuals filing personal injury claims were actually on the bus at the time of the incident. Furthermore, the surveillance video contradicts specific details of the claims that were filed by the defendants who were on the bus at the time of the incident.

Unnecessary epidural, trigger point and facet joint injections done by medical doctors may constitute medical fraud if a patient does not have pathology which warrants any or all of these injections.

Workers compensation insurance protects employees who are hurt on the job. This valued employee benefit pays for medical expenses, lost wages and other expenses while a worker heals. Workers compensation fraud is a serious crime in America today. Tens of billions of dollars in false claims and unpaid premiums are stolen every year. Free money is the biggest motive for the employee and money for 'treatment' entices doctors, therapists, chiropractors etc. to be a part of this fraud.

23. LOW BACK PAIN

Low back pain has many causes; injury, stress, poor posture, or aging. Many people experience back pain, and there are various treatment methods available. In some instances utilizing proper posture techniques and performing stretching exercises during the day can prevent back pain. Your back consists of a large number of bones called vertebrae that are separated from one another by cushions called discs. These discs act as shock absorbers between each bone in your spine.

The bones stack on top of each other like blocks and form joints called facet joints. The purpose of your spinal skeleton is protects your spinal cord from injury. There are foramina, which are holes in each vertebra. The nerves off of your spinal cord go through these holes and go to your arms, legs, and organs within your body.

Your spine is kept in place by muscles in your back that maintain your posture. Your muscles also make your back stable during movement. You have many muscles in your back. Any one of these muscles can cause you to have lower back pain. In addition to muscles, you have ligaments that attach each bone in your spine to both the one above and the one below. Ligaments also are necessary to give your back stability. Your ligaments contain pain fibers and can be a source of your back pain as well.

Most of your lower back pain is usually mechanical in nature. This means that there is usually an abnormal alignment of your bones and/or joints that can cause you to have back pain. Figure 1 demonstrates the anatomy of your lumbar spine. You should note that the discs separate the vertebral bodies. The discs in this model are of a normal size. The nerves come out of foramina and ultimately go down your leg. The foramina are normal in appearance.

When your back degenerates, all or part of your back anatomy changes. These changes may cause you to experience pain. Disc degeneration however, does not mean that you will experience pain. Patients with degenerative disc disease in many instances do not experience pain. Degen-erative disc disease is a normal aging process. This process may be accelerated by smoking cigarettes. You should note that the discs separate the vertebral bodies. The discs in the model (Figure 1) are of a normal size. The nerves come out of foramina and ultimately go down your leg. The foramina are normal in appearance.

When the discs degenerate, they lose water (desiccate). As a result, your disc height becomes smaller. Your overall height becomes less as well. The loss of disc height places stress on your facet joints which may cause you to experience facet joint pain. The foramina can become smaller as well which can cause pressure on one or more of your nerve roots. This may cause you to experience pain down your leg which is called sciatica.

You have five bones in your lower back that are called lumbar verte-brae. Your spine functions to support you when you are standing, walking, bending, pushing, and pulling. Your back must perform repetitive tasks on a daily basis without failure. Most of your everyday back pains are not serious. Your back pain is most probably related to a muscle strain or a ligament sprain from doing an activity that you are not used to doing. You should however, never ignore your back pain. You should be concerned if your back pain goes down your legs. If your back pain is associated with weakness of your legs or numbness or difficulty walking, you need to see a doctor.

If you have damage to your spinal cord, you may become paralyzed. If this happens, you may lose all control of your bowel and bladder. Back pain is the most common cause of disability for workers younger than age 45. Back pain is responsible for 15 percent of work absenteeism in developed countries. Approximately 5 percent of the work force is disabled by back pain yearly. Attempts to prevent back pain have not been proven to be effective. In 1990 in the United States, there were 15 million office visits to doctors for lower back pain. This accounts for approximately 3 percent of all visits to doctors. The number of visits to chiropractors was even greater.

The rates for surgery in the United States have increased over the past 20 years. The rate of surgery for back pain in the United States is greater than in most other countries. Following the onset of back pain, there can be a recurrence of lower back pain in a person within 1 year and a 75 percent recurrence in a person's lifetime. Sixty-five percent of patients usually recover from an episode of back pain within six weeks. At 12 weeks, 85 percent of those with back pain are essentially pain free. If you have pain for more than 12 weeks, it is unlikely that you will receive significant relief of your back pain.

If you have been off of work for more than 26 weeks because of back pain, you will probably not be able to return back to work. If you receive compensation from a workmen's compensation insurance carrier or compensation following a motor vehicle accident, your chances of returning to work are significantly decreased. If you are over 50 years of age, you can expect to have problems with your back and also have limitations in your activity due to back pain. Back pain from heavy physical work is common by age 50. Back pain is an unavoidable part of your life.

If you do a job that requires physical labor, you can expect to have back pain when you are 50 years of age or older. Even people who have not done heavy physical work can begin experiencing increased back pain by age 50. You should realize that it would be difficult to decrease your back pain if you have become inactive. For this reason, you should do aerobic exercise to prevent back pain. You also can use exercise to treat back pain. The muscles in your back must be strong in order to support your back. This is the reason that you must do regular exercise activity.

You may have a job where you must do repetitive lifting or twisting. This can injure your back as well as place wear and tear on your discs. If you have a job where you sit all day at a computer desk or at a workbench and you slouch, your back can become misaligned. You may have suffered sports injuries to your back. If you enjoy gardening, you can cause yourself to have back pain if you are doing a considerable amount of digging or lifting.

If your back is not conditioned and strong, try to avoid heavy lifting and strenuous recreational activities. As you grow older, your discs lose their elastic properties and they become thinner and can become wafer thin. As the discs in your back decrease in height, your overall height decreases. As your discs begin to shrink, pressure from the bones above and below can cause your discs to press outward. This is called a disc bulge.

Sometimes a disc bulge can press on one of your nerves. A disc bulge is not a disc rupture. However, a disc bulge can press on one of your nerves coming off of your spinal cord and can cause you significant pain. If your pain persists and you develop numbness, you may ultimately have to have surgery to remove a portion of this bulge off of your nerve.

In the very center of your disc is a thick liquid. Liquids cannot be compressed. If you bend a certain way or attempt to lift a heavy object in an awkward position, the fluid inside of your disc can burst through the outer ring of your disc. This is called a disc herniation or disc rupture and can cause you to experience significant pain.

The liquid material that bursts outside of your disc is highly acidic. This acidic liquid can cause your nerves, your ligaments and your muscles to become swollen and inflamed and you can develop severe pain. Most of the origins of your back pain discussed are mechanical in nature. However, injuries to your discs between your backbones can cause you to have pain. Remember that your discs are also made up of cartilage as well.

It is important for you to understand that a herniated disc does not mean that you will have back pain. In fact 37 % of individuals in the United States have disc herniations but never experience any back pain. A disc herniation furthermore, does not mean that you are disabled or will become disabled. A disc herniation does not mean that you will need surgery. Most disc herniations are treated conservatively with medications, physical therapy, chiropractic therapy or epidural steroid injections. If you do require surgery, you should not expect to be disabled after surgery. In most instances you will be able to return to work unless you have to do extremely heavy lifting. Most professional athletes return back to work following disc surgery.

The surgery rate in the United States has increased over the past 20 years. The rate of surgery for back pain in the United States is greater than in most other countries. Following the onset of back pain, there can be a recurrence of lower back pain in a person within 1 year and a 75 percent recurrence in a person's lifetime. Sixty-five percent of patients usually recover from an episode of back pain within six weeks. At 12 weeks, 85 percent of those with back pain are essentially pain free.

If you have pain for more than 12 weeks, it is unlikely that you will receive significant relief of your back pain. If you have been off of work for more than 26 weeks because of back pain, you will probably not be able to return back to work. If you receive compensation from a workmen's compensation insurance carrier or compensation following a motor vehicle accident, your chances of returning to work are significantly decreased. If you are over 50 years of age, you can expect to have problems with your back and also have limitations in your activity due to back pain. Back pain from heavy physical work is common by age 50. Back pain is an unavoidable part of your life.

If you do a job that requires physical labor, you can expect to have back pain when you are 50 years of age or older. Even people who have not done heavy physical work can begin experiencing increased back pain by age 50. You should realize that it would be difficult to decrease your back pain if you have become inactive. For this reason, you should do aerobic exercise to prevent back pain. You also can use exercise to treat back pain. The muscles in your back must be strong in order to support your back. This is the reason that you must do regular exercise activity..

You may have a job where you must do repetitive lifting or twisting. This can injure your back as well as place wear and tear on your discs. If you have a job where you sit all day at a computer desk or at a workbench and you slouch, your back can become misaligned. You may have suffered sports injuries to your back. If you enjoy gardening, you can cause yourself to have back pain if you are doing a consider-ble amount of digging or lifting.

In some situations, activity does not cause back pain. If you sleep on a soft mattress, you may awaken with significant spine pain. A soft mattress will cause your back to become out of alignment. Chiropractictic therapy may be necessary to realign your back which should relieve your back pain.

If you develop spinal stenosis (narrowing of the bones of your spine that choke your nerves that run vertical or foramina stenosis that occurs when the openings for your nerves to your legs become narrow. Activity does not cause this condition, but activity can cause you to experience pain. You have to walk bent over. You will have pain in your calves. Sitting will relieve your pain. This is called neuroclaudication.

Your discs and cartilage are elastic and functions as a cushion between your backbones. These discs absorb the impact of your body motion. If your discs put pressure on the nerves going to your leg, your leg may become numb or you could develop a foot drop. You must seek medical attention if this happens. When your doctor examines you, you may have no reflexes in your leg on the side of your pain.

When you reach age 50, the liquid center of your discs, called the nucleus pulposus, becomes dry and less elastic. Pressure on your discs can cause them to protrude and cause your discs to keep protruding until they may become compressed around one of the nerves going to your legs. When this happens, it can compress your nerve. If your leg becomes numb and weak, you will probably become a candidate for surgery. You will need consultation with a neurosurgeon or an orthopedic surgeon.

Aging also can cause your facet joints to become calcified and the surfaces of your joints can become irregular. Excessive wear and tear over time may make your facet joints become misaligned. If your facet joints become misaligned, one of the joint components can move forward and can again compress one of the nerves going to your legs causing pain and possibly numbness and weakness. A normal spine that has been maintained with exercise, proper posture, and range-of-motion exercises enables you to bend and rotate your back without pain. These exercises will help you maintain adequate range of motion for your back. These movements also can help increase blood flow to your discs.

Increased blood flow can encourage your discs to heal and can even prevent scar tissue from forming around your nerves that were temporarily injured. In some instances, you may need to seek chiropractic therapy to realign your back. If the bones in your back are properly aligned, your nerves should be able to transmit normal impulses to your muscles to allow your muscles to function in an optimal fashion.

If there is some entrapment of your nerves by pressure from adjacent body structures, your nervous system cannot function properly. If you are overweight and do not exercise and do not use proper posture, your back muscles and discs will become progressively weaker. Your discs can decrease is size. This occurrence is referred to as degenerative disc disease (figure 3). This is not a disease but normal aging. You will then be prone to a disc rupture if you perform a strenuous activity. This is the reason why you need to maintain a healthful lifestyle that includes exercise.

Cigarette smoking can cause your discs to degenerate. This may be a reason why cigarette smokers have a higher incidence of back pain. Cessation of smoking will not allow your discs to regenerate however. Nicotine can also interfere with the absorption of pain medicines into your blood stream from your stomach and your small intestine. Many smokers who stopped smoking have noticed that their pain medications became more effective. You should also be aware that if you are a smoker and need back surgery, you might not heal properly.

Many surgeons will make you stop smoking at least 4 weeks before doing back surgery. Your discs and cartilage are elastic and functions as a cushion between your backbones. These discs absorb the impact of your body motion. If your discs put pressure on the nerves going to your leg, your leg may become numb or you could develop a foot drop. You must seek medical attention if this happens. When your doctor examines you, you may have no reflexes in your leg on the side of your pain.

When you reach age 50, the liquid center of your discs, called the nucleus pulposus, becomes dry and less elastic. Pressure on your discs can cause them to protrude and cause your discs to keep protruding until they may become compressed around one of the nerves going to your legs. When this happens, it can compress your nerve. If your leg becomes numb and weak, you will probably become a candidate for surgery. You will need consultation with a neurosurgeon or an orthopedic surgeon.

Aging also can cause your facet joints to become calcified and the surfaces of your joints can become irregular. Excessive wear and tear over time may make your facet joints become misaligned. If your facet joints become misaligned, one of the joint components can move forward and can again compress one of the nerves going to your legs causing pain and possibly numbness and weakness.

A normal spine that has been maintained with exercise, proper posture, and range-of-motion exercises enables you to bend and rotate your back without pain. These exercises will help you maintain adequate range of motion for your back. These movements also can help increase blood flow to your discs.

Increased blood flow can encourage your discs to heal and can even prevent scar tissue from forming around your nerves that were tempo-rarily injured. In some instances, you may need to seek chiropractic therapy to realign your back. If the bones in your back are properly aligned, your nerves should be able to transmit normal impulses to your muscles to allow your muscles to function in an optimal fashion.

If there is some entrapment of your nerves by pressure from adjacent body structures, your nervous system cannot function properly. If you are overweight and do not exercise and do not use proper posture, your back muscles and discs will become progressively weaker.

Your discs can decrease is size. This occurrence is referred to as degenerative disc disease. This is not a disease but normal aging. You will then be prone to a disc rupture if you perform a strenuous activity. This is the reason why you need to maintain a healthful lifestyle that includes exercise. In degenerative disc disease, your discs decrease in height and the ends of your bones become irregular. The disc spaces are where the discs are located between the bones.

Every patient who has low back pain does not need a MRI or CT scan. A plain X ray is cheaper and provides significant information about your back. In degenerative discs, the spaces between the discs are somewhat narrow. Osteophytes are present on the vertebral bodies. This finding indicates that some wear and tear of your back is occurring.

Preventative pain medicine is just as important as the treatment of many pain problems. Where your backbone and pelvis meet, they form a joint called the sacroiliac joint. Your sacroiliac joint can be a source of your back pain as well. This joint has a thick capsule that has strong ligaments both in the front and the back of your joint. Other ligaments also help to form and support this joint. The joint is C shaped.

As you become older, the cartilage that attaches to your pelvic bone degenerates faster than the cartilage in your sacrum. As a result this joint which is called the sacroiliac joint can become unstable. It can be a cause of your pain as well. Related to hormone changes that occur during pregnancy, the ligament becomes loose. This is the reason that many pregnant women experience pain in their sacroiliac joints that can last after the birth of their baby until the ligament becomes stronger. Sometimes the pain from your sacroiliac joint can cause pain to go down your leg. In other instances the pain will be referred to your hip or may just be present in your sacroiliac joint. The gluteal muscle over this joint may hurt as well.

You may notice pain in your back when you roll over in bed or when you get out of a car. Furthermore, you can have pain when you go up or down steps. If the muscle over your sacroiliac joint is tight, it can cause you to have pain. A bone scan is helpful in diagnosing sacroiliac arthritis.

During this procedure, a very small dose of a radioactive dye is injected into your veins. After the radioactive dye has had time to go to your joints, pictures are taken with a camera of your sacroiliac joint. If you have arthritis, there will be darkened areas in your joints that will show up on the scan. Usually plain x-rays are not sufficient to diagnose problems with your sacroiliac joint. The treatment of this problem consists of physical therapy.

A type of Velcro belt called an SI belt can be used to hold your joint in place. Stabilization of your joint can decrease your pain. If you have no relief from these methods, your pain-medicine doctor can inject a steroid and local anesthetic into your joint under X-ray needle guidance. These methods should rid you of your pain. If your pain does persist, destruction of the nerves that goes to your joint can be done with either heat or cold. This is called a rhizotomy.

Occasionally, a surgeon may have to stabilize your joint surgically. Nonsteroidal anti-inflammatory medications also can be very helpful for the management of pain in your sacroiliac joint. Because the pain involves a joint, muscle relaxants may not be of any benefit.

If you have a disc herniation, a CAT scan or an MRI can diagnose your pathology. Your lower back is made up of five bones called lumbar vertebrae. The lower part of your back below these bones is called the sacrum. It is made up of five fused bones. Your pelvis anchors here. Your tailbone is called a coccyx.

If you sit in a chair correctly or in the seat of your car correctly, you are keeping all of these bones properly aligned. Each bone then bears the full weight of the bone above it. It is reported that proper alignment of your back can help build bone mass. This is important if anyone in your family has a history of osteoporosis.

Discography is a way of diagnosing whether or not that you have disc-related pain. An MRI and CT scan can show a disc herniation. However, these imaging studies cannot define pain. A discogram is an injection of material into your disc. The pressure in your disc is then measured. You should have a relatively high pressure when material is injected into the center of your disc. If your disc leaks, the leakage of the acidic nucleus pulposus can cause you to have pain.

When your nucleus pulposus leaks out of your disc it hardens just like glue out of its tube. Sciatica is a pain that is felt in your back and the outer side of your thigh, leg, and foot. It is usually caused by degeneration of one of the discs between your backbones. When the disc protrudes laterally off to the side, it can compress the nerves in your lower back. Usually the last two or three nerves are compressed on the side of your pain. The onset of sciatica can be sudden. Furthermore, it can be brought on if you are performing an awkward lifting position or if you are doing a twisting movement such as raking the leaves.

Patients who have sciatica usually have stiff backs and have pain when they attempt any movement. You may have numbness in your leg as well as weakness associated with your sciatica. Bed rest for 24 hours may decrease your pain. If you have significant weakness and pain, nonsteroidal anti-inflammatory medication can help. If this medication does not provide you with relief, your pain-medicine doctor may want to inject the sciatic nerve with some numbing medicine and a steroid.

If you still have pain after conservative treatments have been tried, a surgeon may need to do a surgical procedure to get either a muscle or disc off your nerve to relieve your pain. In addition to degenerative changes in the back and joints as being common causes of back pain, the most common cause of back pain is muscle tension in the lower back. Approximately 80 percent of people living in the United States will experience one incident of an aching back at some time in their lives.

Be aware that stress can play a major role in the origin of your lower back pain. If you are frightened or nervous, your muscles become tense. When your muscles tighten, the tightness of the muscle can progress to muscle spasms where the muscles contract and pull.

You should know that the muscles in your back are not under your control when they become tense. Misalignment of your back due to poor posture or other mechanical strains such as slouching in a chair can cause you to have back pain. If you sit over a computer desk with your back rounded, your muscles are going to adapt to that position. Often the muscle fiber length will change to conform to your improper position. When this happens, your spine is going to adapt to these positions as well.

You must remember that hunching over a desk or slouching in a chair can press some muscles and elongate other muscles. Also, tendons, joints, and ligaments that support your back are affected. Some of the ligaments are stretched while some are compressed. When you slouch or when you sit rounded over, you can compress some of the facet joints while opening other facet joints. You must remember that your lower back supports your body.

Your lower body extends from your ribcage to your pelvis. Not only does your lower back include muscles of your lower back, it also includes muscles around your stomach. Muscles in your back, includ-ng the muscles around your stomach, attach the front of the spine to the hips. At the attachment of the hips, the muscles are anchored. Persistent slouching will eventually affect your posture. When your posture causes your back to be misaligned, you will develop pain.

As previously mentioned, the discs in between the bones in your back can be a source of back pain. Again, you must be aware that slouching puts more excessive pressure and stress on your discs than does any other posture. Slouching can, therefore, decrease the blood flow to your discs and cause your discs to lose their height and begin to calcify, which is called degeneration. This condition can cause you chronic pain.

You can have chronic pain following back surgery. This is usually a result of how your body heals and is not something caused by your surgeon. Scar can form around your nerves that go from your back to your hips and legs. This is called a failed back syndrome. Repeat surgery is usually ineffective. If medications do not provide you with sufficient pain relief, you may need a dorsal column stimulator that is discussed elsewhere in this book.

Slouching in a chair and at a desk also can cause you to have chronic pain by compressing the nerves that come off of your spinal cord and go to your legs. Your lower back has a natural C curve at the lower end of your back. This normal curve is called a lordodic curve.

Chronic slouching can straighten this normal C curve in your back. This misalignment will affect your discs, muscles, ligaments, and joints. Look at your posture in your mirror. If your posture is abnormal, you must correct it. If you cannot do it yourself, you may want to visit a chiropractor or physical therapist to help you with this problem.

Be aware that as you age one of the first consequences of aging is unfortunately in your discs. Before your hair turns gray or before you lose hair and develop wrinkles, changes usually occur in one of both of the two lower discs in your back. The lower discs in your lumbar spine essentially do not have a blood supply from arteries to your disc after age . The blood supply of your discs must come from the ends of your vertebral bodies. Most of the oxygen and sugar that goes to your discs comes from the ends of your vertebral bodies. Your discs need these nutrients. If you smoke, you decrease these important nutrients to your disc that accelerates the degeneration of your discs.

After your discs have begun to age, the joints around your vertebral bodies will degenerate. Remember that your bones stack up on top of each other and that the back of your bones forms joints with the bones above and below your discs called facet joints. As your disc narrows as a result of degeneration, the space between your discs narrows. Not only do you decrease your height, you also compress your facet joints.

Disc compression causes your discs to wear out faster. The facet joints in your spine work to stabilize your spine. As your joints deteriorate, you will lose motion as your age increases. Spondylolisthesis can be another cause of your back pain. This occurs when one of your bones slips upon the one below it. This is usually hereditary in origin.

Trauma can also cause this disorder. However, when one bone slips over the other, it can cause pain in your facet joints and sometimes it can compress the nerves coming off of your spinal cord going to your legs. Vertebral body slippage can put stress on your ligaments that can cause pain as well. Usually surgery is not needed for minor slippage. Your pain can be frequently controlled with NSAIDs. Occasionally a steroid injection into your epidural space or a steroid into your facet joint can help you control your pain. Sometimes chiropractic therapy can help you in the management of your pain if you have this syndrome.

There are many causes of low back pain. Fortunately, most low back pain can be managed with conservative treatment. Preventive care is extremely important. You should be aware of your posture. You should exercise. If you smoke, you should begin a smoking cessation program. A walking program can strengthen your back. You should have a firm mat-tress.

Alignment of your spine may need to be done on occasion. If your muscles become tight, you should do relaxation exercises. Biofeedback can help relax your back muscles. If you are going to lift a heavy object, you should keep your back straight and bend your knees.

Inversion therapy doesn't provide lasting relief from back pain, and it's not safe for everyone. Inversion therapy involves hanging upside down, and the head-down position could be risky for anyone with high blood pressure, heart disease or glaucoma.

In theory, inversion therapy takes gravitational pressure off the nerve roots and disks in your spine and increases the space between vertebrae. Inversion therapy is one example of the many ways in which stretching the spine (spinal traction) has been used in an attempt to relieve back pain. Well-designed studies evaluating spinal traction have found the technique ineffective for long-term relief. However, some people find traction temporarily helpful as part of a more comprehensive treatment program for lower back pain caused by spinal disk compression.

Low back pain is the number one health care expense in the U.S., costing $80 billion a year. It's the second most common ailment seen by general health care practitioners. Spinal disc surgery is the third most frequently performed surgery. CBS News has previously reported that there are 80,000 unnecessary disc surgeries done annually in the U.S.

A wide variety of treatments are being used for low back pain, some good, and others bad, if not outright dangerous. It also criticized surgeons for doing excessive disc surgeries. According to a recent lawsuit, companies tied to a spinal fusion equipment company made improper payments to doctors for using the company's medical devices in their spinal fusion surgeries. Per a federal complaint, some of these major back operations were medically unnecessary and/or excessive.

One of the major concerns in the medical field at the moment is some doctors not having enough training when it comes to various pain management techniques. Quite a few doctors are learning how to give these shots through weekend courses. ABIPP/FIPP Board Certified Pain Management Doctors go through years of training to master these procedures. It is important for patients to choose the most qualified and experienced doctor when considering treatment. A qualified doctor will only administer an Epidural Steroid Injection (ESI) in a Hospital or Outpatient setting such as Ambulatory Surgery Center (ASC) with the use of X-Ray guidance tools to lessen the risk of serious complications and improve the accuracy of the procedure.

Injections of corticosteroids into the space around the spine (known as epidural steroid injections or ESIs) given to the right patient by the right doctor will usually yield a positive result with extremely low complication rates.

Steroid injections into the spine have also long been used for lower-back pain and it might make sense in a few cases, such as for people who have tried other treatments and still have back pain with leg pain or numbness and tingling. But last year the Food and Drug Administration warned that the shots can cause rare but serious side effects, including loss of vision, stroke, paralysis, and death.

Before consenting to one of the procedures you can consider a second opinion.

24. WORKMAN'S COMPENSATION

A patient should be aware that fraud addressed to an injured worker can occur on occasion. If a patient suspects deception he/she should consult an attorney. Workers' compensation generally is supposed to provide injured workers with full medical insurance coverage, rehabilitation costs, and two-thirds of regular weekly pay during disability caused by a workplace injury (or a specified death benefit in case of fatality) without regard to the fault of workers or employers.

If a patient are injured on the job and making a workers' comp claim, a patient must be medically evaluated and treated by doctors who are approved by a patient employer's insurance company. In workers compensation cases, there is always the possibility that a doctor will find nothing wrong with a workers comp client. Treating doctors are very important witnesses in every kind of injury case.

Workers Compensation Insurance is a state run program. A patient's employer, and most of the time a patient, pay premiums each month (a patient's comes out in payroll taxes), and those premiums are set according to the degree of hazard and the number and costs of claims a patient employer experiences on average in a a patient state. They desire to keep these premiums, and their costs, low and this can lead to conflicts over coverage, allowance and sometimes even the handling of a patient claim.

State workers' compensation laws are administered by what is usually called the "workers' comp commission" in each state, appointed by the governor. The commission decides disputed cases when employers contest workers' claims that their injuries are work-related and deserving of compensation. Administrative law judges hear evidence in disputed cases, and their decisions can be appealed to the state commission for review

Navigating the workers' compensation medical process can add even more discomfort to a painful work injury. Each state has its own rules and regulations regarding workers' comp claims, but one rule is common to all: Injured workers seeking benefits must be evaluated and diagnosed by workers' compensation doctors hired by the employer's insurance company.

Treating doctors, and what their opinions are, are of utmost importance to a workers comp client. That's because only a doctor can testify about the nature and extent of injury as well as causation. In workers comp cases, causation refers to a doctor's opinion as to whether the injury is work related. Doctors have various reasons for deciding to work for an insurance company and his/her ultimate goal is money.

Virtually all state regulations permit a patient to be treated by a patient own doctor, but a patient's claim is highly dependent on the medical opinion of the doctor(s) a patient choose from the insurance company's approved list. Doctors have various reasons for deciding to work for an insurance company, but like most people in the workforce, their goal is a paycheck. Whether they are seeking to augment their private practices or are retired and need additional income, most are financially motivated.

Workers' compensation doctors know insurance companies don't like spending money on diagnostics. They are expensive and complicate the entire claim.

As a result, a many insurance company approved doctors are more likely to treat injuries with pain medication. Medications are less expensive than an MRI. Too often doctors don't believe patients' accounts of their pain and discomfort. To remain on the list for workers' comp referrals, some doctors may classify patients as malingerers, rather than diagnosing real pain issues. That's why second opinions are so valuable

There is no such thing as a true IME. Doctors hired to perform IMEs are usually paid by the same workers' comp insurance company handling a patient claim. In most cases, the adjuster working a patient claim chooses the doctor a patient will be required to see. If requested by the insurance company, a patient must submit to an IME. A patient refusal may allow the adjuster to deny a patient claim. Most doctors who perform IMEs have little incentive to take the necessary time to study all the medical documentation related to a patient claim. Fees are based on the number of patients examined , not on the time spent on each case

Nurse case managers are registered nurses whose job is to facilitate communication between the doctor and the insurance company. A patient may have a nurse case manager assigned to help a patient with a patient claim. The nurse may present herself as a patient advocate who is acting in a patient's best interest. Although most nurses are honest and hard-working, do not forget that she is employed by the insurance company.

In most states a patient can refuse to have the nurse in the examination room with a patient while a patient is seeing the doctor. A patient should seek a second opinion if a patient feel the workers' compensation doctor a patient chose isn't addressing a patient's medical issues. Most workers' comp insurance companies permit an injured worker to have a second evaluation from another doctor on their approved list.

While second opinions may seem helpful, the other doctors rendering those opinions are under the same conflict of interest as the primary one After a specified time, usually 30 days or more after filing a patient's claim, a patient will be permitted to have an evaluation and treatment from a physician a patient choose, whether on the approved list or not.

Not seeking treatment right away tells insurance that a patient wasn't hurt that seriously. A consultation visit regarding a claim will always be paid for by the employer or a patient's self-insured employer. A patient's employer may recommend a physician who will save them money by minimizing a patient injury. An injury on the job can cause anxiety, depression, and even a post-traumatic stress disorder. If a patient is not experiencing these symptoms, the insurance company implies that here is nothing wrong with the patient. The patient is deemed "normal" after the accident.

An injured worker should talk to a workers' compensation lawyer and get a second medical opinion. Too many workers compensation doctors would rather satisfy the workman's compensation insurance adjustor rather than provide a patient with good medical care.

Employers and insurance claims adjusters commonly send injured workers for second opinion exams by an "independent" doctor. This is called an IME, which stands for an insurance medical exam, or independent medical exam. The independent insurance doctors are selected by a patient's employer or a workers compensation insurance company, and in some instances they are paid to find nothing wrong a with seriously injured worker.

If a patient receives a letter requesting a patient's presence at an independent medical examination, a patient is required by law to attend. The IME gives a patient employer or its insurance company an opportunity to have a patient examined by a doctor of their choice. Iif a patient do not attend this examination, a patient faces losing workers compensation benefits.

It is common for an independent medical examination to conclude that a patient's condition is not work-related or that a patient can go back to work without restrictions. Many IME consultations find no evidence of injury. Insurance companies use the same doctors over and over again, because they know what to expect from these individuals. Some of these doctors make a career out of testifying for insurance companies.

If a patient has been injured on the job, the insurance company may hire a private investigator to watch a patient. The goal of this action is to do try to observe a patient doing something a patient's doctor told a patient not to do or something a patient told a patient's doctor that the patient could not do. A video of a patient doing something a patient told a patient's doctor he/she could not do is unfavorable to a patient's case. Surveillance is most commonly ordered when a hearing or settlement mediation is approaching.

Private investigators need an opportunity to "pick a patient up." That's what they call it when they start following a patient. Commonly they will do this at a patient house or at a patient's doctor's visit. Because the insurance company knows when a patient will have a doctor's appointment it is easy for them to tell the private investigator where and when they will be able to find the patient in question.

Frequently investigators will park down the street and watch a patient's house. A patient should not be in the yard doing yard work if a patient's doctor told a patient not to so. Taking out the trash is another investigator favorite. They want to catch a patient taking out trash when a patient has lifting restrictions and assume it must have been over the doctor's prescribed limits.

When a doctor releases a patient to return to work, with or without restrictions, a patient's employer or its workers' compensation insurance carrier must send a patient a form entitled a Notice of Ability to Return to Work with the doctor's release before they can offer a patient a return to work. If a patient receives a return to work offer before a patient receives a Notice of Ability to Return to Work form, the patient must contact a workers' compensation lawyer immediately.

The meat and poultry industry have been alleged on occasion to administer workers' compensation programs by steadily failing to recognize and report claims, delaying claims, denying claims, and threatening and taking reprisals against workers who file claims for compensation for workplace injuries.

An administrative law judge previously sued the Arkansas Workers' Compensation Commission for wrongful dismissal after the commission fired her. The judge said her firing was a response to pressure from businesses because of her decisions favoring injured workers.

Insurance companies frequently contest workers' compensation claimed for injuries which are musculoskeletal as separate from injuries which are traumatic and visible. If it's not something obvious with witnesses, the insurance company may state that it is not a job related injury and deny the workers' compensation claim. These companies have an incentive to deny claims or to direct workers toward their regular medical insurance program.

Many workers are fearful of losing their jobs if they request compensation for a workplace injury. Such retaliation is unlawful in every state (except Alabama, which allows employers to fire workers for filing compensation claims). Most states permit employers to have a worker claiming compensation see a company selected physician in addition to the employee's own physician, with provisions for a third opinion in case of a dispute between physicians. Workman's compensation doctors do not need special training to evaluated injured workers and only need to have a state license and be authorized in a specialty.

Most injured workers do not realize that with respect to workers' compensation, it is not enough to prove that a worker was hurt on the job. A patient has to show that he/she suffered an accidental injury at the time he/she was hurt or that an injury was caused by a specific traumatic event or that a patient suffered from an occupational disease.

Federal workers' compensation is entirely different from state's workers' compensation, and there are few attorneys who have specialized experience in the field. The U.S. government provides benefits to civilian federal workers who become injured or ill because of their job duties. The Federal Employees Compensation Act (FECA) is the governing law over federal workers' compensation, is administered by the U.S. Department of Labor, Office of Workers' Compensation Programs (OWCP).

If a patient is injured at work, a patient will initially file a claim with the OWCP and a claims examiner will be assigned to review the patient's file. In cases of traumatic injuries, a patient may receive a continuation of full pay for the first 45 days of disability. Otherwise, if a patient sustain a disabling, job-related injury or illness, a patient may be eligible to receive $2/3$ of the patient's pre-disability wages, or $3/4$ if an injured worker has dependents.

If a patient suffers from a specific job-related permanent partial impairment, such as the loss of the use of a limb, after a patient has exhausted temporary total disability benefits, a patient may be entitled to schedule award. A schedule award consists of monetary payments for a prescribed number of weeks set by statutes and regulations.

There are also cases where a patient may have a pre-existing injury or medical condition, which is aggravated by an event that occurred on the job. A key difference between federal and state workers' compensation is the matter of apportionment. In states' workers' compensation, an aggravated injury or condition may only be partially covered by a patient's employing agency.

In contrast, federal workers' compensation claims only take into account the employee's current state of wellbeing. If a patient had suffered from a back injury years ago, but heavy lifting required by a patient's current job duty aggravates the condition, then the OWCP may cover all of a patient required medical needs, rather than just a portion of it.

MMI (Maximum Medical Improvement) is addressed to any worker injured who is actively being treated and symptomatic for a duration of more than 6 months and is required to be rated for permanent impairment utilizing the AMA Guides To Impairment. Different stated will use different editions of these guidelines. In Colorado, this book provides workers' compensation physicians charts that assign a numeric impairment rating utilizing both diagnosis and range of motion determinations.

These ratings then convert to money benefits required to be paid to the worker under the law. A rating on simply a strained back, with some limited range of motion can mean upward of $60,000 or more in money paid to a worker (depending on age and pay rate). However, the Guide often requires both active care and ongoing symptoms for a duration of greater than 6 months in order for a rating to be given.

Doctors whose source of revenue depends on keeping employers and insurance companies content are finding more and more resourceful ways to justify releasing workers compensation patients back to work just shy of the six month mark in an effort to cheat the employee out of a much deserved and substantial money recovery.

The initial denial of a claim is a major issue in workers' compensation cases. Insurance companies are under pressure from their clients to keep premium costs as low as possible. They carefully scrutinize claims for opportunities to deny or reduce benefits. Because of this behavior the injured worker should have the right to have video recording of compelled medical exams as a matter of an injured worker's right.

25. FIBROMYALGIA

Fibromyalgia is a chronic pain syndrome that affects muscles, tendons, and fascia (a tissue area over your muscle) throughout your body. This disease is also referred to as fibromyositis. It affects about 5 percent of the population, 90 percent of which are women of childbearing age. You and your physician must function together as a team to properly treat this entity. Fibromyalgia causes you to have muscle pain through-out your body, and is associated with joint stiffness and fatigue.

Fibromyalgia is one of the most elusive diseases that affect the human body. Given its many vague symptoms – numbness, anxiety, insomnia, irritable bowel syndrome, depression and more – it's very hard to diagnose, which explains why the cause of FMS is currently unknown. Like any idiopathic disease or medical condition, not fully understanding the cause and treatment can be the most devastating part.

Some experts believe FMS is related to hormonal disturbances and chemical imbalances affecting the nervous system. Others link the condition to illness, trauma or just plain stress. Still other researchers blame genetics or claim there is no explanation at all. Indeed, even today, fibromyalgia is often labeled as a somatoform disorder,

You also may experience sleep disturbances and depression if you have fibromyalgia. It can cause many places on your body to become extremely tender. You are only diagnosed with fibromyalgia after other pain-causing conditions have been eliminated as the reason for your pain. Fibromyalgia is a condition that can be painful, but it is benign and will rarely cause you to be totally disabled. Only you can let it become disabling.

The diagnosis of fibromyalgia includes a history of aches, pains, stiffness in 11 or more tender areas above and below your navel and to the right and left of your navel. You may have a history of irritable bowel syndrome and depression as well. You may be de-pressed and suffer from sleep deprivation in addition to muscle pain. In 2010, the American College of Rheumatology published a new set of preliminary guidelines. These guidelines include a widespread pain index that assesses the number of painful body regions, and a scale that assesses the severity of symptoms such as fatigue, sleep problems, comprehension problems, and others in the body.

By using one or both of these sets of guidelines, along with tests to rule out other possible conditions, it is possible for your doctor to make a fibromyalgia diagnosis. The following diagram shows common body sites where you might experience tender areas associated with fibromyalgia. You muscle will not feel contracted but will feel soft and tender to light touch. Tender areas can also occur in your arms and legs. You should note from the diagram that these tender points occur above and below your navel and occur in a plane to the right and left of your navel.

If you are like other patients with fibromyalgia, the muscle pain that you experience is probably more common in your neck and lower back. However, it can affect any muscle throughout your body. Your pain can range from sharp or cramping to a burning sensation. Your pain may be worse in one specific area, even though the pain can be felt all over your body. You also will notice that fibromyalgia pain affects tender areas on your body that are symmetrical, or located in the same places on the opposite side of your body.

Tenderness and swelling of your hands or feet are also common. Other common areas where you may notice tenderness include the areas under the base of your skull; above the shoulder blade, elbows, the buttocks (gluteal muscle); the front of the neck midway from the chin to the collar bone; the chest; the sides of the body over the hip regions; and the inner aspects of the knees.

It is more common for women to have fibromyalgia than men. Be-cause of this, researchers are trying to find gender-specific causes of fibromyalgia. In general the amount of pain that women can withstand is lower than the amount of pain that men can withstand. Fibromyalgia is seen mostly in women between 20 and 50 years of age. However, it can affect children and elderly people as well.

Fibromyalgia may develop after an injury, a motor vehicle accident, infection (viral or bacterial), or after an onset of rheumatoid arthritis. Stressful situations, cold weather and over exertion can worsen your fibromyalgia. As a fibromyalgia sufferer, you may not be getting enough deep sleep. Even in normal people, not getting enough sleep can produce symptoms of fibromyalgia. It is not currently known if a lack of deep sleep is a cause of fibromyalgia. Some doctors think the loss of deep sleep can hasten the onset of fibromyalgia.

Serotonin and norepinepherine are two chemicals in your central nervous system (brain and spinal cord) that decrease pain signals that travel to your brain. Not having enough serotonin in your brain and spinal cord can cause you lose sleep, which can cause symptoms of depression as well as fibromyalgia like pain. Fibromyalgia also affects your levels of norepinepherine, which is another chemical in your central nervous that also modulates the number of pain signals that go to your brain. Another chemical in your body that causes pain is substance P.

Substance P is found in all of the neurons of your central nervous system as well as nerves that go to your muscles and joints. When your muscle tissues have been injured, substance P is released. This event can trigger burning pain sensations throughout your body. High substance P levels have been noted in the spinal fluid of patients with fibromyalgia. Endorphins, substances produced by your body and deposited in the spinal cord to decrease pain transmission to your brain, are known to slow down the pain-causing effects of substance P. The low levels of endorphins in your brain and spinal cord when you have fibromyalgia may be another cause of pain associated with this condition.

It is well known that vigorous exercise can produce endorphins that are then released in your body. Along with decreasing the pain signals that are sent to your brain, endorphins can affect your mood. It is thought that a lower than normal blood level of endorphins may be another cause of fibromyalgia. People with and without fibromyalgia who do physical exercise have noted a decrease in their pain following aerobic exercise. Normal people usually have an increase in endorphins in their bloodstream following exercise. However, you may show no increase in endorphin levels after you exercise.

There is increased evidence that fibromyalgia can be genetically inherited. You may even know of a relative who has symptoms similar to yours. The exact gene that causes fibromyalgia has not been isolated, but several genes have been proposed as a possible explanation for the genetic inheritance of fibromyalgia and they are being studied. Research into the causes of fibromyalgia must continue.

It is a good idea for you to keep a daily diary of your activities and pain levels. When you visit your doctor, be sure to take your diary with you so your doctor can see your daily activities such as exercise, sleep, and eating habits. Also be sure to write down any medications you have taken and what their effects were. This will help your doctor determine what areas you need help in the most, and can help the doctor prescribe an effective treatment to relieve your pain symptoms. Let your pain-management doctor know if your primary care doctor diagnosed any new disorder or prescribed any new drug since your last visit with your pain doctor.

It is important that you do exercise or some type of low-impact aerobic activity. Aerobic exercise is extremely helpful in decreasing your pain and improving your sleep pattern. Swimming and water aerobics are excel-lent ways for you to accomplish this goal. They are some of the best exercise activities for patients with fibromyalgia.

These types of nonimpact activities will help strengthen and condition your muscles, unlike high-impact exercise that can actually do more damage to your muscles. A study published in 1996 said that following physical exercise, almost 50 percent of people had a significant decrease in their signs and symptoms of fibromyalgia. Exercise will improve your muscle range of motion.

Most doctors agree that medications, injections, and therapy alone will not be able to eliminate your pain, but rather it will help you to manage your pain and cope with it better. Taking steroids to treat your fibromyalgia will not improve your symptoms of pain. People with other muscle or bone conditions such as rheumatoid arthritis do respond well to steroids. However, nonsteroidal anti-inflammatory medications such as ibuprofen may relieve or at least decrease your muscle pain.

The primary goal in treating your fibromyalgia is to attempt to break the pain cycle. One way of accomplishing this goal is to correct any disturbance in your sleep pattern. Amitriptyline (Elavil) can be an important drug in restoring your sleep. Numerous studies have shown that getting enough sleep can significantly reduce your pain.

If you are allergic to amitriptyline, cyclobenzaprine (Flexeril) can be substituted. In some people, nonsteroidal anti-inflammatory medications such as ibuprofen can be successfully used. Amantadine hydrochloride (Symmetrel) also may be used. This medication is an antiviral as well as an anti-Parkinson medication. Serotonin reuptake inhibitors (Paxil) may also have a positive effect on reducing your pain. There are new two drugs approved by the FDA for the treatment of fibromyalgia; Lyrica (an anticonvulsant) and Cymbalta (an antidepressant). Savella or Celexa may also be helpful. In fact, pregabalin has shown enough efficacy, that it is the first and only drug approved by the FDA for the treatment of fibromyalgia.

Nerve stimulation is another method of relieving pain that you may find helpful. A TENS unit (Transcutaneous Electrical Nerve Stimulator) is useful in managing fibromyalgia pain in many patients. This small battery-powered instrument has two to four patches that are placed over your painful muscle areas. Electrical impulses will stimulate the nerves around your areas of pain. This stimulation will cause the production of the pain-relieving chemical enkephalin into your spinal cord. Enkephalin will diminish the intensity of your pain signals that ultimately reach your brain.

Another useful device that is gaining in popularity is a muscle stimulator. This device has six to eight patches that are placed over your painful muscle areas. The muscle stimulator machine will stimulate and work your muscles until they are fatigued and weakened. It is possible for your muscles that have been weakened by the fibromyalgia to be strengthened this way.

Be aware of the "leaking gut" theory as a cause of fibromyalgia. If large proteins leak into your gastrointestinal circulation, your immune system may become overactive. You can then experience an antibody response that causes you to have generalized body pain. Some individuals that have fibromyalgia from this cause can be treated successfully with a gluten free diet, colostrums supplements or hyperimmune eggs.

The FDA has approved only three drugs: Cymbalta, Lyrica and Savella for the treatment of fibromyalgia. Although they generate billions of dollars in annual sales for Pfizer, Eli Lilly, Forest Laboratories and other drug makers, most who have tried the medications say they don't work.

Sixty-two percent of patients who have tried cannabis said it was very effective at treating their fibromyalgia symptoms. Another 33% said it helped a little and only 5% said it did not help at all. Massage, swimming, acupuncture, muscle relaxers and other alternative treatments also helped relieve their symptoms.

A psychologist can help you deal with the suffering aspect of your pain. Your psychologist also may want to teach you biofeedback. This is a good way for you to learn relaxing techniques that can significantly reduce your pain. Your psychologist may want you to listen to a CD or cassette tapes at home. Aromatherapy also could be effective for helping you manage your pain. This method is more effective in women because their scent perception is better than a man's. You may also find that hypnosis can decrease your pain intensity as well. You may want to try self-hypnosis as another modality for the management of your chronic pain.

Insomina is common in fibromyalgia. Chronic insomnia alone impacts 10% to 15% of adults. Epidemiologic data indicate that pain, fatigue, and mood disturbance are common correlates of persistent insomnia. Your physician must try to correct your insomnia. A good night's rest increases norepinerpherine and serotonin in your central nervous system. These are two biochemicals that can decrease your pain.

Given that no two people are alike, if you are taking any medications and begin to take nutritional supplements you should be aware that potential drug-nutrient interactions may occur and are encouraged to consult a health care professional before using any natural product. Combining certain prescription drugs and dietary supplements can lead to undesirable effects such as: diminished prescription drug effectiveness, reduced supplement effectiveness and impaired drug and/or supplement absorption.

Coenzyme Q10 (CoQ10) deficiency has been implicated in the pathophysiology of fibromyalgia. All patients in one study with fibromyalgia showed CoQ10 deficiency. After treatment, all patients showed an important improvement in clinical symptoms in all evaluation methods. According to these results, and evaluated by three methods, patients with FM are candidates for treatment with CoQ10.

Many people suffer from fibromyalgia (FM) without an effective treatment. They do not have a good quality of life and cannot maintain normal daily activity. Vegetarian diets could have some beneficial effects probably due to the increase in antioxidant intake2

The results of a pilot study suggest that dietary Chlorella supplementation may help relieve the symptoms of fibromyalgia in some patients. Moreover, it seems reasonable to eliminate some foods from the diet of FM patients, for example excitotoxins. Non-celiac gluten sensitivity is increasingly recognized as a frequent condition with similar manifestations which overlap with those of FM. The elimination of gluten from the diet of FM patients is recently becoming a potential dietary intervention for clinical improvement.

Fraud can occur in fibromyalgia treatment. A South Lake Tahoe chiropractor Paul Whitcomb was claimed to have discovered the cause of fibromyalgia, a chronic pain syndrome, and was charging patients thousands of dollars for his cure. Whitcomb claims the problem is that the top vertebrae of the spine has been knocked out of alignment with the skull, usually in some kind of accident. The "Whitcomb Method", which consists of a neck manipulation three times a day, five days a week, for at least two months. Several former patients told us that all they got out of Whitcomb's treatment was a stiff neck and an expensive bill.

Patients suffering from fibromyalgia should seek help from reputable medical centers to avoid potential scams.

26. HEADACHES

Headaches can have many causes. Most headaches are caused by emotional stress or fatigue, but some headaches are a symptom of a disease within the brain. Of the many pains that you can feel through-out your body, pain in the head region is usually the most distressing. Pain in your head can arise in your head itself or can be referred from your neck as well.

There are two general classes of headaches, primary and secondary. Primary headaches are those that occur from structures within your brain while secondary headaches can be caused by tumors, infections, etc. Primary headaches have no structural, infectious or other abnormality that could cause your headache. Examples of primary head-aches are migraine head-aches and tension-type headaches. Secondary headaches have underlying abnormalities like a tumor, hemorrhage, blood clot, etc.

Some pain receptors exist outside your skull, and other pain receptors exist within your skull. Structures outside of your skull that can cause pain in your head include the skin and scalp over your head, muscles about your head and neck, and the outer wrapper of the bone of your skull called the periosteum.

Your sinuses can also cause you to have head pain immediately above your eyes. Within your skull, you have a lining that can become inflamed and irritated and cause pain called the meninges. Your veins can cause pain as well if they become engorged. You must tell your doctor where the location of your pain is. This will help your doctor determine the source of your headache.

Your doctor will complete a detailed history and neurological examination and may order a MRI or CAT scan to determine what type of head-ache that you have. The purpose of a neurological examination is to exclude any disease or tumor outside of your brain that could be causing your headache. If you have a history of rheumatoid arthritis, make sure that your doctor knows that you have this disorder. Headaches can arise from instabil-ity of the first two bones in your neck.

Because tight muscles can also cause headaches, your doctor will check the muscles in your neck. Your doctor will then press on the arteries in your temples. If you have tenderness around the arteries in your temples, you may have an inflammation of your temporal arteries. This disease is called temporal arteritis. Your doctor will have you lie flat on the examining table. Your doctor will ask whether you have a change in your headache after your head is lifted. If your headache is originating from your neck, there may be some relief by lifting your head relative to your neck.

Skull X-rays can prove useful for the diagnosis of a skull fracture, cancers, bone destruction, or some shift of the structures of the brain. If you have pain in your neck, your doctor may order x-rays of your neck, with your neck bent forward and then bent backward. This is called a flexion-extension X ray. This test can determine whether you have any instability of the bones in your neck. Blood flow studies may be done to determine whether you have any compromise in the blood flow going to your brain. A decrease in blood flow can cause significant headaches.

Sometimes a CT scan is necessary to determine whether you have swelling in your brain or a brain abscess. An electroencephalogram (EEG) study is sometimes ordered to determine whether you have a seizure disorder or a sleep problem. If you have had trauma to your head, your doctor may want a CAT scan, which will show whether you have bleeding within your head.

An MRI scan of your brain can be done to see whether you have loss of myelin, which is a substance in your brain. With loss of myelin, you may develop neurological symptoms that include memory loss and difficulty concentrating and have pain in your legs. This disease is called Multiple Sclerosis.

Occasionally a spinal tap is done to help make a diagnosis of what may be causing your headache. This procedure can investigate whether you have an infection such as meningitis. This procedure consists of placing a needle into your spinal fluid. At the time that the spinal tap is done, a pressure monitor can be used to see whether you have increased pressure in your central nervous system.

Be aware, that the medical history that you give to your doctor is important. Do not leave out any information. Information that is not important to you may be very important to your physician. Your doctor needs to know if you have had a headache with loss of consciousness. Loss of consciousness could indicate seizures or a hemorrhage into your brain.

If you have had no previous history of a severe headache, your doc-tor may need to order tests to see whether or not you have a bleed in your brain from a weakness in one of the arteries (aneurysm) in your brain. A weakness in the blood vessel is called an aneurysm. If you have headaches accompanied by neurological abnormalities during and after your headache, your doctor will want to make sure that you do not have a clot within your brain or a brain tumor.

Tumors can cause headaches with neurological abnormalities such as forgetfulness and dizziness. If you have a headache that first begins after age 50, your pain may be coming from degeneration of the discs in your neck. Hormonal changes that can occur with decreased function of your thyroid gland can cause headaches as well. Depression also can also cause headaches. If someone has told you that your personality changes when you have a headache, your doctor will want to determine whether you have a tumor or even an infection of your brain.

A headache that occurs when you have an increase in your blood pressure can indicate various medical diseases that may be causing a headache. Be aware that headaches can come from the soft tissues in your neck. An x-ray of your neck will not reveal soft tissue problems. An MRI can usually reveal problems in structures that could cause you to have a head-ache.

A common type of headache is the classic migraine headache. By definition a migraine headache is a headache that returns and varies widely in its intensity and frequency of the attacks and the duration. Usually the headaches occur on one side and are associated with nausea, vomiting, and a loss of appetite. Sometimes you may have visual problems associated with this headache. You can have a head-ache with sensations that forewarn you of an attack of an impending headache.

You may have a sensation of flickering lights or blurred vision or weakness in your arms or legs. These sensations are called an aura. Some migraines occur without an aura. If you have migraines with an aura, usually you have visual disturbances. This type of visual disturb-ance is seen in 90 percent of patients who have migraine headaches with an aura. Migraine headaches can be triggered if you have abnormal response to stress. No one knows what exactly causes migraine headaches. When you have one of these headaches, you may experience mood disturbances as well as pain. You may have nausea and vomiting as well.

Migraine headaches usually begin when you are a teenager. However, some migraine headaches can begin at age 40. Before you suffer a migraine headache, you may have changes in your vision or speech and balance. You may notice zigzag lines in front of your eyes or small specks in one eye.

You may notice different lines that come and go in front of your eyes. You may have numbness in your hands. When the headache occurs following these visual disturbances, your headache is usually on one side of your head.

If you are seeing lines only in front of your left eye, usually your headache will be on the right side of your brain. Sometimes you can have migraine headaches that occur several times a week followed by a long period of having no headaches. Sometimes your migraine headaches can be incapacitating. Movements such as bending over, coughing or sneezing can worsen your headache. You will want to lie down. Following your headache, it can take approximately 24 hours for you to feel normal again.

If you have a history of migraine headaches, be aware that some stressful situations such as weddings, funerals, or speaking in front of people can trigger a migraine headache. Be aware that there can be a family history of migraine headaches. Seventy percent of people inherit the tendency to have migraine headaches. If you have migraine headaches, you usually have less than two attacks per month. However, 10 percent of patients have attacks every week.

Some migraine headaches begin with a visual aura of zigzag lines or a blotting out of your vision or both. Furthermore, numbness of one side of your face and hand, weakness, unsteadiness, or altered consciousness may precede your headache. Most however, are not associated with an aura. The aura can forewarn you of an impending headache. This type of headache is called a migraine headache without an aura. Sometimes these headaches occur on both sides of your head but most occur on just one side of your head.

Before your doctor prescribes medicines for your headache, your doctor must tailor your medications to your type of headache and take into account your disability, your medical history, and your psychological profile. Treatment of your migraines can be divided into acute treatment of the attack as well as treatment to prevent the onset of headaches. Whenever possible, the factors that cause your headaches should be avoided. Stay away from foods that could trigger your migraine head-ache. Cheese, chocolate, red wine, and some Chinese foods that contain the additive MSG are commonly considered migraine headache triggers.

If you have an onset of a headache, a mild attack can be treated with aspirin. Nonsteroidal anti-inflammatory drugs can also be used to treat your headache. Ibuprofen is commonly used to treat headaches and can be purchased without a prescription. The nonsteroidal anti-inflammatory drugs called COX-2 inhibitors (Celebrex) can also be effective for the treatment of headaches. If you have nausea and vomiting associated with your migraine headache, you may need to take a nonsteroidal anti-inflammatory drug by the rectal route.

Newer drugs called triptans have been developed and can decrease your headache within a significant time after its onset. Sumatriptan was the first triptan drug to be used for the treatment of migraine headaches. Triptans are much better tolerated than the older caffeine-ergotamine medications. Be aware that the triptans are expensive. When you first suspect that you are having a migraine, take your triptan immediately.

Sometimes stronger drugs are needed for the treatment of migraine headache symptoms. Codeine is sometimes needed. Stronger drugs such as Percocet have been prescribed for the treatment of migraine headaches. If you have frequent migraine attacks and if these attacks are disabling, your physician may consider prophylactic treatment. Because migraine headaches can be activated by stress, it is important that you tell your doctor what situations trigger your head-aches.

You may have to make life adjustments to control your headaches. If you are having too much stress at work, you may need to consider changing your job. If you have significant psychological problems, consider a consultation with a psychologist. Antihypertensive medications such as Nadolol and Verapamil have been used to prevent the onset of migraine headaches. Amitriptyline, an antidepressant, also has been demonstrated to prevent the onset of migraine headache.

Migraine headaches can be hormonally related in females. They are more common in women until age 60 when the incidence is about equal with men. Migraine headaches commonly occur with the onset of menses in women. These headaches may also occur in the first trimester of pregnancy. The headaches can disappear following a complete hysterectomy.

After the onset of menopause, your migraine headaches may disap-pear or at least decrease in intensity and frequency. However, if you receive hormone therapy at the time of menopause, this can prolong your headache symptoms.

Sometimes your migraine headaches can worsen when you begin using oral contraceptives. Concern exists about the use of oral contraceptives by those who suffer migraine headaches, because they run a higher risk of stroke.

Another type of headache that you could experience is called a tension-type headache. This also is called a muscle contraction headache even though muscle tightness is not a common cause of this type of headache. If you have chronic tension-type headaches, you may have headaches 15 days a month. For your doctor to make a diagnosis of your tension-type headache, you should have at least 10 previous headache episodes.

The headaches could last from 30 minutes to 7 days. You will usually have a headache on both sides of your head. Your headaches should not be aggravated by walking or routine physical activity. If you have a tension-type headache, you should not experience nausea or vomiting. You should not have visual disturbances that are associated with migraine headaches.

Migraine headaches and tension-type headaches are experienced more in women than men. Muscle tension-type headaches can start at any age. Tension-type headaches can begin in childhood if a child is physically and emotionally abused. When you have a tension-type headache, you will feel a tight band and pressure around your head in the form of a tight cap. Your neck muscles will feel as if they are in a knot. The location of your pain is usually all around your head on both sides. Usually a tension-type headache is seen in tense or anxious people.

If depression perpetuates your headaches, you can take antidepressants at bedtime to enhance your sleep or take an antidepressant like Cymbalta during the day. Sometimes muscle relaxants can be used to decrease your pain. Antianxiety drugs such as Valium have sometimes been used preventatively to decrease the chance of one of these headaches developing. When your headache occurs, one of the nonsteroidal anti-inflammatory drugs may be helpful in decreasing your headache.

Another type of headache that you should be aware of is called a cluster headache. This severely painful headache is not common and occurs mostly in men. Usually the headache is on one side of your head and can be above your eye or in your temple. Usually the headache lasts 15 minutes to 3 hours if untreated.

Usually you will have tearing of your eye as well as nasal congestion on the side of your cluster headache. You may have forehead sweating. Your pupil may be extremely small and your upper eyelid may droop. These headaches can be extremely painful. The exact cause of cluster headaches is unknown.

A cluster headache occurs more frequently in men than in women. They also occur more frequently in the spring and fall and occur at the same time of the day. There is a 5:1 man-to-woman ratio of cluster headaches. To treat a cluster headache attack, some doctors suggest inhalation of 100 percent oxygen using a face mask.

Usually your headache will settle in 15 minutes. If this does not work, an injection of sumatriptan (Imitrex) may decrease your pain. Some studies have even recommended the use of local anesthetics on a cotton swab placed in your nose.

Steroids in high doses can be used to treat cluster headaches. Medrol (a steroid) can be given in various doses and schedules as directed by your treating physician. This drug must be discontinued slowly after treatment for five to seven days. It may take up to three weeks to taper the drug. Non-steroidal anti-inflammatory drugs may be effective in the treatment of these headaches as well. Sometimes sufferers need to see a neurosurgeon in consultation to see whether there is a surgical procedure that can be done to decrease the frequency of these headaches.

A headache following trauma can be made worse with physical exer-cise. A post-traumatic headache differs from migraine symptoms in that a chronic post-traumatic headache is usually generalized and permanent. However, it can be made worse by physical or mental strain. Usually this type of headache subsides in 8 to 10 weeks.

You can develop a post-traumatic headache with only a minor injury to your head. In fact, the more severe the injury, the less chance you have of developing one of these headaches. Post-traumatic headache is reported more often in women than men. The incidence of a post-traumatic headache can be forty percent following a head injury. If you are over 60 years of age, you could develop a headache related to temporal arteritis. This usually occurs after you have had a fever. You have a burning pain caused by inflammation of your temporal artery on the side of your head. It is usually accompanied by a throbbing headache about your temple.

With temporal arteritis you may have a burning pain about your scalp. Jaw movement such as chewing worsens temporal arteritis headaches. This type of headache can be accompanied by loss of vision, which is a medical emergency. The diagnosis sometimes has to be made with a biopsy of the arterial tissue. Steroids are usually the treatment of choice for this pain.

Pain in your head can come from direct pressure on structures such as nerves, muscles or blood vessels. Traction on your nerves can cause your pain. If your blood vessels become engorged and if the diameters of your vessels become enlarged, the enlarged vessel can compress your nerves in your brain and cause you to have a headache. A prolonged muscle contraction in your neck can cause pain as well.

Psychological distress can trigger your headaches. Sometimes major social trauma or anxiety triggers headaches. Physical trauma can also be a cause of chronic headaches. If you are a woman, your doctor will want to know the effects of your menstrual periods and pregnancy on your head-aches. Menstrual periods and pregnancies change hormones in the blood-stream, and this change can trigger headaches. Hormone changes in both men and women can increase you incidence of headaches.

A headache that begins at the base of your skull is called occipital neuralgia. The pain from occipital neuralgia shoots up to the top of your head. Local pressure on the back of your head will reproduce your pain. Trauma to the back of your head or an infection can cause pain. Degeneration disc disease may also cause occipital neuralgia. Your doctor may order a CAT scan to try and determine what is causing your pain. Treatment may consist of muscle relaxants, non-steroidal anti-inflammatory drugs, and antidepressant drugs, injections with steroids, botulism toxin or local anesthetics. On occasion, freezing the Greater Occipital nerve may relieve your pain. Currently treatment with a peripheral electrical stimulating wire is gaining popularity.

It appears that there is gender specificity with respect to headaches. In men, when their testosterone increases, cluster headaches become frequent. Cluster headaches are can occur at the onset of puberty. In males and females with an increase in progesterone, estrogen, and testosterone, there is an increase in migraine as well as tension headaches.

Be aware that women produce testosterone as well as men. When progesterone, estrogen, and testosterone blood levels increase in your body, pain in general increases in both men and women. In many instances physicians are under the misconception that a detailed biochemical understanding of each individual disease is required before nutritional interventions can be used. Natural remedy is cheap, easily available, nontoxic, and easy to prepare and provides good mental health as compared to other remedies.

A moderate dose of caffeine can also help relieve a headache (especially the type that cause throbbing or pounding) by constricting the blood vessels that go to the head.Given that no two people are alike, if you are taking any medications and begin to take nutritional supplements you should be aware that potential drug-nutrient interactions may occur and are encouraged to consult a health care professional before using any natural product.

Combining certain prescription drugs and dietary supplements can lead to undesirable effects such as: diminished prescription drug effectiveness, reduced supplement effectiveness and impaired drug and/or supplement absorption.

Omega-3 and omega-6 fatty acids are precursors of bioactive lipid mediators posited to modulate both physical pain and psychological distress. In a randomized trial of 67 subjects with severe headaches, it was demonstrated that targeted dietary manipulation-increasing omega-3 fatty acids with concurrent reduction in omega-6 linoleic acid produced major reductions in headaches compared with an omega-6 lowering intervention alone.Riboflavin is a safe and well-tolerated option for preventing migraine symptoms in adults. Dietary sodium may affect brain extracellular fluid sodium concentrations and neuronal excitability.

Another study demonstrated a harmful association between excess dietary salt and all-cause mortality, noncardiovascular and cardiovascular disease mortality, and headache. It has also been shown that Vitamin D supplementation may be useful in decreasing frequency of headache attacks. The ability of CoQ (10) to mitigate headache symptoms in adults has also verified in pediatric and adolescent populations.6

Based on a nationally representative sample, it was found that cigarette smoking was associated with headache in an exposure-response manner. Mentholated cigarette smokers were not more likely to have headache compared to non-mentholated cigarette smokers.

Migraine Treatment Group Migraine Support Formula is an over the counter natural supplement for migraine headache treatment. The manufacturer says this product will help your body build up its defenses against the triggers of migraines internally and will help you defeat most of the triggers of migraines. It actually works by shocking your system into immediately reducing the occurrence of your migraines. Migraine Support Formula has worked to effectively reduce or even eliminate severe migraine headaches. The ingredients are safe and natural with no known side effects yet appear to work for some people better than prescription medication.

Research shows that spinal manipulation provided by doctors of chiropractic may be an effective treatment option for tension headaches and headaches that originate in the neck. A 2014 report in the Journal of Manipulative and Physiological Therapeutics found that interventions commonly used in chiropractic care improved outcomes for the treatment of acute and chronic neck pain and increased benefit was shown in several instances where a multimodal approach to neck pain had been used.

Be aware of possible Botox scams for headache treatment. A Las Vegas physician and his wife have been ordered to serve federal prison sentences following their convictions for fraud after they treated patients with fake Botox. The FBI, Drug Enforcement Administration and Internal Revenue Service are investigating a headache specialist, saying he prescribed unneeded medication to patients and billed Medicare and private insurers for tests he didn't conduct. Be mindful of some Botox treatments for headache treatment. A patient had Botox treatment for persistent migraines and was then charged a total of $4090.00 for a treatment regimen that took less than 15 minutes.

Furthermore, be aware of the use of the phrase, "FDA approved new medicine." Virtually everyone would assume that FDA stands for Food and Drug Administration. The FDA to which some scammers refer to is the Fighting Disease Association. A Web search found no references to such an organization.

In trials that compared Botox to other headache treatments, there was no statistically significant difference in the number of headaches patients reported each month. Most chronic migraine sufferers who used Botox in the studies experienced just two to three fewer headaches each month on average, compared with those getting placebo injections.

For tension headaches, which the American Headache Society declares is the most common type of headache; Botox doesn't seem to be of much help at all. Botox is usually only prescribed for the 3% of adults whose tension headaches occur on 15 or more days a month, at which point they are considered to be chronic tension headaches. In most cases, stress, fatigue, hunger, overexertion or even poor posture can trigger headache onset.

There are unscrupulous people who prey on people with migraine and other diseases. When a person is desperate, he/she is more probable to be vulnerable to sham treatments. A headache sufferer reportedly paid a man over $14,000 for a spiritual cure which provided no pain relief.

Patients must remember that there are unscrupulous people who prey on people with painful syndromes and other diseases.

27. INJECTIONS

Various pain-modifying procedures are available to help alleviate your pain. In recent years a gigantic industry has grown up around invasive but nonsurgical treatments for back problems. It is split across several larger nondrug disciplines: radiology, anesthesiology, physiatry, and neurology that often fall under the guise of "pain management. "These physicians generally refer to themselves as "spine interventionists." Most are better known among medical professionals simply as "needle jockeys," who do other expensive procedures as well:

Epidural steroid injections (ESI) can decrease your pain if it goes from your neck to your arm (cervical ESI), your midback to your chest (thoracic ESI) or your lower back down your leg (lumbar ESI). If you have an injured disc in one of these areas of your spine, some chemical can leak out and affect one or more of your nerves. These chemicals can cause your nerves to swell. When the nerves swell, they may cause you to experience pain.

The ESI takes the swelling out of your nerves and reduces your pain. Epidural steroid injections (ESIs) are a common treatment option for many forms of low back pain and leg pain. They have been used for low back problems since 1952 and are still an integral part of the non-surgical management of low back pain and sciatica. The goal of the injection is pain relief; at times the injection alone is sufficient to provide relief, but commonly an epidural steroid injection is used in combination with a comprehensive rehabilitation program to provide additional benefit.

Most practitioners will agree that the effects of the injection tend to be temporary. The ESI can provide relief from pain for one week up to one year. An epidural injection can be very beneficial for a patient during an acute episode of back and/or leg pain. Importantly, an injection can provide sufficient pain relief to allow a patient to progress with a rehabilitative stretching and exercise program. If the initial injection is effective, you may have up to three in a one-year period.

In addition to low back (the lumbar region), epidural steroid injections are used to ease pain experienced in your neck (cervical) region or in your mid spine (thoracic) region doctors should inform patients that injecting steroids into the epidural space, just outside the spinal cord, has risks . The steroids used in epidural steroid injections are not approved by the FDA for epidural use, although they are approved for injections into joints.

The Food and Drug Administration has just issued what's called a "Med watch Alert" warning that epidural steroid injections or "ESIs" for back and neck pain can be extremely dangerous. The alert says: "Injection of corticosteroids into the epidural space of the spine may result in rare but serious adverse events, including loss of vision, stroke, paralysis, and death."

There is no conclusive evidence that spinal injections were effective treatments for spinal stenosis, facet joints, sacroiliac joints, or non-radicular back pain. It is important to realize that although needle penetration of the spinal cord can produce injuries, with a wide range of severity, injection of any material into the cord is invariably devastating. It is critical, therefore, to insure proper needle placement prior to injecting anything, including contrast dye. The vast majority of serious injuries related to cord trauma are associated with cervical epidurals.

Although many studies document the short-term benefits of epidural steroid injections, the data on long-term effectiveness are less convincing. Indeed, the effectiveness of epidural steroid injections continues to be a topic of debate. This is accentuated by the lack of properly performed studies. For example, many studies do not include use of fluoroscopy or x-ray to verify proper placement of the medication despite the fact that fluoroscopic guidance is routinely used today. Additionally, many studies do not classify patients according to diagnosis and tend to 'lump' different types sources of pain together. These methodological flaws tend to make interpretation and application of study results difficult to impossible.

Research suggests that sedating patients before a nerve block needed to diagnose or treat chronic pain increases costs, risks and unnecessary surgeries, and sedation does nothing to increase patient satisfaction or long-term pain control. Sedation doesn't help, but it does add expense and risk. Patients may need to take extra time away from daily activities after being under anesthesia, and that rest alone could make the patient feel better. The most likely causes of spinal cord injury following epidural steroid injection are epidural bleeding, epidural abscess, direct spinal cord trauma, and embolization of particulate matter into the arterial supply of the cord.

The clinical argument against deep sedation stems from the fear of undetected harm when a needle makes contact with neural tissue. It is claimed that a patient's conscious ability to communicate about pain or paresthesia is needed to let the clinician know whether a neural structure is in danger of compromise. In this view, a heavily sedated and unaware patient poses a risk that could lead to harm and medical liability.

While many physicians may use sedation in a sincere effort to make the procedure less traumatic for patients, there is also a perverse financial incentive to use it. Unfortunately, medicine has become a business. The fact is, your doctor gets paid more money to do the procedure with sedation. The costs of anesthesia can be more than the fee for the procedure itself. And patients are getting harmed. as a result of this behavior.

On May 7, 2013 Dr. Oz expressed his concern about the use of Epidural Steroid Injections (ESIs) to treat back pain. For those suffering from back pain, Epidural Steroid Injections (ESIs) sound like a dream come true since they can potentially alleviate pain and help patients regain function and mobility for months at a time. This one cortisone shot, for many individuals, can give back significant quality of life. It can also reduce the potential need to use addictive and dangerous pain killers. With Epidural Steroid Injections (ESIs) becoming more popular with many doctors, Dr. Oz suggested that their ability to alleviate back pain might not be worth the potential side effects.

Dr. Oz is concerned about the use of epidural steroid injections, their side effects and efficacy. The number of epidural steroid injections performed has surged, rising 271% from 1994 to 2001 according to an analysis of Medicare claims. Today, general practitioners, physician assistants – even some dentists and chiropractors have started offering ESIs. All three major pain societies, The American Pain Society, The American Society of Interventional Pain Physicians, and the American Academy of Neurology, stated that ESIs are best suited for a diagnosis of radiculopathy, a pinched or inflamed nerve root with pain radiating down your leg. This diagnosis only fits a small minority of patients.

Some doctors spend just one weekend learning the delicate procedure at training centers that teach cosmetic injections like Botox and fillers, but also teach doctors how to poke around people's spines. One weekend training center advertises epidural steroid injections as "lucrative specialty options" that "create dramatic earnings for your practice." These procedures are not FDA approved,.

Epidural steroid injections are being used too often to treat back pain, in part because of an insurance compensation system that encourages doctors to generate more income by using the procedure, several leading experts in pain management have told Pain News Network.

An estimated 9 million epidural steroid injections (ESI's) are performed annually in the U.S. Epidural shots with an analgesic have long been used to relieve pain during child birth, but in recent years injections of a corticosteroid into the epidural space around the spinal cord have become an increasingly common procedure to treat back pain.

Critics say epidural injections are overused and patients risk permanent damage to their spinal cords if they get the shots too often. More studies are needed to properly define the role of epidural steroid injections in low back pain and in sciatica as well as pain in the neck and midback. Despite this, most studies report that more than 50% of patients find measurable pain relief with epidural steroid injections. They also underscore the need for patients to enlist the services of professionals with extensive experience administering injections, and who always use fluoroscopy to ensure accurate placement.

Epidural steroid injections deliver medication directly (or very near) the source of pain generation. With X ray guidance the needle tip can be placed where your discs are disrupted. In contrast, oral steroids go throughout your body may have unacceptable side effects. They also work for the pain from spinal stenosis, degenerative disease (arthritis) and from post lumbar surgery syndrome, whether just in the low back or also in the leg.

The effect of the ESI tends to be temporary. ESI is most helpful if you have severe pain in your spine and extremity. An ESI can provide sufficient pain relief to allow you to progress to physical therapy. Inflammatory chemicals and immunologic substances can generate pain and are associated with common back problems such as lumbar disc herniation. This condition can cause inflammation that in turn can cause significant nerve root irritation and swelling.

Steroids inhibit the inflammatory response caused by chemical sources of pain. Steroids furthermore work by reducing the activity of the immune system to react to inflammation associated with nerve or tissue damage. A typical immune response is the body generating white blood cells and chemicals to protect it against infection and foreign substances such as bacteria and viruses. This response makes your tissue red and swollen.

When you have an epidural injection, you are placed face down on an x-ray table with a small pillow under your stomach. The skin over your back area is cleaned with a surgical scrub solution and then your skin is numbed with a local anesthetic. Using x-ray a needle is inserted into the skin and directed toward the epidural space.

Once the needle is in the proper position, contrast dye is administered to confirm the needle location. The epidural steroid solution is then injected. Following the injection, you are monitored for 15 minutes to make sure that you do not have an allergy to the steroid before being discharged home.

You will follow-up with your doctor in two weeks after your procedure. If you did not have complete pain relief with your injection, your ESI may be repeated two more times until you have had three. You may have 3 injections every 6 months. Occasionally following an ESI you can develop a headache. This is from loss of spinal fluid. This is a complication and is remedied by injection some of your blood into the epidural space to patch up any leak of spinal fluid. You may have facet joint pain. Lumbar facet joints are small located in pairs on the back of your spine. They provide stability and guide motion in your back.

If your joints become painful they may cause pain in areas away from the location of your joints. The facet joint is the moveable joint of the spine that connects one vertebra to another. On April 23, 2014, the U.S. Food & Drug Administration issued a warning for the use of corticosteroid epidural injections for treating back, neck, and radiating pain in the arms and legs. Some rare but serious reactions were reported that cause the agency to issue this warning. Corticosteroid epidural injections used for these purposes can cause vision loss, strokes, paralysis, and sudden death.

Problems resulting from epidural corticosteroid injections are generally associated with physicians that have undergone minimal training in the procedure. Always ensure that your doctor is board-certified to ensure that he or she has sufficient training in the procedure to do it safely.A facet injection is a nonsurgical treatment that can temporarily relieve pain in your spine from inflammation or irritation of the facet joints in your spine. The procedure has two purposes as it can be used as a diagnostic test to see if the pain is actually coming from your facet joints and it can be used as a therapy to relieve inflammation and pain. Just like an epidural injection, facet joints are temporary. Medicare Part B payments for facet joint injections have increased from $141 million in 2003 to $307 million in 2006. Over the same period, the number of Medicare claims for facet joint injections increased by 76 percent. Sixty-three percent of facet joint injection services allowed by Medicare in 2006 did not meet Medicare program requirements, resulting in approximately

$96 million in improper payments. Medicare allowed an additional $33 million in improper payments for.

The OIG report of 20081 showed that Medicare paid over $2 billion in 2006 for interventional pain management procedures. This report also showed that the Medicare payments for facet joint injections increased from $141 million in 2003 to $307 million in 2006. Further, 63% of facet joint injection services allowed by Medicare in 2006 did not meet Medicare program requirements, resulting in approximately $129 million in improper payments. The OIG report also illustrated that over 50% of Medicare facet joint injections were performed by non-interventional pain physicians. The frequency of errors was higher in in-office settings.

Medial Branch Blocks (MBB) and Facet Joint Injections are provided to confirm that the facet joints are indeed, the pain generator for back or neck pain. Each vertebra in the spine is connected by two facet joints. A local anesthetic numbs the skin and tissue down to facet joint. Percutaneous radiofrequency (RF) facet denervation is used to treat neck or back pain originating in facet joints with degenerative changes. Diagnosis of facet joint pain is confirmed by response to nerve blocks. The goal of facet denervation is long-term pain relief. However, the nerves regenerate, and repeat procedures may be required.

After a nationwide medical review of transforaminal epidural injections in 2007, a physician was identified as a person who warranted further investigation because a medical review team suspected most of the injections performed by this physician were not medically necessary and lacked proper documentation. On one patient, whose claim was part of the medical review, the physician in question is said to have filed claims with Medicare for 90 facet joint injections and 96 transforaminal epidural injections in one year, according the to an affidavit.

If these procedures do provide you with relief, a long acting neruodestructive block can be done using heat, chemicals or freezing cold. This procedure is an injection of both steroid and an anesthetic (numbing agent) into a painful facet joint of your spine. The injection can be placed inside the joint capsule (intraarticular) or in the tissue surrounding the joint capsule (median branch nerve block). Steroids reduce inflammation, and they're very effective when delivered directly into the part of your back that is causing pain. Steroids are different than the steroids that athletes use and these steroids will not cause weight gain.

When you have a facet joint injection you are placed face down on an x-ray table. The skin over your back area is cleaned with a surgical scrub solution and then your skin is numbed with a local anesthetic. Using x-ray, a needle is inserted into the skin and directed toward the painful facet joint. Once the needle is in the proper position, contrast dye is administered to confirm that the needle location is accurate. The facet local anesthetic/ steroid solution is then injected. Following the injection, you are monitored for 15 minutes to make sure that you do not have an allergy to the steroid before being discharged home.

You will follow-up with your doctor in two weeks. If you did not have complete pain relief with your initial injection, your facet injection may be repeated another time until you have had two. Usually the painful facet joint and the one above are injected. If your pain persists, one of the long-term facet injections mentioned previously can be done. About 50% of patients experience some degree of pain relief. The pain may be relieved for several days to several months. It is not unusual to have physical therapy or chiropractic therapy after these injections are performed.

Sacroiliac joint pain is not uncommon. This joint is between your backbone and your hipbone. The sacroiliac joint is the largest joint of your lower spine in your buttock region. This joint occasionally becomes painful and inflamed. Steroid medication injected into your joint can reduce the inflammation and thus alleviating your pain. Sacroiliac (SI) joint injections are commonly used to determine what is causing your back pain. You will have pain over your joint when your doctor presses over this area. Analogous to facet joint injections these injections can be diagnostic and/or therapeutic. These injections eliminate pain by filling the SI joint with a local anesthetic medications well as a steroid that numbs the joint and deposits steroid within the joint.

If your SI joint is injected with a numbing medicine and your pain goes away for several hours, it is likely that this joint is causing your pain. These injections are an adjunct treatment, which facilitates participation in an active exercise program and may assist in avoiding the need for surgical intervention. When sacroiliac joint injections are employed, they should be performed with X ray using contrast medium to ensure proper needle and medication placement are done. Following an injection a comprehensive exercise program should be done.

When this procedure is performed you will be placed on your stomach on the x ray table. The area over your pain will be cleaned with surgical soap. Once X ray has identified your joint your skin over this area will be numbed with a local anesthetic. You will then receive the local anesthetic and steroid. If you have pain relief with several injections but if the pain recurs, you can have a rhizotomy of your SI joint. Fraudulent pain clinics will not use X ray or ultrasound needle guidance to do these injections. Image needle guidance is necessary for correct placement of the needle into the joint.

If you have had a whiplash injury and have chronic neck pain and headaches, an occipital-atlantal injection may provide you with pain relief. The atlanto-axial joint is the joint formed by the uppermost cervical vertebrae. It is a common cause of pain at the base of the scalp that can radiate all the way behind the eye. Treatment of pain from this joint with injection therapy can provide long-term relief of these frequently under diagnosed or misdiagnosed headaches.

The occipital-occipital joint is the joint formed by the joining of the skull with the cervical spine. Although a more unusual cause of headaches, it can be a cause of upper neck pain and headaches that occur with rotation of your head. These injections are performed into the uppermost portion of the spine to treat and diagnose headaches and neck pain. This procedure is performed with x ray. You will be placed on your side or face down on the X ray table. The skin over your upper neck will be cleaned with surgical soap. A needle will be guided into this joint with x ray. Contract dye will be administered. Once proper needle tip confirmation has been done, you will receive a local anesthetic and steroid.

Headaches originating at the base of your skull may be seen in arthritis or trauma. You might benefit from an occipital nerve block. Occipital nerve blocks may be of benefit in migraine headache treatment. Occipital nerve block is a procedure where local anesthetics are injected near the occipital nerve on the back of your head near the base of your skull on the side of the headache.

If you have RSD affecting your arm, you may need a stellate ganglion block. The stellate ganglion is part of the sympathetic nervous system. The infiltration of local anesthetic around the ganglion is used to treat reflex sympathetic dystrophy. These injections are frequently performed with X ray. Indications for stellate ganglion blocks include reflex sympathetic dystrophy of the upper extremities, Raynaud's syndrome of the upper extremities, herpes zoster of the face or neck and upper extremity pain due to arterial insufficiency.

For reflex sympathetic dystrophy of your leg, a lumbar sympathetic block can be done. The sympathetic nerves are a chain of nerves that run on the front side of the spinal column. They are part of the autonomic nervous system that controls many bodily functions such as sweating, heart rate, digestion, and blood pressure.

A celiac plexus block is a pain treatment procedure used to numb nerves in your upper abdomen if you have intolerable abdominal pain. The celiac plexus block procedure is most frequently used if you have pancreatic cancer. Celiac plexus block procedure the use of x-ray to allow for the precise placement of the needle. A local anesthetic is administered through this needle. In some instances, two needles may be placed. This block can provide pain relief for the liver, gallbladder, omentum, mesentery, stomach, small intestine, as well as the ascending and transverse portion of your colon.

Spinal cord electrical stimulation is used for pain management in cases of chronic pain following back surgery, reflex sympathetic dystrophy and vascular insufficiency. In this therapy, electrical impulses are used to block pain from being perceived in the brain. Instead of pain, you feel a mild tingling sensation from a catheter placed in your back. A lawsuit claims that a spinal stimulator company committed multiple illegal acts in relation to its Precision Plus SCS spinal cord stimulation system, including submitting fraudulent Medicare and Medicaid billing claims, concealing defects and denying replacement devices, engaging in a kickback scheme and retaliating against employees who raised the red flag about such practices.

There are many options available to you for pain management. Your treatment should be tailored to your problem and your overall health. A "one size fits all approach" cannot be used when addressing chronic pain problems. Implantable Neurostimulation Systems and other spinal-devices are a huge business for the medical implant device industry. The global market for spinal-devices is currently over $ 3 billion per year and is expected to increase to over $5 billion per year by 2018.

Neurostimulators have been used for a variety of types of chronic back pain situations including heriniated disks, post laminectomy pain, Complex Reginal Pay Syndrome, unsuccessful disk surgery, Degenerative Disk Disease, and Failed Back Syndrome. The Medtronic implantable neurostimulation system is indicated for spinal cord stimulation (SCS) as an aid in the management of chronic, intractable pain of the trunk and/or limbs including unilateral or bilateral pain associated with several different conditions. Unfortunately, because of the profits to be made from implanting a spinal stimulator, many people have received spinal stimulators for off-label or non-approved indications.

A Minnesota-based medtech company, has agreed to pay $2.8 million to resolve allegations that the company promoted its neurostimulator device for unapproved chronic pain treatment. According to the complaint, originally filed by former Medtronic sales rep Jason Nickell, Medtronic sales staff were directed to sell the device at discounted prices to pain management doctors. Nickell also alleged that sales reps promised physicians could "make upward of $10,000 profit on each patient, while adding only minutes to the procedure" by using a billing code meant for an FDA-approved use.

Neurostimulation provides pain relief by blocking pain messages before they reach the brain—instead of pain, patients feel a tingling sensation. According to the complaint, the procedure and intended use of neurostimulation devices at issue, referred to as Sub-Q, subcutaneous targeted neurostimulation ("STN"), or peripheral nerve field stimulation ("PNFS"), was a new application of an older device first developed around 2005 and still in an experimental stage as the company was promoting it.

It has been reported that medical device maker Medtronic Inc. (NYSE: MDT) says 14 patients have died from complications caused by its SynchroMed implantable pain pump. The pump is used to deliver analgesic drugs directly to the spinal fluid in patients with intractable pain or severe spasticity.

Although the Synchro Med pump has been classified by the Food and Drug Administration as a Class I recall, meaning there was a "reasonable probability" that it could cause serious health problems or even death, the company is not recommending that the pump be removed. Over 200,000 Synchro Med devices have been implanted worldwide, according to Medtronic.

Class-I-recall-issued-on-Medtronic-SynchroMed-drug-infusion-pumpsThe company has identified four issues with the pain pump that cause the improper mixing of medications prior to their injection into patients.

It is reasonable to expect that the resulting unintended drug delivery is a contributing factor to adverse events involving overdose and underdose. These adverse events will vary depending on the drug being infused, but could include lack of therapeutic effectiveness, confusion or altered mental state, sleepiness, nausea, respiratory depression, coma or death," the company said in a warning letter to physicians last month. Two patient deaths were caused by a drug blockage and one is blamed on an electrical short in the device. The deaths occurred between 1996 and April of this year.

Injection therapy can provide a patient relief if it is done by a fellowship trained board certified pain management specialist.

28. INFLAMMATION

Arthritis is a degeneration of your joints that causes you to experience joint pain. Arthritis can be caused wear and tear of your joints (osteoarthritis) or from inflammation of your joints (rheumatoid arthritis). Approximately one out of seven people has some form of arthritis, and there are many different types. More than 35 million people in the United States suffer from this disease, and every year the treatment costs the United States billions of dollars.

Inflammation that occurs in your joints can cause you to have pain as well as swelling of your joints. Cartilage is a tough, slippery layer of tissue that covers the surfaces where bones contact each other in joints. In degenerative arthritis, the cartilages in your joints wear out. A joint liner called a synovium lines the inside of your joints. The synovium contains a multitude of pain fibers. When the synovium swells, it causes release of pain signals in the area where the swelling occurs.

Approximately 25 percent of people with arthritis are unable to carry out their normal activities of daily living. This means that they have difficulty shopping, driving, and dressing. If you suffer from arthritis, your pain may come and go. More than 50 percent of people with arthritis however, report that they have pain that is constant. If you have osteoarthritis arthritis, you will experience stiffness of your joints in the morning but that the stiffness progressively decreases as you become more active.

With rheumatoid arthritis, your pain will be constant. If you have the rapid onset of joint pain that involves one joint such as the joint in your great toe, this usually signifies gout. If you have a relative who has a history of rheumatoid arthritis, you run the risk of developing this type of arthritis. If you have had weight loss as well as chronic fatigue, you must include this in your pain diary. Weight loss and fatigue can be associated with rheumatoid arthritis.

Your doctor may use a needle and syringe to extract fluid from your joints. Your doctor will look at the fluid to see whether it is clear. Normal joint fluid should be clear. If you have osteoarthritis, the fluid can be straw colored. Other types of arthritis that you may have include rheumatoid arthritis or gout. Your fluid may be yellow. Your doctor will examine your fluids for cells. Your doctor also will obtain blood from you. Your blood will be examined for any elevation in your white cells (a sign of inflammation) and a test for rheumatoid arthritis can be done at the same time.

Your doctor may also order x-rays or even a CAT scan or MRI of your painful area. Furthermore, it is not unusual for your doctor to eventually order a bone scan if your pain persists in spite of conservative treatment. A bone scan consists of injecting a very small and harmless dose of radioactive dye into your vein. After this has been done, a special camera takes a picture. If you have arthritis, there can be an increased uptake of the radioactive material into your painful joint, showing that the joint is inflamed.

Osteoarthritis is the most common arthritic disease. It also is called degenerative joint disease. Most of us will eventually develop osteoarthritis as we experience wear and tear of our joints. Osteoarthritis occurs when your cartilage is worn down and damaged by overuse, sometimes allowing the rigid and brittle bone ends to come into direct contact with each other.

Your bones can wear out and develop irregular growths called osteophytes that can interfere with the proper movement of your joint and cause pain. Your joints provide you with range of motion and do support your body as well. To have normal range of motion, you must havecartilage between your bones. This is why you have difficulty moving when your cartilage wears out. Osteoarthritis progresses with age. Osteoarthritis can cause not only pain in your arms and legs, but also in your spine.

Osteoarthritis can affect the elastic cartilage in your discs between your bones. These discs between your vertebra in your back act as cushions between each vertebra. You also have joints in the posterior aspect of your vertebra where each joint stacks on top of one another. These joints are called facet joints. These joints can degenerate, which will cause you to become stiff and will decrease your range of motion. Osteoarthritis can occur in your neck, lower back, or n your mid back.

Degenerative arthritis can affect your hips and knees as well. Your knees may become warm as well as swollen. Osteoarthritis also can affect the joints in your hands. You may notice a bony growth about the joints in your fingers. Joint pain associated with osteoarthritis usually begins gradually and progresses slowly over years. Initially, you may have degeneration but not experience pain. With the passage of time, symptoms may begin. You may notice an increase in your pain when it rains or when the weather becomes cold. Your pain may become severe to the point that it keeps you up at night. Osteoarthritis usually occurs in older people.

Approximately 85 percent of people over 65 develop osteoarthritis. However, only half of these people experience any symptoms. Obesity puts increased pressure and stress on your joints in your legs. Obesity is an abnormal increase in your body fat resulting in excessive weight. Obesity is measured by your body mass index (BMI). There must be a 20 percent weight gain greater than the ideal for your height and body build. If you are obese, you have an increased chance of developing osteoarthritis. Any excess weight that you carry may cause deterioration of the joints in your hips and knees.

Nonsteroidal anti-inflammatory medications are commonly used to treat osteoarthritis (for example, Celebrex, Mobic, etc.). Steroids injections into your joints can also decrease the inflammation of your knee joints, which will decrease your pain. Your doctor can also inject hyaluronic acid into your joints for pain modification. Glucosamine, which is available without a prescription, has been demonstrated to decrease pain associated with osteoarthritis. If you persist with chronic pain and disability, consultation with an orthopedic surgeon may be indicated to see if you would benefit from a total joint replacement.

Rheumatic arthritis is characterized by redness, warmth, swelling, and painful joints. If you have rheumatoid arthritis, you will have decreased range of motion of some of your joints in your body. You also may complain of stiffness. This disease attacks the synovial linings of your joints as well as the tendons about your joints.

If you develop rheumatoid arthritis, you may suffer generalized weakness and weight loss. The exact cause of rheumatoid arthritis is unknown, but approximately 43 million people in the United States suffer from rheumatoid arthritis. Rheumatoid arthritis affects men and women, all races, and all ages. Family history plays an important role in the development of rheumatoid arthritis.

Rheumatoid arthritis may result from an abnormality in your immune system. Your antibodies may attack your joints to cause significant degeneration within your joints. It can usually have a slow onset. However, be aware that it can have an acute rapid onset as well. The onset of rheumatoid arthritis occurs more often in the winter. You probably have rheumatoid arthritis if you have four of the following seven criteria: 1.morning stiffness around your joints, 2.arthritis of three or more joints, 3.arthritis of your hands, 4.arthritis that occurs on both sides of your body, 5.boney nodules over your bony joints, 6.an elevated rheumatoid factor in your bloodstream, 7.X-ray determination of your joints.

The treatment of rheumatoid arthritis is to relieve your pain, preserve joint range of motion and decrease your joint inflammation. In addition, your doctor will want to maintain as much range of motion about your joints as possible. Splinting, range of motion exercises and strengthening exercises can be extremely beneficial to you. Occasionally, you may need a brace on one of your extremities.

Usually nonsteroidal anti-inflammatory drugs are prescribed for the management of your arthritic pain. As mentioned with regard to osteoarthritis, the COX-2 inhibitors are safer for your gastrointestinal system than the older nonsteroidal anti-inflammatory drugs. Some doctors prescribe medications such as gold compounds, antimalarials, and sulfasalazine. However, each of these drugs has the potential to cause serious side effects. Steroids also may be necessary to decrease the inflammation of your joints. Steroids typically decrease pain and swelling in your joints and can be very effective.

If these methods do not relieve your pain, you may be a candidate for immunosuppressive therapy. Immunosuppressive therapy is the administration of a drug that eliminates or lessens an immune response. Methotrexate is used frequently for the treatment of your rheumatoid arthritis. Methotrexate can cause liver pathology. Surgery is the last resort for the treatment of rheumatoid arthritis and consists of total joint replacement. If your pain becomes intolerable and if you have significant limitations in joint function, surgery can provide you with relief. Joint replacements are now available for hips, knees, shoulders, elbows, and ankles.

Disease-modifying antirheumatic drugs (DMARDs) can substantially reduce the inflammation of rheumatoid arthritis. DMARDs can reduce or prevent joint damage, preserve joint structure and function, and enable a person to continue his or her daily activities. Drugs in this class include hydroxychloroquine (Plaquenil), methotrexate (Rheumatrex), gold salts (Ridaura, Solganal), D-penicillamine (Depen, Cuprimine), sulfasalazine (Azulfidine®, azathioprine (Imuran), leflunomide (Arava), and cyclosporine (Sandimmune, Neoral).Several weeks to months of treatment are often necessary before the effects of DMARDs become evident.

Ankylosing spondylitis is an inflammatory disease that predominantly affects men. Pain usually begins in the back and sacroiliac joint (the joint where the back and hip bones meet) early in life. An x-ray of the spine of a male with ankylosing spondylitis appears as bamboo and is called a bamboo spine. This pattern is also seen on MRI imaging studies.

Ankylosing spondylitis usually affects men before the age of 40. If you have ankylosing spondylitis, you may develop arthritis of your spine as well as the large joints in your body. Ankylosing spondylitis is present in 8 percent of Caucasians and 3 percent of African American men. A marker in the bloodstream called HLA-B27 is present in 90 percent of patients who have ankylosing spondylitis. Ankylosing spondylitis has been observed in rats when the HLA-B27 gene is expressed.

Usually ankylosing spondylitis will become manifest in a male around age 20. This arthritic disease does occur in women, but the symptoms are more prominent in men. If you do suffer from ankylosing spondylitis, your primary symptoms may be pain in your hip joints. You may have progressive decrease of your back range of motion. You may have some pain in the joints of your arms and legs as well. X-rays have shown arthritis in sacroiliac joints. Over time, your spine will continue to stiffen. The onset of ankylosing spondylitis is gradual. You have a normal curve in your lower back that will become straight. You may have difficulty expanding your chest to take a breath.

If your ankylosing spondylitis worsens, your entire spine may become fused, which restricts your motion about your spine in all directions. The earliest x-ray changes usually occur in your sacroiliac joints. Erosion of these joints becomes evident. The outer rings of your discs in your spine become calcified. Furthermore, calcification of the vertical ligaments that run in front and back of your vertebral bones occurs. When this happens, if you have an x-ray of your spine, it will appear as a bamboo stick. Remember that rheumatoid arthritis affects mostly small joints. Ankylosing spondylitis affects large joints. Osteoarthritis does not usually affect your sacroiliac joints.

If you have ankylosing spondylitis, physical therapy and nonsteroidal anti-inflammatory drugs are important for the treatment of the pain associated with this disease. No treatment is currently available that will eradicate ankylosing splondylitis. Occasionally stronger analgesics such as opioids are needed to control your pain. Sulfasalazine is sometimes useful for pain for arthritis in your arms and legs. The problem with ankylosing spondylitis is that you can have pain that is severe over decades of your life. The severity of the pain associated with this disease varies greatly. Approximately 10 percent of patients have disability so severe that they are unable to return to work after 10 years.

Gout is one of the most painful arthritic diseases. Gout results from the formation crystals of uric acid that are deposited into joint spaces between your bones. These uric acid crystals deposited into your joints cause inflammation with swelling, redness, and warmth about your joint. Gouty arthritis comprises 5 percent of all cases of arthritis. We all have the formation of uric acid in our bodies.

Uric acid is formed in your body from the breakdown of chemicals called purines that are found in many foods. You should avoid foods that will elevate your uric acid blood level. If you have a history of gout, avoid excessive meat and seafood in your diet. Do not eat gravies. Avoid yeast products, including beer and other alcoholic beverages. You must also avoid oatmeal, asparagus, cauliflower, and mushrooms.

Uric acid is dissolved in your bloodstream and is excreted through the kidneys. If your kidneys do not eliminate enough uric acid from your bloodstream, the uric acid will increase in your bloodstream. If you eat a lot of liver, beans, or peas, you may increase the uric acid in your bloodstream. If the uric acid forms crystals and deposits these crystals into your joints, gout will develop. In many people, the uric acid deposits affect the joints in their great toes. The big toe is affected in approximately 75 percent of people suffering gout. The ankles, heels, knees, wrists, and fingers may also be affected by gouty arthritis.

If you have a family history of gouty arthritis, you run the risk of developing this disease. Gout is more common in men than in women and is more common in adults than in children. Obesity increases the risk of developing gout. An excess consumption of alcohol also interferes with the excretion of uric acid from your body. The increased uric acid that occurs from excessive alcohol consumption can form crystals and deposit these crystals into your joints. Adult men between the ages of 40 and 50 are most likely to develop gout. Gout is occasionally seen in women. It rarely occurs before menopause. For some reason, people who have had organ transplants are more susceptible to gout.

A diagnosis of gout can be made by withdrawing fluid from your painful joints and analyzing the fluid for uric acid. When your gout attack is severe, you may be totally incapacitated. If your gout is not treated, you may develop severe pathology of your affected joints. The prevalence of gout for men is approximately 14 cases per 1,000 men, whereas the prevalence in women is approximately 6 cases per 1,000 women. Estrogen hormones noted in women can help the body eliminate uric acid. For this reason, gout is rarely seen in premenopausal women.

When a gout attack occurs, the maximum pain associated with the gout usually occurs in approximately the first 10 hours. In general, attacks resolve in less than 14 days. Uric acid crystals can not only be deposited in your joints, they can also form in your soft tissues. A collection of uric acid crystals in your tissues can form a lump (called a tophi), often noted on the outer edges of your forearms. Be aware that if you have gout, you have an increased risk of developing kidney stones. These stones are usually composed of uric acid. If you have gout, you also have a higher risk of developing a kidney disease. Finding uric acid crystals in the fluid of your joints makes the diagnosis of gout.

Uric acid crystals are usually formed when your uric acid level exceeds 6.8 mg/dL. Sometimes overproduction of uric acid is related to a genetic disorder. Excessive exercise can also increase uric acid, as can obesity. Starvation or dehydration can increase uric acid, too. Thyroid disease can also increase uric acid. Diuretics (medications that make you urinate, such as furosemide [Lasix] and hydrochlorthiazide [or HCTZ], a common blood pressure medicine) and cyclosporine A (an immunosuppressive medicine) can increase the uric acid concentration in the bloodstream.

The initial treatment of gout may include nonsteroidal anti-inflammatory medications or steroids or colchicine. The use of COX-2 inhibitors is under investigation. Steroids can be used to treat gout and can be given orally or by injection into your muscle.

Symptoms of arthritis tend to come and go so it's easy to fall prey to so-called "treatments", such as magnets, copper bracelets, chemicals, special diets, and electronic devices. Many supplements offer health benefits, but claims to treat or cure diseases are unproven and not allowed by law. Increasingly, so called "dietary supplements" are found to contain hidden illegal drugs and other chemicals that could cause serious harm.

Promotions for fraudulent health products are frequently found on the Internet, and you might even receive them in unsolicited emails. Fraudulent health products are also sold in stores and through mail-order catalogs. Be wary of personal testimonials by "real people," or "doctors," played by actors claiming amazing results. Testimonials are not a substitute for scientific proof and can be a tip-off that it's a scam.

The Arthritis Foundation recommends seeing a doctor if you have joint pain, stiffness, or swelling which persists for two or more weeks, whether or not your symptoms began suddenly or gradually. Only a doctor can diagnose arthritis. An accurate diagnosis is needed so appropriate treatment can begin.

If you prefer a natural approach to treating arthritis, it's still imperative that you tell your doctor what you are taking or what you want to try. There are many natural treatment options, also referred to as alternative treatments, which are popular but not fully endorsed for effectiveness and safety. People spend billions of dollars a year on health-related products and treatments that not only are unproven and often useless, but also sometimes are dangerous. The products promise quick cures and easy solutions for a variety of problems, from obesity and arthritis to cancer and AIDS.

29. ACUTE PAIN

Acute pain begins suddenly and is usually sharp in quality. It serves as a warning of disease or a threat to the body. The approach to patients with acute pain begins by identifying the underlying cause and a disease-specific treatment. Acute pain can be controlled using short-term pharmacologic treatment (with or without nonpharmacologic treatments). Regular evaluation of pain control using a pain scale allows the physician to monitor treatment effectiveness and to determine when changes are warranted.

Scheduled, rather than as-needed dosing provides more consistent drug levels and therefore more consistent pain control. The World Health Organization pain relief ladder recommends a nonopioid such as acetaminophen or a nonsteroidal anti-inflammatory drug (NSAID) for the initial management of pain. There is a ceiling to the analgesic effects of NSAIDs but not to their anti-inflammatory effects.

Pain is the most common symptom encountered in the hospitalized patient. Acute pain management is necessary following surgery, in burn patients and in sickle cell disease. Acute pain is mentioned in this book because the manner in which acute pain is treated can affect chronic pain occurrence and its management. Acute pain is the pain experienced after tissue injury from surgery, cancer or trauma. Chronic pain is pain that continues after tissue has healed. Pain that is under treated in the hospital can lead to an increase in your blood pressure and heart rate.

If you have severe acute pain, you can suffer psychological distress as well as demoralization. The treatment of your acute pain must be provided on an individualized basis. Under treated acute pain may make the management of chronic pain difficult, as you may be skeptical of pain care from other physicians. You may as a result of improperly acute pain management exaggerate your symptoms to insure that you receive an adequate dose of pain medications.

The acute pain specialist must be responsive to your needs. Effective pain management is fundamental to quality care, and good pain control speeds recovery following surgery. Advantages of good acute pain management can be shown by increases in patient mobility and cough suppression. Effective relief can be achieved with oral non-opioids and non-steroidal anti-inflammatory drugs. These drugs are appropriate for many post-surgical and post-traumatic pains, especially when you go home on the day of the operation.

There is an old adage that if patients can swallow it is best to take drugs by mouth. There is no evidence that non-steroidal anti-inflammatory drugs given rectally or by injection perform better than the same drug at the same dose given by mouth.. These other routes become appropriate when patients cannot swallow. Topical non-steroidal anti-inflammatory drugs are effective in acute musculoskeletal injuries.

A patient's perception of pain varies among individuals. A person's first experience with severe pain may be after surgery. At one time post-surgical pain was managed with shots of narcotic into your muscle. Postoperative pain management is now more advanced. The goal of acute pain management is to keep your patient comfortable while avoiding opioid addiction. Inadequately treated acute pain may result in patient depression and/or anxiety. Depression can decrease your pain tolerance. This means that mild pain may be perceived as severe pain by the depressed patient. There is an ethical and humanitarian need to treat patients suffering with acute pain.

Barriers to effective pain management involve prejudice on the part of the physicians and/or patients. Patients and some physicians are afraid of opioid addiction. Addiction usually does not occur when an opioid is used short term. When considering the use of opioids for acute pain, the treating physician must consider the risks and benefits of opioid administration. The physician must however, consider the ethical responsibility of relieving a patient's pain and suffering. For severe acute pain opioids are the first line treatment.

Intermittent opioid injections can provide effective relief of acute pain. Unfortunately, adequate doses are withheld because of traditions, misconceptions, ignorance and fear. Doctors and nurses fear addiction and respiratory depression. Addiction is not a problem with opioid use in acute pain. Irrespective of the route, opioids used for people who are not in pain, or in doses larger than necessary to control the pain, can slow or stop breathing. The key principle is to titrate the dose against the desired effect.

There is no evidence that demonstrates that one opioid is better than another. Morphine is commonly used for the treatment of acute pain. Morphine has an active metabolite, morphine-6-glucuronide. Morphine also has a metabolite; morphine-3-glucuronide that does not provide pain relief In renal dysfunction morphine-6-glucuronide can accumulate in your body and result in a greater effect from a given dose, because it is more active than morphine.

Less morphine will be needed to control your pain. Tapentadol (Nucynta), a Schedule II controlled substance, is a muopioid receptor agonist and norepinephrine reuptake inhibitor that can be used orally for relief of moderate to severe acute pain.

Accumulation of morphine can be a problem with unconscious intensive care patients on fixed dose schedules when renal function is compromised. Opioid adverse effects include nausea and vomiting, constipation, sedation, pruritus (itching), urinary retention and respiratory depression. There is no good evidence that the incidences of these side effects are different with different opioids.

Aggressive pain management can decrease postoperative recovery time. This aggressive management can decrease the incidence of developing chronic pain. Patient controlled analgesia is a method of pain relief that allows you to self-administer small amounts of narcotics on demand into your vein. The patient presses a button and receives a pre-set dose of opioid, from a syringe driver connected to an intravenous or subcutaneous cannula. This device delivers opioid to the same opioid receptors as an intermittent injection, but allows you to prevent delays for pain treatment.

There is little difference in outcome between efficient intermittent injections. You can select how much medication is necessary to control your pain. This method of pain relief avoids delays in your pain management. You have control over your pain. This method of pain relief is safe because the drug delivery machine only allows you to get a specific amount of drug each hour. When it is time to discontinue your medicine, you will be given a pill. You will still have access to your drug delivery machine.

Another method of pain relief is administration of a drug under your skin. This method is called glysis. If your veins are not readily accessible, this method of pain relief can be effective. Epidural analgesia is another method for managing your pain after surgery. A small tube is placed in your back. A pump is connected to this tube to give you medicine when you need it. This pump can be programmed to give you medication like the patient controlled drug delivery system. Narcotics, local anesthetics and muscle relaxants can be placed into your body by this method.

Narcotics can also be placed into your spinal fluid. This is called intrathecal therapy and is used for acute cancer pain management. If you are having surgery on your arm or leg, s small tube can be placed in your extremity that will give a continual dose of local anesthetic. For example if you are having surgery on your leg, a tube can be placed at the nerve that causes your pain to numb it. You can then have physical therapy without any pain. Other routes of opioid administration include intra-articular, nasal, active transdermal and inhalational administration.

Pre-emptive analgesia is used when patients have established pain prior to surgery. For example, if you have severe chronic hand and wrist pain prior to scheduled surgery, your anesthesiologist may do a nerve block to stop your pain prior to hand surgery. The advantage of regional analgesia with a local anesthetic is that it can deliver complete pain relief by interrupting pain transmission from a specific area, so avoiding generalized drug adverse effects. This advantage is more obvious when it is possible to give further doses via a catheter, extending the duration of analgesia.

Be aware that established pain is harder to control than new pain. When chronic pain occurs, changes occur in your brain and spinal cord. These changes enhance pain perception after surgery. Placement of a hollow tube (epidural catheter) with the administration of a local anesthetic (numbing medication) can significantly decrease your postoperative pain and may decrease your chance of developing chronic pain. Epidural infusion via a catheter can offer continuous relief after trauma or surgery, for your lower limb, spine, abdominal or chest.

The risks of associated with an epidural injection include a spinal headache, infection, hematoma or nerve damage. Some epidural infusions contain local anesthetics. Side effects of local anesthetics include a decrease in your blood pressure, motor block of your muscles, seizures, and heart rhythm disturbances. If opioids are used, side effects can include nausea and vomiting, sedation, urinary retention, respiratory depression and generalized itching.

Post-operative treatments include patient control analgesia (PCA) where you press a button that controls an intravenous infusion of opioid. This gives you control of your postoperative pain. Epidural morphine with or without local anesthetics can provide pain relief as well. Oral opioids can provide relief as well.

The modality for acute pain management will depend on the skill and expertise of the treating physician. Prior to having any invasive procedure, you should discuss postoperative pain management with your surgeon and anesthesiologist prior to any surgical procedure. You must know what to expect so that your hospital experience will be pleasant.

There other types of acute pain besides post-surgical pain. Burn pain can be a result of medical treatments like dressing changes or from the thermal destruction of the tissue itself. The dead tissue must be frequently removed. This procedure is painful. Narcotics and anesthesia drugs like ketamine are necessary to control the pain.

Sickle cell disease pain can be profound. Acute bone destruction associated with this disease can be extremely painful and may require the administration of strong narcotics. Common sites of pain include the back, joints chest and abdomen. Narcotics may be given by mouth, but most patients require intravenous narcotics.

A former chief of acute pain at a medical center has agreed to plead guilty to falsifying medical research and must pay $420,000 in restitution to a pharmaceutical company, federal court records show. This doctor prompted a furor in the medical community when he was accused of making up research results in at least 21 published studies and inventing patients in certain instances.

The charge issued in U.S. District Court in Boston states that Reuben was a noted anesthesiologist and "regular on the medical lecturing circuit" focusing on post-operative pain management. This doctor was on one side of a debate in the anesthesia community over whether there was an effective alternative to easing post-surgical pain with opioids, including morphine.

Prosecutors say he proposed research studies to pharmaceutical companies, accepted grant money and published articles in medical journals on phony research. In 2005, this doctor received a $74,000 research grant from a pharmaceutical company, and agreed to test a medication as a component of the multimodal therapy.

He claimed to have treated 200 patients, 100 with the drug company's product and 100 with a placebo. This physician in fact had not enrolled any patients into that study and the results reported both to the pharmaceutical company r and to a prestigious medical journal and in turn to the public were wholly made up by this physician. This case demonstrates the fact that pain management can occur in academic pain management environments as well as in the private sector.

Prolozone is a treatment method for acute pains that seem to be gaining popularity by the day. It is the use of oxygen and ozone to treat affected areas of the body. These substances are delivered into the body using an injection. Unlike the earlier forms of treating body pains, the prolozone therapy brings almost immediate relief to the pains, with some quarters also saying that it can repair tissues permanently, ending chronic pain in totality.

The fact that scientists have not been able to establish a study or review of the long-term effect of prolozone requires that one is cautious of opting for this form of treatment. One major side effect to using prolozone treatment besides the fact that it is not covered under health insurance is that some patients complain of having increased pain around the treated region.

The Pain Gone Pen is a Piezo Electric Therapy stimulator which works much like a TENS device. The device has been clinically tested to be safe and fast working. In fact, many claim that it is years ahead of its time in respect to the current TENS field.

It is not a TENS machine. The Pain Gone Pen basically treats pain using small bursts of controlled electronic frequencies. The Pain Gone Pen is a Piezo Electric Therapy stimulator and delivers a small, controlled electric current every time the button is click. These currents are not created by batteries, but rather by small crystals within the pen itself.

There may be reasons to believe that Pain Gone Pen is actually a legitimate pain relief device and not just some sales gimmick. The first is the clinical trials that the device has gone through. In one particular study, it was actually tested on 50 different patients suffering from chronic pain in the lower back and large joints. These patients were recruited from the pain clinic at the Northern General Hospital Sheffield, and 90% of sufferers reported improvement

The name Airrosti stands for Applied Integration for the Rapid Recovery of Soft Tissue Injuries. The providers are chiropractors who have been trained by the company in their special methods. the Airrosti website claims to have evidence. Airrosti according to the website has been proven, through extensive third-party research and analysis, to be the most effective, efficient, and affordable option for resolving musculoskeletal conditions. Furthermore they claim measurable prevention of surgeries, hospitalization, MRIs, injections, and pharmaceuticals for back pain and other musculoskeletal conditions. Further controlled studies from an academic center are necessary to verify these claims.

30. URINE DRUG TESTING

Drug screening emerged a decade ago when pain doctors ordered tests for chronic pain patients as a precaution to protect against overprescribing charges, but said a second wave of claims has been from a profit seeking-period. Fraud experts have said drug screening has become a "money spigot,"

Urine drug testing (UDT) is an important component of the treatment plan for patients who are prescribed opioids for chronic pain. While there is not enough information so far to support a specific testing protocol for patient-centered clinical urine drug testing, experts in the fields of pain and addiction and pharmacology have developed recommendations for the use of UDT as an initial assessment and for ongoing monitoring in this population

The question of whom to test is made easier by having a uniform practice policy either in a pain or primary practice that would help reduce individual stigma. Any risk of patient profiling based on racial, cultural, or other physical appearances is eliminated. Careful explanation of the purpose of testing normally allays patient concerns.

UDT must be done routinely as part of an overall best practice program in order to prescribe chronic opioid therapy. This program may include risk stratification; baseline and periodic UDT; behavioral monitoring; and prescription monitoring programs as the best available tools to monitor chronic opioid compliance.

Evidence suggests that predictors of aberrant behavior are not completely reliable, however, and that a substantial number of individuals using illicit substances will be missed if clinicians restrict urine testing to those they deem to be at high risk. Thus, UDT may be a valuable tool for low-risk patients on chronic opioid therapy, as well.

A drug test is a technical analysis of a biological specimen, for example urine, hair, blood, breath, sweat, or oral fluid/saliva to determine the presence or absence of specified parent drugs or their metabolites. Urine analysis is primarily used because of its low cost. Urine drug testing is one of the most common testing methods used.

The rationale for performing UDT will depend on the clinical question(s) to be answered; for example, to assist in medication adherence, seeking an initial diagnosis of drug misuse or addiction, as an adjunct to self-report of drug history, to encourage or reinforce healthy behavioral change, or as a requirement of continued treatment.

Doctors frequently order patients to take urine drug tests to safeguard against prescription pain-pill abuse but federal investigators and Medicare say these routine tests designed to ensure patients properly use opioid drugs have led to questionable billing practices by some for-profit labs, doctors, and addiction-treatment centers. Urine tests can show doctors whether their patients are taking extra pain drugs and whether they are taking their prescribed drugs.

Patients may need urine drug screening tests for a variety of reasons including monitoring of their pain medication regimen or simply as a screening tool to look for the presence of drugs. It's important to understand the types of drug screens and why one would need them prior to investigating any issues involving these tests. There is often a legitimate need for such drug tests, to determine whether an addict has relapsed or to ensure that patients prescribed painkillers are taking them rather than selling them.

There are two types of urine drug testing procedures: qualitative and quantitative. Qualitative drug screens are testing for the presence or absence of a particular drug. Quantitative drug screens are testing for how much of that substance is present. In 20 years' the number of prescriptions written for pharmaceutical drugs in the U.S. has climbed abruptly; more than six-fold, which has consequently driven up demand for urine drug testing services by doctors trying to monitor their patients' drug intake habits.

With this explosion in the urine drug testing industry has come a wave of fraud and corruption allegations. In 2011, the average number of older Americans misusing or dependent on prescription pain relievers grew to about 336,000, up from 132,000 a decade earlier, according to the Substance Abuse and Mental Health Services Administration. Medical guidelines encourage doctors who treat pain to test their patients, to make sure they are neither abusing pills nor failing to take them, possibly to sell them. Now, some pain doctors are making more from testing than from treating.

The FBI has arrested doctors for receiving kickbacks from laboratories for ordering drug testing. This behavior violated federal anti-kickback laws by giving away urine collection cups and testing strips to doctors, who says there is a growing incidence of giving workers' compensation claimants' urine drug tests even when doctors have not prescribed opioid pain medications.

Spending on the urine tests took off after Medicare cracked down on what appeared to be abusive billing for simple urine tests. Some doctors moved on to high-tech testing methods, for which billing wasn't limited. They started testing for a host of different drugs including illegal ones that few seniors ever use and billing the federal health program for the elderly and disabled separately for each substance.

Medicare's spending on 22 high-tech tests for drugs of abuse hit $445 million in 2012, up 1,423% in five years. The program spent $14 million that year just on tests for angel dust,. For dozens of pain doctors, Medicare payments for drug testing have eclipsed their income from treating patients. Routinely testing specimens for many different drugs is a red flag

Safe prescribing now requires expertise in approaches that minimize the risk of unintentional overdose, drug abuse, addiction, and diversion. These approaches include urine drug testing, and while there is yet no consensus among pain specialists about the patients who should be tested and how often to test, there is broad and unqualified agreement that clinicians who treat patients with opioid drugs should be able to use urine drug testing as a tool in the assessment of drug-related behavior. There also is agreement that urine drug testing, like all tests, will yield useless information unless the indications, practicalities, and interpretation of the data are appreciated by those who order it.

Some labs encourage doctors to refer more patient specimens for drug testing by giving physicians an ownership stake or cut of test revenue, according to doctors and documents from several labs. There are some good reasons to do confirmation testing. It eliminates the risk of false-positives.

The initial screening tests are very sensitive, so sometimes they incorrectly say a specimen contains evidence of drug use; the confirmation test is specific. Another reason is to measure not only whether someone is misusing drugs, but also whether they are taking therapeutic medications at the prescribed levels. There is a need for maintenance screening to determine if someone has relapsed.

There are two focal categories of urine drug testing screening: point of care followed by confirmation. Screening tests are initial, qualitative drug tests conducted to identify classes of drugs present in the urine and typically are done using immunoassay. They rely on a set threshold above which a positive result is produced and therefore do not detect lower concentrations of a drug. Confirmatory tests are used for further analysis of a sample to confirm a positive or negative, result and typically are done using gas chromatography/mass spectrometry or high performance liquid chromatography.

Confirmatory testing can identify a specific drug. If the goal is to detect a synthetic or semisynthetic opioid, this testing should be used as immunoassays do not typically detect these opioids. Due to the possibility of false positives and the qualitative nature of screening tests, confirmatory testing is recommended to affirm positive or unexpected results and to identify the presence of a specific drug

It is important to be sure that the drug testing occurs at a reputable and certified laboratory. A credible drug screening program will involve a two-step process. Initial (immunoassay) and confirmatory gas chromatography-mass spectrometry (GC-MS) analysis testing are the methods most commonly utilized to test for drugs. Using a combination of both tests allows a high level of sensitivity and specificity, meaning there is an extremely low chance for false positives or false negatives.

The immunoassay is performed first and is often used as a screening method. If the immunoassay is negative, no further action is required, and the results are reported as negative. If the sample is positive, an additional confirmatory GC-MS analysis is performed on a separate portion the biological sample. The more specific GC/MS is used as a confirmatory test to identify individual drug substances or metabolites and quantify the amount of the substance. Confirmatory tests, such as GC-MS should be utilized prior to reporting positive drug test results

Many drugs stay in the system from 2 to 4 days, although chronic use of marijuana can stay in the system for 3 to 4 weeks or even longer after the last use. Drugs with a long half-life, such as diazepam, may also stay in the system for a prolonged period of time. Drugs can be detected in hair samples up to six months

False positive drug tests are very rare in licensed, reputable laboratories. However, certain prescription medications, over-the-counter drugs, and herbal remedies can be mistaken for drugs of abuse in drug tests. For example, some decongestants might lead to a positive drug test for amphetamines

In general, one can expect a urine test to detect drugs for the following times substances: Amphetamine: 2 days, Barbiturates: 2 days-3 weeks, Benzodiazepines: 3 days (therapeutic dose); 4-6 weeks (habitual use), Cocaine: 4 days, Ecstasy: 2 days, Heroin: 2 days, Marijuana: 2-7 days (single use); 1-2+ months (habitual use), Methamphetamine: 2 days, Morphine: 2 days, PCP: 8-14 days (single use); 30 days (chronic use). Be aware that an individual can do the following to an urine sample: dilution is the process of reducing the concentration of drug or drug metabolites in the sample. This is accomplished by adding fluid to the sample, and some sites online may recommend it. However, drug testing laboratories all routinely test samples to detect dilution.

One method of diluting the sample involves adding liquid to urine. However, the temperature of the urine is measured by drug tests, and diluted urine is easily detected. Substitution is a method that involves substituting your urine with that of another person's or a synthetic sample. There are many companies that sell devices for urine substitution over the internet, as well as companies that sell synthetic urine.

Point of Care cups (POC) are enzyme mediated immunoassay (EIA) devices. These are cups with strips that change color and are similar to urine pregnancy tests. They are the least expensive, and least accurate, of all the urine monitoring tools. To use these, the doctor needs no special equipment or training.

In 2009, the American Pain Society and the American Academy of Pain Medicine convened an expert panel that developed Clinical Guidelines for the Use of Chronic Opioid Therapy in Chronic Noncancerous Pain. The panel concluded that UDT has a central role in monitoring patients receiving chronic opioid therapy to avoid its potential harms. Specifically, the panel recommended that UDT should be used periodically in all treated patients who are at high risk for abuse or diversion, and that UDT should also be considered even for patients who do not have known risk factors in order to confirm adherence to the chronic opioid therapy plan of care.

In the panel's opinion, UDT should be considered in all patients, including those without apparent elevated risk, as part of the protocol of practices, especially when controlled substances, such as opioids, are prescribed. The literature is clear that when aberrant behavior alone is used as a trigger for UDT, a significant proportion of patients who would benefit from this technology will be missed. Therefore, a consistent clinical approach in performing UDT will optimize the use of this technology for both patient and practitioner alike.

Provider fraud may occur with respect to drug testing. A Dallas health care provider has faced allegations that it paid millions in kickbacks to physicians and others for patient referrals. The number of federal health care kickback cases is spreading nationwide. The Justice Department has targeted labs, pharmacies, physicians, chiropractors and hospitals in recent years. The company paid sales brokers to find medical providers willing to engage in the illegal kickback scheme, the lawsuit said.

The kickbacks were disguised as payment for administrative, marketing or consulting services.

A minority of drug screening laboratories received nearly $100 million from Oklahoma's Medicaid program over the last five years, prompting an investigation from state officials. Between 2011 and 2014, Oklahoma's annual reimbursement to urine testing laboratories increased more than 700 percent, from $3.7 million to $32 million, and threatened to drain the state's healthcare budget. The labs often billed for medically unnecessary tests, or billed for more expensive quantitative panel tests that cost as much as $800, according to the Oklahoma Health Care Authority. Several labs also engaged in kickback schemes, compensating physicians in exchange for referrals.

A physicians group has agreed to pay $7.4 million to the federal government to resolve allegations that it violated the False Claims Act by performing medically unnecessary drug screen procedures, the U.S. Department of Justice said Wednesday. The settlement relates to the business' use of tests that identify and count particles of illicit drugs in patients' urine.

The DOJ said the quantitative drug tests, which are very specific and expensive, are appropriate only if there is reason to doubt the more general and cheaper qualitative drug test screens. However, the DOJ said regardless of results of the less expensive test, Coastal performed and billed all patients for the quantitative drug tests.

A laboratory in California allegedly billed Medicare, Medicaid and other federal health care programs for medically unnecessary urine drug and genetic testing, and for providing free items to physicians who agreed to refer expensive laboratory testing business to this laboratory.

Another physician group was approached by a laboratory sales consultant with an opportunity to offer, and profit from, lab tests. As the representative explained to the physicians, his organization would help the physicians set up and run a lab in which the physicians would own a 40% minority share.

Presumably the lab would have been based in a small local hospital which would perform the billing. The purpose of the minority ownership was to conceal the fact that physician-owned laboratories are illegal and unethical. The reason for billing through the local hospital was because many of the insurance companies have caught on to the fact that laboratory companies have been charging despicable amounts for unnecessary tests for their patients. But few insurance companies haven't discovered that the billings for these tests are now coming from small, previously reputable hospitals.

Patients need to be aware of possible fraudulent laboratory practices and if these practices are in question, the patient should notify his/her insurance carrier.

31. OSTEOPOROSIS

Osteoporosis is a reduction in bone mineral density that leads to fractures. The most serious are hip fractures, which require surgery, have complications like blood clots, and carry a high mortality. Many of those who survive never walk again. Vertebral fractures are common in the osteoporotic elderly and are responsible for dowager's hump and loss of height. There is also an increased risk of wrist and rib fractures. An estimated $18 billion is spent annually on direct health care services related to osteoporotic fractures, making it an attractive market for pharmaceutical companies that produce drugs to help manage the disease.

If you suffer from osteoporosis, you will have a progressive reduction in the density of your bones. The normal composition of your bones is preserved. Osteoporosis affects 20 million Americans and results in more than 1.3 million bone fractures in the United States every year. In a lifetime, women lose more than half of their spongy bone, which comprises the center of bones, and approximately 30 percent of the nonspongy (compact) bone, which composes the outer aspect of these bones.

Bone density tends to decrease with age. Postmenopausal women are particularly susceptible to osteoporosis when their production of estrogen declines. The risk is increased in people taking corticosteroids and in people with certain diseases like rheumatoid arthritis. Other risk factors are European or Asian ancestry, smoking, excess alcohol, a family history of fractures, vitamin D deficiency, too much or too little exercise, malnutrition, and low body weight. Approximately 30 percent of all postmenopausal Caucasian women will suffer from fractures related to osteoporosis. More than one third of all women and one sixth of all men over 65 years of age will sustain a hip fracture.

During your lifetime, bone is constantly being made and is constantly being lost. In normal circumstances, the production and reduction of your bone is balanced. Osteoporosis can result if you do not make enough bone or if you have an accelerated decrease in your bone minerals and the matrix structure (the components of your bone which make your bones hard) of your bone or both.

Genetics can affect differences in bone density and these differences are the result of a gene that is linked to your vitamin D receptor gene. Variations of the vitamin D receptor gene result in differences in bone density changes of 10 percent to 12 percent in osteoporosis-prone individuals. Your bone density will continue to increase throughout your life until you reach an age where your bone density becomes stable.

When you approach 40 years of age, your bone density can begin to decline. Bone density decreases are noted in women before menopause. In men, a decrease in their bone density occurs somewhere between 20 to 40 years of age. In women, after menopause has occurred, the rate of bone loss accelerates.

Osteoporosis is usually diagnosed when a fracture occurs. Fractures may occur in your vertebra (compression fracture). However, your wrists, hips, ribs, pelvic bone, and your leg bones can sustain fractures. The bones in your spine can have a loss of height, which is called a compression fracture. If you have osteoporosis, your bones become more porous. This means that the bones in your body develop holes, which in turn weaken the structure of your bones.

All of your bones can be affected, and each of your bones can be at an increased risk for a fracture. If you have a low calcium intake and are not physically active, you are also at risk of developing osteoporosis.

Hyperthyroidism and hyperparathyroidism in addition to excessive cortisone (a steroid) may be causes of osteoporosis. It is important for your body to absorb calcium through your gastrointestinal system. If you have a history of a gastrectomy (removal of a portion of your stomach), cirrhosis of the liver, or any other gastrointestinal malabsorption syndrome, you are more prone to develop osteoporosis.

If you have a history of multiple myeloma or leukemia, you may de-velop osteoporosis. The exact cause of this finding is presently unknown. Alcohol can contribute to your development of osteoporosis. Chemotherapy can also cause osteoporosis. Steroid use has been implicated as a cause of osteoporosis as well. A plain X-ray cannot make a diagnosis of osteoporosis. You will need a DEXA test for a true diagnosis.

Osteoporosis can cause your vertebra to compress. This is called a compression fracture. Essentially your vertebra collapses. This disease can be very painful. If you have a vertebral compression in your mid back, for example, there will usually be a decrease in the height of your affected (compressed) bone that can be seen on X-ray. Sometimes a bone scan is needed to diagnosis osteoporosis. If you have a bone scan, a doctor will inject a radioactive material into your vein. You will have a picture of your body taken by a special camera.

Compression fractures, which were not diagnosed by other means, can be detected by a bone scan. Osteoporosis can also be diagnosed by measuring your bone mineral density. Your bone density value will be compared to a normal value that is noted for young adults of your same sex. A bone density test can predict the probability of you developing a fracture related to your bone density value.

Quantitative computed tomography can also be used and is effective for diagnosing osteoporosis because it will not only measure your bone mineral density, but this test can also measure the density of your spongy bone within your back and hip bones. However, this test is expensive and will expose you to radiation.

Different types of tests are being used and being developed to diagnosis osteoporosis. Bone scanning can be useful for the diagnosis of compression fractures. If you have a decreased bone density, your doctor should attempt to determine the cause of your osteoporosis.

Sometimes your doctor needs to obtain blood samples from you for further testing. Your doctor may take some blood from you to be sent to a lab to measure the calcium, organic phosphate, and alkaline phosphatase in your bloodstream. These minerals are usually normal if you have osteoporo-sis. However, your alkaline phosphate may be higher if you have a fracture. Vitamin D can help you increase your calcium absorption through your gastrointestinal tract by up to 65 percent.

Smoking on the other hand, increases the rate of bone loss. Hip and spinal bone fractures are higher in men and women who smoke. Nicotine can inhibit absorption of calcium that is needed for bone health. Osteoporosis in men can be diagnosis by a bone mass measurement. This is a special type of x-ray that emits a trace amount of radiation. Middle-aged men who have complaints of back or hip pain may be candidates for a bone mass measurement as well as a measurement of the testosterone in their blood-stream. You should avoid steroid injections.

As previously stated, the absorption of calcium from your gastrointestinal system decreases with age. The United Stated recommended dietary allowance of calcium is up to 1,000 milligrams per day. Calcium can retard your osteoporosis but cannot completely stop it. An increase in calcium in your bloodstream may not protect you from compression fractures of the bones in your spine.

Calcium therapy can help you if you are a woman and postmenopausal. Some endocrinologists have recommended that if you are postmenopausal that you should consume 1,500 milligrams per day of calcium.

Calcitonin is another drug that you could possibly take to prevent bone loss in your vertebral bodies throughout your spine. Calcitonin is most effective in early and late menopause. Calcitonin is available for intranasal use. Calcitonin has been shown to produce pain-relieving effects. Calcitonin is most useful if you have a history of osteoporosis and have chronic pain related to fractures related to your osteoporosis.

If you have had a fracture of one of the bones in your spine, treament that puts bone cement into your bone can be used to treat any compression fracture that you may have. The techniques that use this cement are called vertebroplasty and kyphoplasty.

Vertebroplasty involves the injection of bone cement into your vertebral bones. Kyphyplasty introduces a surgical instrument into one of the bones in your spine with intent to elevate the compressed bone. When this instrument is withdrawn, the space left is filled with bone cement. Each of these procedures remains to be studied.

Bisphosphonates are an important class of drug for the treatment of osteoporosis. These drugs can increase the minerals in the bones throughout your body. Furthermore, the chance of you having a vertebral fracture is decreased if you are in late menopause. Examples of these drugs include etidronate and alendronate. Further research is being done with respect to these drugs in the prevention of bone fractures.

However, these drugs will not reverse osteoporosis. There are other drugs available for women who have osteoporosis. Fosamax and Actonel are two of the drugs commonly used to decrease the progression of osteoporosis. Fosamax slows the cycle of bone breakdown. If the rate of bone breakdown is decreased, there is a reduced chance of you having a fracture.

Given that no two people are alike, if you are taking any medications and begin to take nutritional supplements you should be aware that potential drug-nutrient interactions may occur and are encouraged to consult a health care professional before using any natural product. Combining certain prescription drugs and dietary supplements can lead to undesirable effects such as: diminished prescription drug effectiveness, reduced supplement effectiveness and impaired drug and/or supplement absorption.

The prevalence of vitamin D, insufficiency is high. Vitamin D in the food supply is limited and most often inadequate to prevent deficiencies. Supplemental vitamin D is likely necessary to avoid deficiency, especially in winter months. Most cells and tissues in the human body have vitamin D receptors that stimulate the nuclear transcription of various genes to alter cellular function. Vitamin D, appears to have an effect on numerous disease states and disorders, including osteoporosis.1

Tridax procumbens flavonoids could be a potential anabolic agent to treat patients with bone loss-associated diseases such as osteoporosis. Vitamin D (cholecalciferol) sufficiency is essential for maximizing bone health. Vitamin D enhances intestinal absorption of calcium and phosphorus. sun exposure or ingesting at least 800-1000 IU of vitamin D daily. Patients being treated for osteoporosis should be adequately supplemented with calcium and vitamin D to maximize the benefit of treatment.

Fortification of bread and cereals is a feasible way to improve vitamin D nutrition in elderly nursing home residents. The diet of a large part of society is not properly balanced which can cause abnormalities in achieving proper bone mineralization. Long-term deficiencies in calcium and vitamin D in daily diet are the cause for taking dietary supplements. Unfortunately, some preparations on the market do not have adequate storage. It happens that these preparations are poorly absorbed and the amount of active compound is too low.6

Onion juice consumption showed a positive modulatory effect on the bone loss and bone mineral density by improving antioxidant activities and thus can be recommended for treating various bone-related disorders, especially osteoporosis. Furthermore, coffee consumption may have protective benefits on bone health in Korean postmenopausal women in moderate amounts.

An individual claimed to have identified foods containing specific "multi-functional proteins" and "organic chemicals" that, when taken in specific combinations, promote new bone tissue growth and work as a completely natural and 100% effective way to heal osteoporosis forever. In fact, the Osteoporosis Protocol is claimed to consist of just 3 simple steps, and its ingredients cost about $17 and can be found at your local grocery store. Unfortunately, due to the pharmaceutical industry, this individual claims that this method of stopping your bone deterioration at the source has been suppressed.

Bisphosphonate drugs like Merck's Fosamax and Boniva were intended to reduce the risk of fractures in patients with osteoporosis. They are effective in reducing spine fractures and in increasing bone density measurements, but some studies have shown no reduction in non-spine fractures, which are more common, and in the case of hip fractures, more significant.

The FDA has approved twice-a-year Prolia (denosumab) injections to treat osteoporosis in patients at high risk of fracture. The clinical trials on which Prolia approval is based lasted for three years. Over that time, postmenopausal women taking Prolia had fewer fractures and increased bone density.

Teriparatide (Forteo) is a synthetic version of the human parathyroid hormone, which helps to regulate calciummetabolism. It promotes the growth of new bone, while other osteoporosis medications improve bone density by inhibiting bone resorption, or breakdown. It is the only osteoporosis medicine approved by the FDA that rebuilds bone.

An estimated $18 billion is spent annually on direct health care services related to osteoporotic fractures, making it an attractive market for pharmaceutical companies that produce drugs to help manage the disease. Drug companies advertise but it is the doctors who write the prescriptions: when drugs are over-prescribed, only the prescribers are to blame. Doctors should be recommending preventive lifestyle changes to all their patients. They should stick to the best science-based practices and evaluate the evidence for themselves rather than being influenced by Big Pharma propaganda. They should prescribe drug treatments only when fracture risk is significant, when a fracture has already occurred, or when they think bone density is significantly low.

The U.S. Food and Drug Administration raised concerns about the potential for some serious side effects in women taking bone-building drugs called bisphosphonates, specifically Fosamax, Actonel and Reclast. In 2011, the agency voiced concerns that taking the drugs long-term may actually make bones weaker and increase the risk of rare but serious side effects such as atypical fractures of the thigh bone, esophageal cancer and osteonecrosis of the jaw, a rare but painful condition in which the jaw bone crumbles.

Women without osteoporosis seem to get few to no benefits to their bones from taking the drugs beyond five years. In light of the concerns about the potential side effects, the authors said some patients should be able to safely stop taking the drugs after that time. it is older women who have a history of fractures or are at an increased fracture risk, particularly of spine fractures, who stand to benefit from taking the drugs for longer than five years.

Medicare, which covers most health costs for those over 65, has a particularly large impact on the osteoporosis market due to the overlapping demographics of the patient population. While Medicare currently covers most osteoporosis treatments, changes in osteoporosis coverage will affect both pharmaceutical and health insurance companies.

32. TMJ

Facial neuropathy and neuralgias or pathology and pain of the nerves of the face have been recognized for centuries. These types of pain, especially trigeminal neuralgia, can be severe. The pain associated with trigeminal neuralgia has been well defined. A common type of pain syndrome is pain related to temporal mandibular-lar joint disorders. This usually involves the joint between the mandible, and the maxilla. When these two bones meet, they form a joint called the temporomandibular joint.

The trigeminal nerve, which has three branches: ophthalmic, maxillary, and mandibular. Other nerves also can cause facial pain. The facial nerves, glossopharyngeal nerve, the vagus nerve, and some cervical nerves go to various parts of the mouth areas and facial areas and can cause pain. Trigeminal neuralgia affects mainly adults, especially the elderly. If the pain is coming from a nerve, typically the pain is sharp and stabbing. On the other hand, if the pain is coming from the muscles, it is generally continuous and dull. Pain from the blood vessels is usually of a throbbing nature.

The TMJ is a complicated joint that connects the lower jaw to the temporal bone at the side of the head. It has both a hinge and a sliding motion. When the mouth is opening, the rounded ends, or condyles, of the lower jaw glide along the sockets of the temporal bones. Muscles are connected to both the jaw and the temporal bones, and a soft disc between them absorbs shocks to the jaw from chewing and other jaw movements.

TMJ problems were originally thought to stem from dental malocclusion, upper and lower teeth misalignment and improper jaw position. That prompted a focus on replacing missing teeth and fitting patients with braces to realign their teeth and change how the jaws come together.Later studies revealed that malocclusion itself was an infrequent cause of facial pain and other temporomandibular symptoms. Rather, as the Boston specialists wrote recently in The New England Journal of Medicine "the cause is now considered multifactorial, with biologic, behavioral, environmental, social, emotional and cognitive factors, alone or in combination, contributing to the development of signs and symptoms of temporomandibular disorders."According to the American

Academy of Orofacial Pain, the disorder "usually involves more than one symptom and rarely has a single cause."

Among the "mechanical" causes that are now recognized as distorting the function of the TMJ are congenital or developmental abnormalities of the jaw; displacement of the disc between the jaw bones; inflammation or arthritis that causes the joint to degenerate; traumatic injury to the joint (sometimes just from opening the mouth too wide); tumors; infection; and excessive laxity or tightness of the joint. Patients may have popping noises in the jaw, or have difficulty opening or closing the mouth. Simple acts like chewing, talking excessively or yawning can make the symptoms worse.

Jaw-irritating habits, like clenching the teeth or jaw, tooth grinding at night, biting the lips or fingernails, chewing gum or chewing on a pencil, can make the problem worse or longer lasting. Psychological factors also often play a role, especially depression, anxiety or stress But the most common TMJ problem is known as myofacial pain disorder, a neuromuscular problem of the chewing muscles characterized by a dull, aching pain in and around the ear that may radiate to the side or back of the head or down the neck. Someone with this disorder may have tender jaw muscles, hear clicking

Trigeminal neuralgia is also called tic douloureux. Tic douloureux is defined as a sudden stabbing pain felt in the face. It usually occurs on one side of the face. One of the nerves that supplies sensation to the face is the trigeminal nerve. This is the nerve that comes off of the brain stem. This trigeminal nerve is the cause of the trigeminal neuralgia. If the exit of the trigeminal nerve from the brain stem is depressed by a blood vessel or other tissue, this can be the cause of the pain. Compression of the trigeminal nerve with blood vessels occurs in approximately 80 percent of trigeminal neuralgia.

The trigeminal nerve is a nerve which provides sensation to the face, teeth, mouth and nose. Symptoms can be triggered by touching the face, brushing the teeth, feeling a breeze of air, putting on makeup, shaving, or merely touching certain parts of the face. The trigeminal nerve, has three branches:1. Ophthalmic (around the eye); 2. Maxillary (around the upper jaw); and 3. Mandibular (around the lower jaw). The pain may be limited to one or more of these branches.

Trigeminal neuralgia is one of the most common causes of facial pain with the highest incidence in individuals greater than 60 years old. Trigeminal neuralgia (TN) refers to sharp, lancinating pain in the areas supplied by trigeminal nerve. Both pharmacological and surgical lines of treatments are available for the treatment of TN.

Trigeminal neuralgia is a severe neuropathic pain in the distribution of one or more branches of the trigeminal nerve, which occurs in recurrent episodes, causing deterioration in quality of life, affecting everyday habits and inducing severe disability. The pain of trigeminal neuralgia comes from the trigeminal nerve. This nerve carries the feelings of touch and pain from the face, eyes, sinuses, and mouth to the brain. Trigeminal neuralgia may be part of the normal aging process. Trigeminal neuralgia may be caused by: Multiple sclerosis or pressure on the trigeminal nerve from a swollen blood vessel or tumor. Often, no cause is found.

One of the most common neuralgic pains affecting the face is the pain of TN. Although numerous lines of treatment options are available for its treatment, all these have one or the other drawbacks. Trigeminal neuralgia is a serious health problem, causing brief, recurrent episodes of stabbing or burning facial pain, which patients describe as feeling like an electric shock. The consequences of living with the condition are severe.

Infratentorial arteriovenous malformations (AVM) associated with the trigeminal nerve root entry zone are a known cause of secondary trigeminal neuralgia. Although microvascular decompression (MVD) has become the best surgical treatment for trigeminal neuralgia, it does not achieve 100% cure rate. Repeat Gamma Knife radiosurgery (GKRS) is an established option for patients whose pain has recurred after the initial procedure, with reported success rates varying from 68% to 95%.Tests that are done to look for the cause of the problem include: Blood tests MRI of the head and Trigeminal nerve reflex testing.

Local subcutaneous injection of botulinum toxin-A for TN treatment has considerable therapeutic effects lasting several months and is safe for this indication. At least one-quarter of patients in one study maintained complete analgesia. The first-line treatment for the management of in adults is an antiepileptic-carbamazepine or oxcarbazepine. There is a lack of research on the use of antiepileptics in the elderly however. The use of antiepileptics raises a number of problems due to the polypharmacy therapy common in older patients. Other medicines include: gabapentin, lamotrigine, phenytoin, valproate, and pregabalin. Muscle relaxants including baclofen, or clonazepam may be beneficial. Tricyclic antidepressants (amitriptyline, nortriptyline, or carbamazepine) may also be beneficial.

The three primary surgical options for the treatment of trigeminal neuralgia are: Trigeminal Glycerol Rhizolysis (TGR). Microvascular Decompression (MVD) and Gamma Knife (GK) treatment. With Trigeminal Glycerol Rhizolysis, a needle is advanced under X ray until it reaches a small pocket of fluid surrounding the trigeminal nerve. Glycerol will destroy the nerve which will eliminate or decrease the pain. TGR is the preferred surgical approach for elderly patients with some medical issues who are in such extreme distress that they need urgent and immediate relief.

With microvascular decompression , a small incision will be made behind the ear on the same side as the trigeminal neuralgia pain. The surgeon will expose the trigeminal nerve. Once the nerve is exposed a careful inspection is done for vascular compression of the nerve (the nerve is compressed by the blood vessel). After detecting the vascular compression, the surgeon will elevate the blood vessel off of the nerve and place pledgelets of Teflon under the nerve. Gamma Knife treatment itself is silent, completely painless and lasts roughly 30 minutes. In the majority of patients take six to eight weeks to notice major improvement in the trigeminal neuralgia pain.

Micro vascular decompression continues to be the procedure of choice for the treatment of trigeminal neuralgia in patients reluctant to medical treatment, including elderly patients because age is not a contraindication.1   The incidence of trigeminal neuralgia in elderly patients is high. However, for those with poor fitness, the optimal surgical treatment for those refractory to medical treatment is controversial. CT-guided percutaneous radiofrequency thermocoagulation is safe and effective for classic TN patients 70 years or older, including poor-fitness patients.8

Trigeminal neuralgia related to multiple sclerosis (MS) is more difficult to manage pharmacologically and surgically. Gamma Knife surgery has been proved safe and effective in this special group of patients. A high percentage of patients that are surgically treated for trigeminal neuralgia consult their dentist first and receive possibly unjustified dental treatment. Differential diagnoses include odontogenic pain syndromes as well as atypical orofacial pain.

TN is one of the most common causes of facial pain. A higher prevalence of psychiatric co-morbidities, especially depressive disorder, has been proven in patients with TN might increase the risk of subsequent newly diagnosed depressive disorder, anxiety disorder, and sleep disorder, but not schizophrenia or bipolar disorder.

Carotidynia is a form of vascular neck and face pain in which the vascular change occurs in the carotid artery in the neck. The disorder is not uncommon, and most patients have a prior history of migraine. They present with pain in the neck and face, and are often thought to have a disorder such as chronic sinusitis or trigeminal neuralgia. The diagnosis can be made from the type and location of the pain and the finding of a tender and swollen carotid artery on the same side.

If a patient has a history of arthritis, he/she can have joint problems within the temporal mandibular joint (TMJ). This pain is caused by dislocations of the small discs within the TMJ. This can result in inflammation as well as dysfunction of the joint and cause persistent and chronic inflammation, which in turn will cause chronic pain.

TMJ not only manifests itself as pain and discomfort but defines the conditions that have developed in seniors that leads up to being dizzy or having vertigo. Aging causes a lack of normal motion in the bones of the skull. The bones in the skull are not rigid. Two of the bones, the temporals, affect balance. When these bones lose motion ability, it can affect the balance. This happens as one ages and wears the teeth down. The lower jaw shifts due to this wear and many seniors end up with this as a contributing factor to some component of dizziness.

Muscles involved in chewing can refer pain to the sides of the head. Sometimes heat and muscle relaxants can relieve some of the pain. The TMJ muscle pain can originate from psychological causes. Stress, which can cause a patient to grind the teeth, leading to dental irritation, can cause the muscles to become overactive. This can cause the muscles about the jaw to become spasmodic and can fatigue easily.

Temporomandibular joint disease (TMJ), is a complex health condition that affects the mandible, or jaw bone, of anyone at any age. For older adults, especially those who are at-risk for developing arthritis, the onset of TMJ is a risk that can often lead to secondary health complications. TMJ disorders occur in 12 percent of individuals in the United States. The actual cause of TMJ remains unknown. One's facial pain may have led to changes, which may affect an older patient's nutrition.

Unlike traditional types of arthritis, where physical therapy and medications are effective, TMJ often does not respond to medications and, instead, requires more aggressive forms of treatment. For many elderly adults who have TMJ, there is a need for facial massages, home warm compresses, and even the use of steroid blocks in the neck and face to alleviate facial pain. Without proper treatment of the TMJ arthritis, older adults have a greater tendency to fall into a process of not eating and, ultimately, this can lead to malnutrition.

If a patient has an abnormal mouth bite, a patient can develop pain in the TMJ joint. When the teeth are properly aligned, especially during chewing, the muscles will be of a normal tone. If a patient has an abnormal bite, the muscles around the jaw can develop areas of spasm. Sometimes the muscles that are involved in chewing fail to relax. This muscle behavior causes a patient to have myofascial trigger points in the muscles involved with chewing. Not only will a patient have pain in the muscles and the TMJ; a patient also will eventually have TMJ dysfunction. The dental specialist can make a special orthotic device for a patient that can be placed intermittently, which will allow the jaw muscles to relax. This modality will ultimately decrease the myofascial trigger points.

If a patient has TMJ, a patient can have ringing in the ears and hearing loss as well as pain around the ear. Heat and massage as well as analgesic medications can reduce the TMJ pain. The nervous habits can result in TMJ pain as well. There have been reports of TMJ pain related to individuals holding their telephone on their shoulder for hours at a time. These maneuvers compress some of the muscles, leading to myofascial pain and trigger points. It has been shown that women are more prone to TMJ than men.

The discs in the joints can displace or wear out and cause a patient TMJ pain. This is called intra-articular TMJ pain. If the disc is displaced forward, a patient may develop clicking, popping noises when a patient open and close the mouth. A patient can also have pain as well as the limitation of the jaw movement. Over time, a patient will develop wear-and-tear changes, leading to osteoarthritis of the joint. The capsule around the TMJ can become inflamed as well as deranged.

In the central nervous system, there are areas that exist in the spinal cord and the brain that inhibit painful impulses from reaching the pain center in the brain. It is possible that TMJ may be associated with impairment in the inhibitory system. This allows pain impulses from the jaw to reach the brain without being filtered or decreased in intensity.

If a patient has a decrease in the inhibition in the spinal cord, a patient will have exaggerated responses to both painful stimuli and psychological stimuli. For some reason, increased pain sensitivity throughout the body is more prevalent in patients with TMJ. The enhanced pain sensitivity noted among patients with TMJ was done in a clinical laboratory setting.

TMJ patients in general have a lower pain threshold than normal subjects for an unknown reason. TMJ patients in general can have more physical and psychological symptoms of stress. TMJ individuals report greater stress than healthy individuals. This finding is important because stress can cause a patient to clench the teeth. This clenching of teeth can affect the muscles for chewing as well as the TMJ joint.

Both fatigue as well as psychological distress can increase the pain. As time progresses, the pain will become constant. X-rays can identify changes in the TMJ space. Traumatic injuries can also cause a patient to experience TMJ pain as well. If a patient has rheumatoid arthritis, a patient can develop TMJ pain. Rheumatoid arthritis is usually on both sides of the body, whereas osteoarthritis is usually confined to one side.

If a patient has rheumatoid arthritis, this disease can progress to the TMJs on both sides of the head. In addition to x-rays, a patient may need a magnetic resonance image (MRI). A CT can also be used to examine the TMJ. At present, MRIs are the most effective tool for diagnosing TMJ problems. The TMJ specialist can also inject to dye into the joint. This injection of dye, called an arthrography, can help diagnose the disc displacement.

If a patient has a displacement of the TMJ disc, the mouth will deviate to one side as a patient open the mouth. If a patient has a popping or clicking in the jaw, a patient may have disc pathology. If an injection into the TMJ provides a patient with significant relief, the pain is intra-articular or coming from within the TMJ itself. However, if injection into the muscle provides a patient with pain relief, this tells the health-care provider that the pain is coming from outside the joint. Furthermore, by injecting around the nerve that goes to the TMJ, this maneuver can provide information as to whether the TMJ is the source of the chronic pain.

These injections are safe. Since most TMJ sufferers are missing pieces of their actual jaw bone or cartilage that helps keep the jaw in place, the muscles actually have to work harder to chew. When these muscles get fatigued, the jaw pops out of place, the TMJ joints get inflamed, and the headaches and jaw pain occurs. A patient should avoid chewy foods as well as crunchy foods.

Surgery is sometimes indicated for the management of a TMJ problem. When less-invasive procedures fail to alleviate TMJ pain, oral surgery procedures can be done. These include using a scope to reposition the discs. The oral surgeon can also remove the discs. Implantations can be done into the TMJ. Using a scope is less invasive than opening the

TMJ joint. A patient need to remember that the most conservative therapies are usually the best therapies.

TMJ prevalence peaks between the ages of 25 and 44. After age 44, the chance of a patient developing TMJ decreases with increasing age. For some reason, female patients who develop TMJ were more likely than males to have chronic pain. Studies have shown that sex is a definite risk for the development of TMJ. TMJ is most noted in women during their reproductive years. The reason for this finding is not known. The problem with doing gender-specific studies on TMJ patients is that only a small number of males actually seek treatment for TMJ. A study in 1994 demonstrated that women have more physical and psychological symptoms with TMJ than males. However, in the study, males had greater psychological-related symptoms.

Studies have also been done to determine whether TMJ psychosocial symptoms were different from women when compared to men. Higher levels of stress, depression, and anxiety have been reported in the TMJ population in general when compared to healthy individuals who do not suffer from TMJ. It was previously reported that if a patient suffers from TMJ that the patient has a higher rate of psychopathology than normal control individuals. A patient must be aware that psychopathology is strongly associated with generalized muscle pain throughout the body. The psychological disorders reported in TMJ patients are higher in females than males. If a patient has a history of sexual abuse or trauma, a patient has a higher risk of developing TMJ.

Close to 50 percent of TMJ patients have a history of sexual or physical abuse. An abuse history makes a patient more prone for depression and anxiety. An abuse history in general is associated with increased physical as well as psychological symptoms if a patient suffers from chronic pain. An abuse history is related to the increased pain complaints as well as the psychological disturbances. Sexual abuse has been noted to be associated with an increased risk of generalized muscle pain in females but not in males. Be aware that females are more often the victims of sexual and physical abuse. As a result, the effect of abuse on pain response is more likely to be noted by females than by males.

Pain in the mouth and face can come from the teeth, jaws, the temporal mandibular joints, the muscles involved in chewing, and from the salivary glands. The nose and sinuses can also be a source of pain.

One person gets migraine headaches, another ringing in the ears, a third clicking and locking of the jaw, a fourth pain on the sides and back of the head and neck. All are suspected of having a temporomandibular disorder. Up to three-fourths of Americans have one or more signs of a temporomandibular problem, most of which come and go and finally disappear on their own. Specialists from Boston estimate that only 5 percent to 10 percent of people with symptoms need treatment.

Popularly called TMJ, for the joint where the upper and lower jaws meet, temporomandibular disorders actually represent a wider class of head pain problems that can involve this pesky joint, the muscles involved in chewing, and related head and neck muscles and bones.But too often, experts say, patients fail to have the problem examined in a comprehensive way and undergo costly and sometimes irreversible therapies that may do little or nothing to relieve their symptoms. "Less is often best in treating TMJ disorders."

Resting the jaw is the most important therapy. Stop harmful chewing and biting habits, avoid opening your mouth wide while yawning or laughing (holding a fist under the chin helps), and temporarily eat only soft foods like yogurt, soup, fish, cottage cheese and well-cooked, mashed or pureed vegetables and fruit. It also helps to apply heat to the side of the face and to take a nonsteroidal anti-inflammatory medication, for up to two weeks.

Other self-care measures suggested by the orofacial academy include not leaning on or sleeping on the jaw and not playing wind, brass or string instruments that stress, strain or thrust back the jaw.Physical therapy to retrain positioning of the spine, head, jaw and tongue can be helpful, as can heat treatments with ultrasound and short-wave diathermy. Some patients are helped by a low-dose tricyclic antidepressant taken at bedtime, or antianxiety medication. Stress management and relaxation techniques like massage, yoga, biofeedback, cognitive therapy and counseling to achieve a less frenetic work pace are also helpful, according to the findings of a national conference on pain management.

If you clench or grind your teeth, you can be fitted with a mouth guard that is inserted like a retainer or removable denture, especially at night, to prevent this joint-damaging behavior. It is important to remember that, at present, there is no cure for TMJ disorder. Any article, blog, doctor, or person claiming that there is, could be pushing remedies like the ones above. Most patients find that the best course of action is one of conservative, non-invasive treatment with adequate pain management and self-care.

An ethical issue is the harm that can be caused to the patient by treatments that have not undergone scientific scrutiny. Today, it has been realized that TMD is a group of highly complex diseases involving many genes, hormones and a myriad of complex biologic factors. It's also important to note that over 36 million Americans are affected and the majority is women in their childbearing years. The issue of why women are more affected by TMD has stimulated increased endocrinology research in this area.

So in essence the buyer must beware and not be fooled by advertisements that claim they can easily fix a TMJ problem.

33. SHINGLES

According to the Centers for Disease Control and Prevention, nearly one million Americans experience shingles each year, and the disease is most common in older adults. A vaccine, which can help prevent shingles, is available to people ages 50 and older, and it is recommended by dermatologists. Because the Shingles always displays in a Dermatomal Pattern that is related to the individual nerves (see picture at left or click the previous link), they tend to manifest in rather clear cut and delineated manners, whether on the head or body.

Although the Shingles themselves tend to last 2-4 weeks, about 50% of the people over 50 years of age who get Shingles end up with what is called Post-Herpetic Neuralgia (PHN). This means that the Herpes Virus stays in the nerve causing pain long after the visible signs of the disease itself are gone.

Shingles is a painful disease that is caused by the same virus (herpes zoster virus) that caused chickenpox when you were a child. This virus is rendered dormant by your immune system when your body has healed from the chicken pox infection. This same virus may affect some of the nerves that go out of your spinal cord to your chest or face. One or more nerves can be affected. Shingles occurs in those patients who have had chickenpox. Usually the shingles pain stays on one side of your body.

The shingles virus will remain in a nerve after your chickenpox has healed. This area is called your dorsal root ganglia. This virus is dormant but typically reactivates when you age. This reactivation usually occurs after your immune system has been weakened, usually by another viral infection such as the flu or common cold. If you have cancer, you may be prone to develop shingles as well.

Sometimes there is no known reason why you develop shingles. If you have had contact with an individual who has active chicken pox, there is a chance that you could develop shingles. However, this scenario is rare. You need to be aware that shingles does not increase during seasonal chicken pox outbreaks. When the virus is reactivated in your dorsal root ganglia, it goes along your nerves to your nerve endings. The virus at this time will cause your skin to develop painful skin lesions.

You need to be aware that this virus can affect any part of your central nervous system. In rare cases, this virus can even affect your brain; this is called encephalitis. The virus has been reported in some cases to affect the sympathetic ganglia as well, which can cause severe burning pain. This will cause you to have symptoms that mimic reflex sympathetic dystrophy.

Following a chicken pox infection, antibodies are made in your body to fight the chicken pox virus. This is the reason why you usually do not get chicken pox again. However, if your immune system is compromised for any reason, your body's ability to combat the virus is greatly reduced. This is the reason why you may develop shingles. If your immune system appears to be attacked, your body will immediately fight the shingles virus by producing antibodies to the virus.

After you have had the onset of shingles, you may develop post-herpetic neuralgia. This is a chronic pain syndrome that occurs following the onset of shingles. When you have the onset of shingles, you will have blisters as well as burning sensations in your skin where the infected nerves run. When you develop post-herpetic neuralgia, which can persist for years, after your skin lesions have healed.

If you are between the ages of 40 and 60, the chances of you developing post-herpetic neuralgia are 20 percent. If you are over 60 years of age, your chance of developing post-herpetic neuralgia will increase to 50 percent. Post-herpetic neuralgia is a difficult entity to treat. Post-herpetic neuralgia can cause you to have agonizing pain as well as suffering. Some individuals have even committed suicide to escape this terrible pain. Sometimes you can develop burning pain associated with the herpes zoster virus. However, it may be some time before your skin lesions appear.

Before you develop a skin rash, the diagnosis of herpes zoster is difficult to make. After your skin lesions erupt, the diagnosis is easier to make. If you have pain in your mid chest, you may be incorrectly diagnosed with a coronary artery disease or pneumonia. If your doctor wants to confirm your diagnosis, the virus should be isolated from your pustules no later than seven days after they erupted. Be aware that if you have severe burning pain that develops on one side of your body, you may or may not have a skin eruption but you can have shingles.

Sometimes the lack of a skin eruption confuses doctors as to whether you actually have the onset of shingles, because skin lesions are so common. If you do develop skin eruptions, the lesions will begin as redness. The redness over your skin will turn to blisters. The blisters can form pus. Eventually these lesions on your skin break down. A crust then forms. If the virus affects your skin, in addition to your nerves, you may develop scars as well as loss of skin pigment about the infected site.

Be aware that the virus can travel to your eyes. If you or anyone in your family has developed shingles and begins to complain of eye pain, this is a medical emergency. You must contact an ophthalmologist immediately. If left untreated, the virus may blind you. Shingles may be preceded by other events. Be aware that psychological stress can also trigger the onset of shingles. If you have a history of a prolonged use of steroids, you may also be prone to develop shingles. For reasons yet unknown, the Caucasian race appears to have a higher incidence of shingles than other races. Your chest will be most affected by shingles.

A nerve coming off of your brain that distributes branches to your face called the trigeminal nerve is the next most common nerve affected. Next the nerves off of your neck (called the cranial nerves) are affected, followed by the nerves coming off of your spinal cord that go to your legs (called the lumbar nerves). As you can see, shingles can affect nerves all over your body.

After you have been diagnosed with shingles, your doctor will probably treat you with an antiviral drug.. Acyclovir, famciclovir, and valacyclovir can be used for the treatment of your viral infection. Antiviral medications are used to decrease the intensity and duration of your shingles and are used to prevent the chronic pain associated with post-herpetic neuralgia.

Be aware that you can still have the onset of post-herpetic neuralgia even after treatment with these antiviral agents. Pain associated with post-herpetic neuralgia can be described as aching, burning, or stabbing. The worst pain is pain that is triggered by light touch such as clothing, bathing, or lying on a mattress. Sometimes cold weather or cold water can worsen your pain. Post-herpetic neuralgia is a dreaded complication of shingles.

If you develop shingles and if your pain lasts longer than six weeks after your skin lesions have disappeared, you may have developed post-herpetic neuralgia. Be aware that a certain proportion of individuals who develop post-herpetic neuralgia will improve over time with no treatment. If you have post-herpetic neuralgia, the chances are that you will have improved by 12 months. Approximately 30 percent of individuals who develop post-herpetic neuralgia still complain of pain after one year. Two percent of individuals who suffer from post-herpetic neuralgia will have pain longer than five years.

Doctors of different specialties treat shingles. Your primary care doctor or a dermatologist may treat you. You may have to go to an emergency room because of severe pain and be treated by that doctor.

You may also be referred to a pain-medicine specialist. Psychologists are also valuable in the management of your pain. All of these health-care providers can significantly help you manage your pain. You may find that each of these providers uses a different modality for the treatment of your pain. If your pain is moderate, a mild analgesic such as Ultracet (tramadol) or a mild narcotic such as

Tylenol with codeine may suffice for the management of your pain. If your pain becomes excruciating, these medications will not provide you with any significant pain relief. At this time, you may require more potent opioid medication such as Percocet or Vicodin.

If these stronger narcotic drugs do not provide you with relief, you may require the administration of a strong opioid medication such as morphine. If you develop post-herpetic neuralgia, avoid stressful situations that may worsen your pain. Avoid situations that cause you significant anxiety and/or depression. If you live in a cold environment, dress warmly.

In addition to antiviral agents, your doctor may prescribe steroids. Lotions, different types of patches, nonsteroidal anti-inflammatory drugs, antidepressants, and muscle relaxants may all be needed to control your pain. You may even need injections of numbing medicines into your nerves. Placement of local anesthetics around your sympathetic nerves may be of benefit in reducing your pain, especially if the injection is done soon after the onset of your pain.

Topical agents are frequently used to treat shingles pain. These agents accelerate the healing of your skin and can decrease the pain associated with the shingles virus. However, topical anesthetics administered at the time that you develop shingles will not affect the development of post-herpetic neuralgia. Compresses or Burrow's solution or calamine lotion placed directly over your painful site can decrease the pain associated with acute herpes zoster.

A patch has been developed for the treatment of shingles. This patch called the Lidoderm patch has proven to be extremely useful in the management of shingles and post-herpetic neuralgia pain. A local anesthetic called lidocaine is placed within a patch system. The lidocaine is placed within an adhesive. The adhesive binds to your skin. Another type of transdermal (skin) drug-delivery system is a clonidine transdermal patch. This is placed over the area of your maximal pain. This drug is a drug that controls an individual's blood pressure. Tricyclic antidepressants are frequently used for the management of pain associated with post-herpetic neuralgia. In fact, tricyclic antidepressants are used to treat a variety of chronic pain syndromes.

The exact mechanism by which these drugs decrease your pain is unknown. If narcotics are to be used, mild narcotics should be initiated, as previously stated. Morphine is commonly used for severe pain. Baclofen, Amantadine, and Elavil can decrease your burning pain associated with post-herpetic neuralgia while anticonvulsant medications can lessen your sharp, shooting pain. Another topical drug that is sometimes used is capsaicin cream. It can be purchased over the counter and can also be purchased by prescription at a higher concentration. A newer anticonvulsant drug called Lyrica (pregabilin) is very effective in decreasing your pain.

Shingles pain may be decreased by physical therapy. Heat, cold, and massage are frequently used for the management of your pain. Sometimes a transcutaneous electrical nerve stimulator (TENS) can be helpful. The TENS unit, however, is not frequently prescribed because on occasion it could worsen the pain associated with shingles. Water therapy can be helpful because the warm water can be soothing and may also desensitize the nerves that are causing the severe pain.

If your activities of daily living are limited because of your pain, consult an occupational therapist to learn how to preserve your daily-living activities. Sometimes your doctor may want to put numbing medicine mixed with a steroid around your affected nerve. If you are experiencing pain in your chest wall, for example, your doctor may place an injection into the nerve that provides sensation to your chest. This nerve is called the intercostal nerve.

The type of nerve block used to treat your pain depends on the type of pain that you have. The pain associated with post-herpetic neuralgia can be somatic, sympathetic, or central. The somatic pain follows a certain nerve that is affected. Sympathetic pain can decrease the blood flow to your tissues and causes you to have a burning pain. Central pain is a result of rewiring of your central nervous system. For this type of pain, you need a different type of block.

Sympathetic nerve blocks, if done early, can relieve pain associated with shingles and can also decrease the incidence of developing post-herpetic neuralgia. To be effective, they should be performed within the first two months after the onset of your symptoms.

Stellate ganglion blocks are used for pain in your head, neck, and arms. Thoracic epidural blocks are used for pain in your mid back and chest wall, whereas lumbar sympathetic blocks are used for the management of post-herpetic neuralgia pain in your lower extremities. The purpose of nerve blocks is to interrupt your pain impulses and to facilitate therapy and to help you increase your daily-living activities. Nerve blocks should be used if your pain is becoming too severe and cannot be controlled by non-narcotic medications.

If you have sympathetic pain that does not respond to the previously mentioned modalities, more permanent blocks of your sympathetic nervous system can be done using a modality called radiofrequency thermocoagulation. This device provides some heat about your sympathetic nerves. This device does not burn your nerves, but the heat essentially puts your nerves out of commission. The procedure is done on an outpatient basis with only minimal discomfort. Radiofrequency thermocoagulation can provide you with a long-term interruption of your pain fibers and pain impulses.

Occasionally a dorsal column stimulator can be placed in your epidural space to manage your pain. The dorsal column stimulator is essentially an epidural catheter that has electrodes on it. The number of electrodes that are used depends on the pattern of your pain. The dorsal column stimulator is placed within your body on a trial basis. The catheter is placed on an out-patient basis with x-ray. The end of the catheter attaches to a battery pack which can be placed under your skin. How the dorsal column stimulator actually works is debated.

It is believed that the electrical interference with ascending pathways may be the mechanism for decreasing your pain impulse transmission. The use of this device has been demonstrated to be effective for the management of post-herpetic neuralgic pain that is refractory to all other modalities. The goal of the stimulation is to decrease your pain by at least 50 percent. If you do obtain adequate pain relief, the stimulator is implanted permanently surgically.

For pain that persists in your arms or legs and is refractory to other treatments, a nerve stimulator can be placed in that extremity to provide you with pain relief. Chemical substances that disrupt nerves have been used since 1930 for the treatment of post-herpetic neuralgia.

Phenol is an alcohol-like drug used to disrupt your nerve impulses. It also has some local anesthetic properties. The first reported use of a neurolitic solution was in 1863 by Luton. Neurolitic blocks for chronic pain management were further developed by neurosurgeons. In 1925, Dr. Doppler used phenol for disruption of nerves. In 1955, phenol was administered in the spinal fluid of patients to disrupt their chronic pain.

Alcohol has also been used to disrupt nerve signals. However, the use of the alcohol can cause post-block pain called neuritis. Whenever neurolitic chemicals are used, the procedure must be done under X-ray guidance to know where the solution is going. Sometimes the phenol must be re-administered to provide you with a good long-term block of your nerves.

If all the previous modalities fail to provide you with relief, a narcotic pump can be placed within your body. The pump consists of a reservoir about the size of a hockey puck. A newly developed snail toxin placed in this pump may give you significant pain relief. The pump is connected to a tube that runs into the fluid that surrounds your spinal cord.

Essentially this pump gives you a drop of a narcotic drug every minute or so and is another way of controlling your pain. The drug-delivery system is refilled approximately every 45 days. Before placing this pump, your doctor will do a trial of morphine or a similar drug and compare it to a salt solution (placebo) to see whether you actually obtain pain relief from this device. A snail toxin placed in the pump may also be effective.

Cold Laser Therapy works on the premise that every single cell in your body has photo receptors (light receptors). When certain frequencies of light stimulate these photo receptors, it turns on the mitochondria to produce the one and only source of energy that cells can use ATP. Specific frequencies of laser light can penetrate deep into injured or diseased tissues and stimulate the production of cellular energy by as much as 8 times. Using Cold Laser Therapy for pain control is that it is not simply masking pain like medications do, but actually healing the tissue. Insurance com are not yet paying for treatment with Cold Laser

The fact is that any time one sees a product or treatment that is a panacea cure for large numbers of incongruent conditions it should spark one's skeptical intuition. The reality of lasers is that a few studies have shown that laser therapy can have some small-localized effects on wound healing by treating the wound edges and some pain reduction in certain situations where tendons are close to the surface of the skin. But pain is highly subjective and several recent studies show that when it comes to pain control, sham laser treatments work just as well as laser treatments. However this treatment appears to be effective in some patients. Further studies are medically indicated.

Aetna considers treatment with low-level infrared light experimental and investigational for the treatment of acne, back pain,

Bell's palsy, central nervous system injuries, chronic non-healing wounds, diabetic peripheral neuropathy, ischemic stroke, lymphedema, neck pain, osteoarthritis, Parkinson's disease, retinal degeneration, and stroke because of a lack of adequate evidence in the peer-reviewed published medical literature regarding the effectiveness of infrared therapy for these indications

CIGNA concludes: Low-level laser therapy has been proposed for a wide variety of uses, including wound healing, tuberculosis, and musculoskeletal conditions such as osteoarthritis, rheumatoid arthritis, fibromyalgia and carpal tunnel syndrome. There is insufficient evidence in the published, peer-reviewed scientific literature to demonstrate that LLLT is effective for these conditions or other medical conditions. Large, well-designed clinical trials are needed to demonstrate the effectiveness of LLLT for the proposed conditions.

The Center for Medicare and Medicaid Services (CMS) has determined that there is sufficient evidence to conclude that the use of infrared devices is not reasonable and necessary for treatment of Medicare beneficiaries for diabetic and non-diabetic peripheral sensory neuropathy, wounds and ulcers, and similar related conditions, including symptoms such as pain arising from these conditions.

The use of infrared and/or near-infrared light and/or heat, including monochromatic infrared energy (MIRE), is not covered for the treatment, including symptoms such as pain arising from these conditions, of diabetic and/or non-diabetic peripheral sensory neuropathy, wounds and/or ulcers of skin and/or subcutaneous tissues in Medicare beneficiaries.

34. HIV

The acquired immune deficiency syndrome (AIDS) is caused by the human immunodeficiency virus (HIV). The virus can replicate itself within a host cell or do nothing once it infects the host cell. When a virus replicates itself in a host cell, thousands or even millions of copies of itself can be released from the cell and then go on to infect other cells. HIV, for example, can enter your body from unsafe sex practices or contaminated blood, enter your cells, and make millions, billions, and even trillions of copies of itself that go on to infect other cells in your body.

A virus, therefore, is a highly effective means of causing you to develop and have an infection. If the virus gets into your body, it can cause a disease unless your antibodies attack it. A virus, on the other hand, can reproduce only by invading one of your cells.

A virus is spread randomly through the wind, in water, food, by blood, or by body secretions. With respect to HIV, blood and body secretions are important mechanisms by which this virus spreads from one person's body into our body. HIV, which is the causative virus of AIDS, is a very complex virus.

When new viruses are replicated, the virus that destroys the outer wall of your cell releases an enzyme. The enzyme destroys the outer wall of your cell. When this wall is destroyed, the new viruses that have been made within your cell are now released into your body. These viruses will go to infect other cells of different tissues within your body. As this process progresses, you will develop fever, chills, joint pain, nerve and muscle pain, and so forth.

Be aware that when the new virus is made from the original virus, your cell that was infected by the virus will then be destroyed. When a new virus infects your cell, it does not cause immediate cellular destruction. This example is the reason why HIV can be present in the body for some time before causing symptoms. You can become infected with the HIV virus by exposure to infected blood products, sexual contact with infected people, or from a mother to her baby.

Infection from this virus appears within two to six weeks following infection. Early symptoms of infection with HIV are much like flu symptoms and include muscle pain, joint pain, headaches, as well as a sore throat and fever. Antibodies to the HIV virus develop in your body within three to six months of your infection. Later symptoms, which take up to 10 years to develop, as those of AIDS, result from the destructive effects of HIV on your immune system and are characterized by unusual types of pneumonia, cancer, central nervous system infections, and other problems.

Changes in your immune system will eventually occur after you have been infected. After the HIV virus enters your cells, each virus can set up a chronic infection in which new virus particles are constantly being produced. You may develop some antibodies to the virus. When the level of your body's antibodies decreases, you can develop AIDS.

Progression to AIDS, which is a syndrome following infection with the virus, can begin with a low red blood cell count. Other factors can be necessary for you to contract the HIV infection and for the development of progression to AIDS.

There are four high-risk groups for acquiring AIDS; homosexual and bisexual men, hemophiliacs and transfusion recipients, intravenous drug abusers and children born to infected mothers. Homosexual and bisexual men account for approximately 37-40 percent of the reported cases of AIDS in the United States. However, this number is increasing. The majority of women with AIDS in the United States are in childbearing years.

The number of individuals with AIDS does not take into account the high number of HIV-infected asymptomatic women. Remember that an HIV infection takes time to develop AIDS. The risks for a woman to expose herself to the HIV virus are through unsafe sex practices, intravenous drug use, and transfusions. A significant number of HIV-infected women have given birth to HIV-infected babies.

There is speculation that pregnancy can accelerate the disease progression of HIV. If you are pregnant and have HIV, you may develop symptoms two to three years after the delivery of your baby. This rate of AIDS development is faster than for homosexual men or intravenous drug users; approximately 40 percent of asymptomatic carriers of the virus in these categories will develop AIDS.

The AIDS virus will decrease your lymphocytes, which are cells that normally exist in your bloodstream. Lymphocytes are important mediators of your immune system. These cells help fight the development of various diseases. The average time of onset of your viral infection to development of AIDS varies months to years with a mean time of approximately 10 years.

Health-care providers cannot test an individual for HIV without permission. To test for an HIV infection, your doctor must obtain an informed consent from you. Informed consent is a legal requirement and means that your doctor must inform you that you will be tested for HIV. You must sign an agreement that gives your doctor the right to do this test. Without your informed consent, your doctor is violating your patient rights.

The name for the initial viral test performed is ELISA (enzyme-linked immune absorbent assay). If you have a positive screening test using ELISA, the infection with the HIV complex is confirmed with a repeat ELISA test as well as another test called a Western blot test. A doctor will usually not report a positive ELISA test to you until your Western blot test has been confirmed to be positive.

The HIV virus induces AIDS by causing the death of the CD4+T cells in your body. These cells are important for the normal function of your immune system. The AIDS virus also interferes with their normal function. When this happens, your ability to fight other infections is diminished. HIV virus is called a slow virus. This means that the course of infection with the HIV virus has a long interval between the initial infection and the onset of the AIDS symptoms.

HIV/AIDS can cause: fever and night sweats, loss of appetite, nausea and vomiting, chest pain related to pneumonia, chronic sinus infection with headache, tumor on your spinal cord, meningitis with neck pain and headaches, painful lesions in your mouth, hepatitis with abdominal pain and/or, burning or piercing pain in your arms or legs

Once infected, you can progress to AIDS in an average of 10 years as previously mentioned. Combinations of three or more anti-HIV drugs called highly active antiretroviral therapy can delay the progression of the HIV disease for prolonged periods. This disease frequently causes a painful neuropathy in many areas of your body. A neuropathy is a lesion in your nerves in your body that are outside of your spinal cord and brain.

AIDS can cause you to have a painful neuropathy. Neuropathy associated with AIDS can be intermittent or constant. The pain can vary in severity from mild to severe. The pain can be burning, shooting, aching, or stabbing. It is believed that the HIV virus causes nerve damage, which causes your painful neuropathy. You can develop headaches from HIV virus meningitis. Also you can have abdominal pain related to gastrointestinal disease and chest pain related to pneumonia.

You may develop headaches as well as fever and have significant changes in your mental status as your infection progresses. To make this diagnosis, your doctor will do a spinal tap by placing a needle into your spinal fluid. The laboratory will identify any abnormal cells in your spinal fluid. Your doctor will measure your spinal fluid pressure by placing a needle into your spinal fluid to see whether you are having excessive pressure on your brain. You may need repeated spinal fluid taps followed by removal of some of your spinal fluid to decrease any pressure that could be affecting your brain.

One of the leading causes of death in individuals with AIDS is the pneumocystis carini pneumonia. This is the most common infection in AIDS patients and is the leading cause of death in this patient population. Not only does this disease affect your lungs, it can affect other parts of your body as well. If you have AIDS, you can also develop tumors associated with AIDS. These tumors include Kaposi's sarcoma as well as Hodgkin's and non-Hodgkins lymphoma.

There is now hope for individuals infected with HIV. It is estimated that if 1 million people in the United States now have HIV or AIDS, approximately 500,000 of them are either untreated or undiagnosed. Drugs for the treatment of AIDS are constantly being developed. Essentially, AIDS has gone from being an immediate sentence of death to a chronic manageable disease. Currently Russia has the fastest growing epidemic of AIDS, thought to be because of intravenous drug use. Epidemics are now beginning in China.

The HIV disease is very complicated. No cure has been developed yet. There are many different treatments and products that claim to help people with HIV disease. Some of these have not been carefully tested, and some might even be harmful. The rate of AIDS cases and deaths did slowdown, which was attributed to successful antiretroviral therapy.

The problem with some of the drug therapy is that some individuals either develop a resistance to the drugs or they experience side effects from the drugs and stop taking them. Some of the vaccines currently being studied provide protection for some individuals but not all. Two anti-HIV drugs have been shown to cause death in some pregnant women. These drugs are stavudine and didanosine. Between 1991 and 1995, there was a 63 percent increase in women diagnosed with AIDS.

Martin Shkreli, the CEO of an American drugs company who hiked the price of life-saving HIV-related drugs from $13.50 to $750, was reportedly arrested on securities fraud charges relating to a firm that he founded. He was charged with illegally taking stock from Retrophin Inc., a biotechnology firm he started in 2011, and using it pay off debts from unrelated business dealings, Bloomberg said.

The fact that AIDS causes great suffering and is deadly has encouraged the marketing of hundreds of unproven remedies to AIDS victims. The alleged cures have included processed blue-green algae (pond scum), BHT (an antioxidant used as a food preservative), pills derived from mice given the AIDS virus, herbal capsules, bottles of "T cells," and thumping on the thymus gland.

Some firms have offered to freeze and store bone marrow, claiming that it could be used to restore an AIDS victim's marrow when AIDS began to deplete the body's supply of bone marrow, which manufactures the body's blood cells. Autohemotherapy is essentially an ineffective procedure in which a sample of the patient's blood is withdrawn, exposed to hydrogen peroxide and then replaced.

Your pain can be treated with narcotic drugs as well as antidepressants and anticonvulsant medications such as Neurontin. Intravenous lidocaine may decrease your pain. Mexilitine, a heart rhythm medication, may also help to control your pain. Exercise therapy is sometimes beneficial for the management of your pain. It is believed that exercise can increase your body's endorphins, which in turn helps to manage your pain.

Endorphins are natural chemical substances that your body produces HIV-related pain becomes increasingly severe as the disease progresses. Drugs used to treat the HIV infection can cause neuropathic pain. It is estimated that 30 percent of the neuropathic pain syndromes suffered by individuals who have the HIV disease are caused by drugs to attack the HIV virus. Neuropathic pain in the HIV-infected patient in most instances can be adequately controlled.

Given that no two people are alike, if you are taking any medications and begin to take nutritional supplements you should be aware that potential drug-nutrient interactions may occur and are encouraged to consult a health care professional before using any natural product. Combining certain prescription drugs and dietary supplements can lead to undesirable effects such as: diminished prescription drug effectiveness, reduced supplement effectiveness and impaired drug and/or supplement absorption.

Food insecurity is defined as a limited or uncertain ability to acquire acceptable foods in socially acceptable ways, or limited or uncertain availability of nutritionally adequate and safe foods. Improvement in life expectancy with the use of combination antiretroviral therapy has come with the recognition of the complications associated with chronic human immunodeficiency virus infection. Vitamin D has been of particular interest because of its effect on bone health and immune functions. Vitamin D deficiency was common among the patients included in this study.

A study was done to determine the effects of nutritional status at the start of highly active anti-retroviral therapy on treatment outcomes. Malnutrition predisposes HIV patients to early death. The response to the HIV infection is situated within complex interactions between host nutritional health and immunologic function, which contribute to the varied phenotypes of immune activation among HIV-infected patients across a spectrum from malnutrition to obesity.

HIV patients who experienced severe food insecurity negatively influenced their mental health and general wellbeing. The inclusion of resources for food assistance in HIV treatment programs may help ameliorate mental health challenges.

HIV fraud is the promotion, advertisement, or sale of products that are supposed to diagnose, treat, or cure HIV when those products have not been proven to be safe and effective for those purposes. According to press reports, Dr. Rodriguez conspired with five other medical professionals to recruit patients, diagnose them with HIV, then forge false records for HIV treatment services that earned them millions of dollars in Medicare reimbursements. From October 2003 through February 2006, the team of doctors bilked Medicare (and taxpayers) for $20 million in false claims.

Regular medicine does not have a cure for HIV. Because it is a serious illness, many people with HIV disease are willing to try almost anything to get healthy. Some unproven treatments may be harmless, but others can be dangerous. For example, one brand of "Brain Wave Synchronizer" caused epileptic seizures.

The product prevents or cures HIV or AIDS. Researchers have been working hard for over 10 years, but there is not yet any known cure for HIV or AIDS. The only sure way to prevent AIDS is to avoid being infected with the HIV virus. Be suspicious if the promoters use key words like miraculous cure, amazing breakthrough, foolproof, suppressed treatments, or secret ingredients.

A 40-year-old Florida resident admitted he pocketed thousands of dollars in kickbacks in exchange for giving the clinics his Medicare number to bill the agency for phony HIV infusion treatments. Manassas is among hundreds of Medicare-licensed clinics in South Florida that defraud the system with fake HIV-drug claims, according to federal claim records and authorities.

The scams are especially outrageous because HIV infusion therapy, which entails intravenous drips of medication to boost a patient's immune system, has been replaced almost everywhere but South Florida by more effective antiretroviral drugs taken orally. Yet Medicare has continued to allow the outdated HIV infusion services and to pay hundreds of millions of dollars for the treatments because the agency still considers them ``reasonable and necessary."

Recruiters arrange for patients to take blood tests at the clinics, which have staff on site, to establish that they are HIV-positive or have full-blown AIDS. With that written designation, the patients can qualify for Medicare services, and the clinic operators can bill for bogus intravenous treatments.

The clinic operators made a fortune by prescribing costly HIV/AIDS drug infusions such as immunoglobulin, billing Medicare for each bogus treatment. The patients sign paperwork saying they receive the treatments. In turn, the clinics pay the patients kickbacks. Clinic owners also pay bribes to physicians for each drug-infusion prescription.

A Virginia man was found guilty of defrauding investors of more than $700,000 from a project aimed at purportedly developing a treatment for Human Immunodeficiency Virus infection/Acquired Immunodeficiency Syndrome (HIV/AIDS). Fraudulent misrepresentations to investors regarding his proposed HIV/AIDS treatment ended in substantial proceeds being misappropriated for his personal use.

Patients need to be aware of fraudulent HIV/AIDS treatment as some could cause bodily harm.

35. BIG PHARMA

Pharmaceutical companies can also be a source of medical fraud. According to criminal complaints, attorneys general reports and other sources accused the specialty pharmaceutical company Insys Therapeutics with the help of several physicians across the country is putting profits before patient care as it makes millions off patients' pain syndromes.

Insys is subject to investigations regarding the sales and marketing practices of its pain product Subsys Fentanyl, a painkiller delivered as an oral spray. The Scottsdale, Arizona-based Insys Therapeutics' company revenue is almost entirely derived from the highly addictive opiate fentanyl, which it markets under the brand name Subsys Fentanyl.

In the six months which ended June 30, 2015, Subsys sales accounted for $147.2 million of $148.4 million in total revenue. The potency of Subsys also comes with a high price tag. One package of 30 sprays can cost between $900 and $3,000, depending on the dosage, and those prices only seem to be increasing. Subsys, according to FDA guidelines, is only meant to be used to treat late-stage cancer pain.

The suit alleges that "the Company's management was aware that about 10% of prescriptions approved through the Prior Authorization Department were for cancer patients. The majority of prescriptions were written for peripheral neuropathy, lower back pain and sciatica. A sales representative admitted that she provided doctors with financial kickbacks in return for them overprescribing Insys.' This drug is a controversial painkiller to insured patients, most of whom weren't approved for the drug under FDA guidelines. Furthemore, a connection could be more readily detected between the volume of Subsys prescriptions and payments to doctors.

Another unfortunate case involved Celebrex. The importance of Celebrex to Pfizer is indisputable. Officials made a strategic decision during the early trial to be less than forthcoming about the drug's safety. It is one of the company's best-selling drugs, racking up more than $2.5 billion in sales, and was prescribed to 2.4 million patients in the United States last year alone. Celebrex is still sold and heavily marketed, as if nothing would have happened. There is still no clinical proof that Celebrex is better at preventing serious gastrointestinal injuries. The truth was that Celebrex was no better at protecting the stomach from serious complications than other drugs.

A person must be aware that fake online pharmacies are scams that are designed to trick you into paying for items you will never receive, or items that do not live up to their claims. Scammers will set up fake pharmacy websites that are designed to look like legitimate retailers. They will offer health products, medicines and drugs at very cheap prices or without the need for a prescription from a doctor. Prescription-only medicine requires a doctor or other qualified healthcare professional to have examined you. Most medicines have at least some side-effects and these can be very serious for some people. They can also have dangerous interactions with medicines you are already taking.

Be aware of some online fraudulent pharmacies. If you take up an offer, and pay the 'retailer', you may never receive the items you ordered. If you do receive the products that you order, there is no guarantee that they are the real thing. In some cases, the medicines or other products may even damage your health. But with the proliferation of counterfeit medicine, a growing number of Americans who use online pharmacies may be at risk for taking fake pills that can result in serious health problems or even death.

According to the Federal Drug Administration, drugs sold on bogus websites may contain the wrong ingredients, incorrect quantities of ingredients, or may be composed of materials like drywall and eggshells. Drugs like Viagra and pain killers were the prime focus for counterfeiters until the last 10 years or so, but now people are involved in faking a variety of drugs, including cancer drugs, blood pressure medicines and cholesterol medicines. According to the FDA, drugs like Ambien, Xanax, Lexapro, and Ativan are also being faked.

Among the sellers of opioids, none has been more successful or controversial than Purdue Pharma, the maker of the No. 1 drug in the class: OxyContin, which generated $3.1 billion in revenue in 2010. OxyContin's bad reputation, however, has obscured a significant step. Last year Purdue began selling a reformulated version that should help reduce the worst form of abuse. The original drug had a time-release mechanism that could be defeated by crushing the pill and snorting it, smoking it, or adding water to the powder and injecting it for a heroin-like high. Purdue's claims that the time-release process reduced the addiction risk were crucial in making doctors feel comfortable prescribing a powerful addictive drug.

By contrast, the new version of OxyContin breaks into chunks rather than a powder. If water is added, the result is the formation of a gelatinous mass. The drug wears off hours early in many people.

OxyContin is a chemical counterpart of heroin, and when it doesn't last a 12 hour duration, patients can experience excruciating symptoms of withdrawal, including an intense craving for the drug. Over the last 20 years, more than 7 million Americans have abused OxyContin, according to the federal government's National Survey on Drug Use and Health. The drug is widely blamed for setting off the nation's prescription opioid epidemic, which has claimed more than 190,000 lives from overdoses involving OxyContin and other painkillers since 1999.

Doctors eventually discovered that the drug lasted around eight hours rather than 12, and that patients would crash, needing more and higher doses. Patients who took moderate amounts for backaches or arthritis could find themselves hooked. Addicts saw they could easily get high by crushing the pills and then snorting, chewing, or injecting them.

Mylan's EpiPen became the focus for scrutiny, as its price increased by nearly 500 percent over seven years. This device is potentially a life-saving device for allergies. The cost of the life-saving drug inside each EpiPen injector is worth a couple of dollars. When pharmaceutical companies face no competition in the market pharmaceutical companies have the power to set whatever price they need, and patients then pay more for health insurance.

In another scenario, It's quite shocking that nearly three-quarters of all retracted drug studies are due to pure falsification of data. Especially when one considers that even well-researched drugs can still have significant side effects. Vioxx is perhaps one of the better examples of what can happen when a drug is manufactured and sold under false pretenses. It killed more than 60,000 people in just a few years' time, before it was removed from the market. In the case of Vioxx, there are lingering questions about the soundness of the original research used to back the drug initially. We are therefore confronted with indisputable evidence that the drug paradigm is about money, not health, and certainly not dependable scientific inquiry.

It's important to realize that all research is not published. It should therefore, come as no surprise that drug studies funded by a pharmaceutical company that reaches a negative conclusion will rarely be published. Drug companies spend far more on marketing drugs which is almost twice as much than on developing drugs.

Until recently, paying bribes to doctors to prescribe their drugs was commonplace at big pharmaceutical companies although the practice is now generally frowned upon and illegal in many places. GlaxoSmithKline (GSK) was fined $490m in China previously for bribery and has been accused of similar practices in Poland and the Middle East.

The rules on gifts, educational grants and sponsoring lectures, for example, are less clear cut, and these practices remain commonplace in the US. Furthermore, a previous study found that doctors in the US receiving payments from pharma companies were twice as likely to prescribe their drugs. This may well exacerbate the problem of overspending on drugs by governments. A recent study by Prescribing Analytics suggested that the UK's National Health Service could save up to £1 bn a year by doctors switching from branded to equally effective generic versions of the drugs.

For two years, federal prosecutors in at least four states, including Texas, have been working with the Defense Department and other agencies to investigate allegations that some of the firms and their sales staff are committing healthcare and prescription fraud, selling expensive pain creams and other drugs not approved by the Food and Drug Administration to veterans and their families.

The use of compounded drugs by current and former servicemen and servicewomen has skyrocketed in the past decade, federal data show. They were paying illegal kickbacks to some doctors and medical professionals to issue prescriptions for compounded medications. Tricare officials say the beneficiaries are receiving calls or direct requests from sales representatives who ask whether patients have certain medical conditions, and, if so, if they are interested in compound medications.

They then ask the patients to complete forms and provide their sponsor's Social Security number to initiate the prescriptions while they bill Tricare. Such medications can range in cost from a few hundred dollars to more than $9,000 per prescription.

In the last few years pharmaceutical companies have agreed to pay over $13 billion to resolve U.S. Department of Justice allegations of fraudulent marketing practices, including the promotion of medicines for uses that were not approved by the Food and Drug Administration. Pfizer was fined $2.3 billion, which was then the largest health care fraud settlement and the largest criminal fine ever imposed in the United States. Pfizer pled guilty to misbranding the painkiller Bextra with "the intent to defraud or mislead", promoting the drug to treat acute pain at dosages the FDA had previously deemed dangerously high. Bextra was pulled from the market in 2005 due to safety concerns.

Merck agreed to pay a fine of $950 million related to the illegal promotion of the painkiller Vioxx, which was withdrawn from the market in 2004 after studies found the drug increased the risk of heart attacks. The company pled guilty to having promoted Vioxx as a treatment for rheumatoid arthritis before it had been approved for that use.

Sanofi-Aventis agreed to pay $109 million to resolve allegations that the company gave doctors free units of Hyalgan (an injection to relieve knee pain) to encourage those doctors to buy their product. Sanofi lowered the effective price by promising these free samples to doctors, but at the same time got inflated prices from government programs by submitting false price reports,

Endo Health Solutions Inc. and its subsidiary Endo Pharmaceuticals Inc. agreed to pay $192.7 million to resolve criminal and civil liability arising from Endo's marketing of the prescription drug Lidoderm. As part of the agreement, Endo admitted that it intended that Lidoderm be used for unapproved indications and that it promoted Lidoderm to healthcare providers this way.

An anesthesiologist Scott Reuben revolutionized the way physicians provide pain relief to patients undergoing orthopedic surgery for everything from torn ligaments to degenerative hips. Now, the profession is in shambles after an investigation revealed that at least 21 of Reuben's papers were false, and that the pain drugs he touted in them may have slowed postoperative healing.

Reuben's studies led to the sale of billions of dollars' worth of the potentially dangerous drugs known as COX2 inhibitors, Pfizer's Celebrex (celecoxib) and Merck's Vioxx (rofecoxib), for applications whose therapeutic benefits are now in question. Reuben was a member of Pfizer's speaker's bureau and received five independent research grants from the company.

Reuben, in his now-discredited research, attempted to convince orthopedic surgeons to shift from the first generation of nonsteroidal anti-inflammatory drugs (NSAIDs) to the newer, proprietary COX2 inhibitors, such as Vioxx, Celebrex, and Pfizer's Bextra (valdecoxib). He claimed that using such drugs in combination with the Pfizer anticonvulsant Neurontin (gabapentin), and later Lyrica (pregabalin), prior to and during surgery could be effective in decreasing postoperative pain and reduce the use of addictive painkillers, such as morphine, during recovery.

Americans now spend a staggering $200 billion a year on prescription drugs, and that figure is growing at a rate of about 12 percent a year Drugs are the fastest-growing part of the national health care bill which itself is rising at an alarming rate. The increase in drug spending reflects, in almost equal parts, the facts that people are taking a lot more drugs than they used to, that those drugs are more likely to be expensive new ones instead of older, cheaper ones, and that the prices of the most heavily prescribed drugs are routinely increased, at episodes several times a year.

Pharmaceutical companies are primarily marketing machines used to sell drugs of sometimes dubious benefit in many instances. This industry uses its wealth and power to label every institution that might stand in its way, including the US Congress, the FDA, academic medical centers, and the medical profession itself. Most of its marketing efforts are focused on influencing doctors, since they must write the prescriptions.

A physician got an inside look at this shadowy mess while examining drug company internal documents as an expert witness in a case against a pharmaceutical company. The voluminous amounts of documents he was given access to showed serious misrepresentation of both the effectiveness and safety of certain drugs, with published articles making the research appear positive, while negative secondary outcomes were deleted.

In 2005, Dr. John Ioannidis, an epidemiologist at Ioannina School of Medicine, in Greece, showed that there is less than a 50 percent chance that the results of any randomly chosen scientific paper will be true.

President Trump has recently stated that "big pharma" is now going to have to address the high drug prices, and he is demanding change. Hopefully patients and physicians will back him in this endeavor.

36. PILL MILLS

A pain management clinic (in the general legal definition) is a facility providing pain treatment options or that has at least one doctor licensed to prescribe controlled medication for pain. Pain clinics are subject to legal rules and standards, such as being licensed, being subject to inspection by the board and the state, employing licensed staff, etc.

Prescription pain medication is regulated by federal law, so doctors who prescribe it without a legitimate medical purpose or outside the usual course of medical practice can be charged with drug trafficking. Pill mills are essentially places where doctors hand out prescription drugs. ..."

A Pill Mill is essentially a term used primarily by local and state investigators to describe a doctor, clinic or pharmacy that is prescribing or dispensing powerful narcotics inappropriately or for non-medical reasons. These pill mills usually: Accept cash only, do no physical exams, No medical records or x-rays are needed to be admitted to the clinic, A patient picks his/her medication, no questions about a patient's medical condition are asked, patients may be directed to a certain pharmacy,

Patients are only treated with pills, a patient gets a set number of pills and the facility will tell a patient a specific date to return. These clinics may have security guards and there may be huge masses of people waiting to see the doctor By contrast, in many "pain clinics," walk-ins are the only method of intake, the office is understaffed, no referral is required, and little or no examination or work-up is done.

A legitimate practice will only accept patients that have health insurance, whereas most "pill mills" will see patients for cash payments without any health insurance. This difference is a giveaway, since most insurance companies will actually require that physicians who provide care to their patients meet certain standards and be board certified in the specialty. Otherwise, care and visits will not be authorized.

To be more specific, a "pill mill" according to the State of Florida is a doctor's office, clinic, or health care facility that routinely conspires in the prescribing and dispensing of controlled substances outside the scope of the prevailing standards of medical practice in the community or violates the laws of the state of Florida regarding the prescribing or dispensing of controlled prescription drugs.

Signs that a facility may actually be a pill mill as previously mentioned include not requiring a physical exam, X-rays or medical records before being prescribed drugs, being able to pick your preferred medication, being directed to "their" specific pharmacy, and treating pain solely with pills. Pill mills also tend to open and close very suddenly, as an attempt to evade law enforcement.

The term "pill mills" is the nickname given for the illegitimate pain clinics that have sprung up in strip malls and office parks nationwide over the past few years. These alleged pain management centers tend to occupy unmarked office spaces or storefronts, may display a misleading or false business name and have armed security guards patrolling the clinic's lobby. Armed security guards are needed to prevent thieves from robbing the pill mill cache of drugs.

The clinics are employed by unlicensed doctors who prescribe massive amounts of powerful narcotic medications to anyone who walks into the clinic off the street. Although they exist nationwide, most pill mills are located in Texas, Kentucky and Florida due to the states' previous looser restrictions on prescription drug monitoring.

All pill mills operate in the same fashion: no medical records, x-rays, or examinations are needed; pain is treated only with prescription medication; patients can request whatever medication they want with no questions asked; only cash is accepted; prescriptions can only be retrieved from their pharmacy and patients must return on a specific date to obtain more prescriptions. The idea is to get patients hooked on these drugs to ensure the sale of more drugs and help physicians quickly profit.

The clinics tend to shut down and open up in new locations to avoid getting caught by law enforcement and face legal prosecution and pill mill owners are hard to trace since clinics are registered with absent doctors or stolen identities. The closing down of many "pill mills" has resulted in "patients" willing to drive a long way to continue receiving prescriptions from other doctors.

Today, pain specialists rarely prescribe strong opioids for chronic pain unless it's cancer-related. From late 1980s through early 2000s, physicians tried to improve the way they treated chronic pain by prescribing opioids for more people. They believed that by taking the highly addictive drugs only as prescribed for pain control, patients wouldn't become addicted. There are growing rates of addiction to heroin. The reason is that the less-expensive opioid is commonly turned to by addicts for cost reasons or when their pill mill gets shut down.

An opioid is any "opium-like" substance that binds to the opioid receptors in the human brain, which includes heroin but also substances like hydrocodone, oxycodone and morphine found in prescription painkillers. These drugs at certain doses can stop a patient's ability to breathe which may ultimately result in death of a patient.

Drug mills cause drug addiction and destruction to livelihoods, families, and communities. Such characteristics can be far easier to spot and investigate when prescription drug databases are used as mandate. Other states have had vast success in reducing illegal prescriptions when implementing mandatory use of their state prescription drug database. Medical board support for the mandatory use of prescription drug database will go a long way to help take drugs off the streets, protect patients and identify impaired or drug-dealing doctors."

Certain legislation, like Tennessee's Intractable Pain Treatment Act, on the other hand has been accused of establishing a realm where pill mills can flourish. Put into effect in 2001, the Tennessee measure was meant to make drugs, like the newly developed oxycodone, more accessible to patients with cancer and intractable pain. What the act ended up facilitating was an "explosion in use" of prescription painkillers in locales like Sullivan County (which saw 11 pain clinics emerge to meet the demand.

It is against Federal law for a doctor to prescribe pain medication without a legitimate medical purpose or "outside the usual course of medical practice." For example, if a prescription is deemed as not valid, a doctor could be charged with drug trafficking. This is a felony with the possibility of up to life in prison. It is also illegal to practice or prescribe medicine without a license.

Pill mills can have a negative impact on some communities. As mentioned previously, a pill mill is an operation in which a doctor, clinic or pharmacy prescribes and/or dispenses narcotics without a legitimate medical purpose. In a typical Kentucky town, complaints started coming in from business owners neighboring a pill mill, complaining that the parking lots overflow with drug seekers, tailgating while waiting for their appointments and snorting pills outside the buildings.

These are just a few typical signs of the establishment of a pill mill in a community, Remember that a pill mill is an operation in which a doctor, clinic or pharmacy prescribes and/or dispenses narcotics without a legitimate medical purpose. Unlike a typical clinic, it is strictly a cash business. There is no insurance plan and no individualized treatment. If a patient's pain could be eased with physical therapy, injection therapy, braces or surgery, it would not be a treatment option offered in a pill mill.\

Recently the DEA conducted Operation "Pilluted', the largest pharmaceutical drug investigation of all time, where across four southern states over 140 people, mostly doctors and pharmacists, were arrested for their participation in dispensing narcotics without a legitimate medical purpose. Local and state authorities across the Deep South have been working closely with the Drug Enforcement Administration and other federal agencies over the past 15 months to stem the flow of prescription medications flooding the streets. Officials with the DEA New Orleans Field Division said the extensive investigation, dubbed Operation Pilluted, led to the arrest of 22 doctors and pharmacists and 280 other individuals across Arkansas, Alabama, Louisiana and Mississippi.

Agents executed 21 search warrants across the four states during the course of the investigation. Those warrants led to the seizure of 51 vehicles, 202 weapons and $404,828 in cash. Agents also executed 73 seizure warrants that netted more than $11 million in currency and $6.7 million in real property. However, as clinics dispensing oxycodone and hydrocodone are being dismantled, new ones continue to spring up.

Buprenorphine, branded under Suboxone or Subutex, is the latest narcotic being churned out by networks of shady clinics. It also happens to be the very drug that is supposed to help opiate users kick their habit. Suboxone Film contains buprenorphine, an opioid that can cause physical dependence with chronic use. Physical dependence is not the same as addiction.

Kentucky state officials also found the use of buprenorphine increased 241% since 2012 which is the same year many of pill mills selling oxycodone met their demise. That same report found one user who was doctor shopping, obtaining prescriptions from nine different prescribers. Buprenorphine came on to the scene where a cash for pills market was already set, and where practices like doctor shopping through networks of certain doctors were in full swing.

Some doctors now prescribe buprenorphine and other opioids in combination with benzodiazepines. The combination of opioids and benzodiazepines greatly increases the risk of a fatal overdose. When the DEA cracked down on pill mills and other systems of prescription drug abuse, it inadvertently caused users to flock to a ready and waiting supply of cheap heroin. Hence the four-fold increase in heroin-related mortality from 2000-2013, reported by the CDC.

It's worth noting, that most of this mortality spike occurred after 2010, around the time prescription painkillers became more tightly controlled. Many opiate users seek Suboxone to ward off withdrawal symptoms in the event their source runs dry, they run out of money, or are sincerely trying to kick.

In Kentucky, prior to the initial prescribing or dispensing of certain classes of controlled substance, the practitioner shall: Obtain a complete medical history and conduct a physical examination of the patient and document the information in the patient's medical record; Query a physician prescribing data base (called KASPER) for all available data on the patient; Make a written treatment plan stating the objectives of the treatment and further diagnostic examinations required; Discuss the risks and benefits of the use of controlled substances with the patient, including the risk of tolerance and drug dependence; and Obtain written consent for the treatment.

In addition, a practitioner must periodically monitor the course of treatment and query the state physician prescribing data base no less than once every three months before issuing any new prescription refills for the controlled substances. The practitioner must also create and maintain detailed records regarding the patient and the controlled substances prescribed.

The bill also mandates that each health care professional licensing board in the Commonwealth establish regulations regarding controlled substances, including establishing mandatory prescribing and dispensing standards, prohibiting a practitioner from dispensing greater than a forty-eight hour supply of certain controlled substances, and establishing procedures for suspending a practitioner's license to protect patients and the public.

The nationwide surge in deaths now places prescription drug overdoses as the second leading cause of accidental death behind traffic crashes and painkillers as the top narcotic contributing to death. A recent National Drug Assessment study shows that prescription narcotics are the second most abused drug (behind marijuana).

Lawmakers and law enforcers have been cracking down recently on clinics, as well as doctors and pharmacies that illegally or irresponsibly dispense prescription narcotics. These clinics sell prescription drugs to those who have no medical need of them, or in excessive amounts, and have directly contributed to many of the recent restrictions that have been placed on the distribution and availability of prescription drugs. Although they can be found all over the country, they have made most notable headlines in Florida, Kentucky and Texas,

Federal law empowers state medical board inspectors to enter any clinic and inspect its books and procedures. It is important for people to be vigilant when buying prescription drugs from clinics and pharmacies. Some of the most common prescription drugs sold in drug mills include Vicodin, Percocet, and Oxycontin. States that have conducted crackdowns on drug mills have experienced considerably fewer deaths from drug overdoses. Crackdowns on drug mills are some of the most effective ways for states to reduce prescription and narcotic drug overdose death rates.

Pill mill clinics accept cash only. Cash leaves no paper trail for the reporting of income. The patient might not even be seen by a physician or have no physical exam during the visit. In a pill mill no diagnostic X-rays are ordered. There are no referrals for physical therapy, but only a monthly supply of a deadly combo of drugs.

The Hippocratic Oath clearly states, "I will neither give a deadly drug to anybody who asked for it, nor will I make a suggestion to this effect." A study conducted by the Centers for Disease Control and Prevention stated that a relatively small number of doctors were responsible for a large proportion of painkiller prescriptions. Dealers obtain the maximum prescription 240 pills and then turn around and sell the pills. On average, a 30-milligram Oxycodone pill has a street value of about $10 to $12.00. Otherwise, the pill runs $1.42 at a pharmacy, according to a Johns Hopkins University website.

A county in Florida established the following pain clinic rule with respect to opioid prescribing: Requirements of the new law include: Pain clinics must be owned by a doctor, group of doctors or registered under the Agency for Health Care Administration. The Department of Health will conduct annual inspections and document any violations. A physical exam must be performed the same day the prescription is prescribed.

If a doctor prescribes more than a 72-hour supply of medicine for pain, the reason must be documented in the patient's medical record. A doctor cannot dispense more than a 72-hour supply for patients who pay with cash, check or credit card instead of insurance. Doctors must use counterfeit resistant prescription blanks.

While many pain clinics and doctors take their position very seriously and only prescribe drugs after carefully determining their patients' needs, many others are simply getting rich off of other people's drug addiction.

The number of people dying because of prescription and narcotic drugs overdose has risen significantly and drug mills are a major source of this problem. Below are the states that had the most providers prescribing 3,000 prescriptions for Schedule 2 controlled substances in 2012 in Medicare Part D, per ProPublica: Florida: 52 providers, Tennessee: 25 providers, North Carolina: 15 providers, Ohio:15 providers, Georgia:14 providers, Pennsylvania: 12 providers, Alabama:12 providers, Kentucky: 11 providers, Oklahoma:, Arizona, Arkansas and Texas 9

There are different ways to curb prescription drug abuse. The first way has already been taking place across the country, which is to arrest and charge doctors that operate pill mills. It is also necessary to more closely monitor patients who use prescription painkillers, through better regulations at clinics or doctors' offices, or through a prescription drug database. Only a small numbers of pain clinics actually fill a very large amount of oxycodone prescriptions compared to those filled at pharmacies.

While legitimate pain management clinics do exist to serve those with chronic pain or terminal illness, other unscrupulous clinics, called pill mills, merely serve only as drug traffickers. Remember that the common characteristics of pill mills as previously mentioned include: cash only/no insurance; no appointments; armed guards; little or no medical records; grossly inadequate physical examinations; and large prescription doses of narcotics that exceed the boundaries of acceptable medical care.

The drug contract patient doctor agreements may require patients to submit to blood or urine drug tests, fill their prescriptions at a single pharmacy or refuse to accept pain medication from any other doctor. If patients don't follow the rules, the agreements often state that doctors may drop them from their practice.

Pain is such a nebulous pathology that it's hard to point a finger and rightfully accuse a pain management doctor for harming a patient by prescribing the medications. It could very well be that the patient really does need that drug in order to function in life, especially in chronic pain patients. However, it could be that patient is an addict and the doctor is reinforcing that behavior for the business. For the latter case, it is a criminal act. However, it's very difficult to prove such intentions.

Before a pain clinic accepts a chronic pain patient, a patient should have to fulfill basic criteria: Be over 21 years old, have pain greater than 3 months in duration and be anticipated to continue on pain management indefinitely. A patient must have a verifiable (laboratory tests, CT or MRI evaluations) and pathological problem that is severe enough to qualify he/she as a chronic pain patient. Furthermore a patient must agree to pursue therapies that can alleviate their pain (e.g. physical therapy, behavioral therapy, weight loss, regular exercise and smoking cessation).

      Patient intake documentation must be completed and verified. The patient must furthermore agree to regular drug testing. Pain medicine is absolutely not about prescribing opioids. It's about treating the whole patient. Anyone who suspects a pail mill should report it to local authorities. Pain management is a delicate balance. It's difficult to help a patent regain his or her quality of life and keep them from becoming addicted. However, this action could save a life.

37. HOSPITAL PAIN MANAGEMENT

Pain is a major barrier to engaging patients during their hospital stay and after they are discharged. Healthcare professionals must be familiar with their hospital policies and openly discuss pain control with patients and their families. They must furthermore, be aware that different cultures have differing tolerance of or willingness to reveal pain. Pain management must address both the physical and emotional symptoms of pain.

Pain medicine may not get rid of all pain. It should keep the pain at a level that lets a patient move around, eat and breathe easily. Pain medicines may be given as a pill or a liquid to swallow, a shot or through an IV line or an epidural catheter in the spine.

Unfortunately malnutrition in a hospital can be a source of a patient's pain as well. A high level of malnutrition has been reported in adults in hospital and is linked to poor clinical outcome. Almost 50% of patients are malnourished on hospital admission. Many others develop malnutrition during admission. Malnutrition contributes to hospital morbidity, mortality, costs, and readmissions. The prevalence of pain on the inpatient medical ward is lower than that of a surgical service, but is still substantial. In one hospital survey, 43% of medical ward patients experienced pain, and 12% reported unbearable pain.

Optimal pain care for hospitalized patients continues to remain elusive. Only 63-74% of hospitalized patients nationwide reported that their pain was well controlled. Pain control in a hospital setting typically involves the use of opioid medications and other pharmaceutical drugs that produce side effects such as respiratory depression, clouded mentation, hypotension, nausea, constipation, dizziness, and falls.

Integrative care reduces immediate pain levels by more than 50% and that it can be provided as part of routine clinical care across numerous patient populations. Malnutrition is an under-recognized problem in hospitalized patients. Nutrition support is recognized as an important cofactor in altering morbidity and mortality of hospitalized patients. Malnutrition in hospitals remains a serious issue. It occurs worldwide and affects patients of all ages. Almost 50% of patients are malnourished on hospital admission; many others develop malnutrition during admission.

The prevalence of malnutrition for older adults (>65 years) in hospital and rehabilitation units has been reported as being as high as 60%; some older patients with good appetites do not receive sufficient nourishment because of inadequate feeding assistance. Malnutrition contributes to hospital morbidity, mortality, costs, and readmissions. The Joint Commission requires malnutrition risk screening on admission. Disease states and acute events predispose patients to malnutrition, the degree of which is usually determined by the severity of the illness.

The Joint Commission is an independent, not-for-profit group in the United States that administers accreditation programs for hospitals and other healthcare-related organizations. The Commission develops performance standards that address crucial elements of operation, such as patient care, medication safety, and infection control and consumer rights. The Joint Commission standards function as the foundation for healthcare organizations to gauge and enhance their performance. These standards focus on quality care and patient safety.

The Joint Commission develops standards criteria based on feedback and interactions with consumers, healthcare professionals and government agencies. The Joint Commission requires malnutrition risk screening on hospital admission. If screening identifies malnutrition risk, a nutrition assessment is required to create a nutrition care plan. The Joint Commission has mandated universal screening and assessment of hospitalized patients for malnutrition since 1995.

The plan should be initiated early in the hospital course, as even patients with normal nutrition become malnourished quickly when acutely ill. Patients with inadequate intake over time may develop potentially fatal refeeding syndrome. Ae hospitalist must be able to recognize the risk factors for malnutrition, patients at risk of refeeding syndrome, and the optimal route for nutrition support. Finally, education of patients and their caregivers about nutrition support must begin before discharge, and include coordination of care with outpatient facilities.

Malnutrition in hospitals remains a serious issue. It occurs worldwide and affects patients of all ages. Patients who are at risk for malnutrition related complications (MRCs) must be identified. The characteristics that correlated best with malnutrition-related complications risk level assignment were occurrence of a wound, poor oral intake, malnutrition-related admission diagnosis, serum albumin value, hemoglobin value, and total lymphocyte count.

A model using four variables (malnutrition-related admission diagnosis, serum albumin value, hemoglobin value, and total lymphocyte count) was almost as good as that using six predictors. The ability of admission information to accurately reflect MRC risk is crucial to early initiation of restorative medical nutritional therapy.

For years, physicians have attempted to improve the metabolic status of patients after surgery or trauma. Currently, major emphasis is placed on perioperative nutritional status and its effect on postoperative wound healing. It is suggested that the issue of nutrition in hospitals is of concern and that there are numerous factors which contribute to this. However, this aspect of patient care is not identified as the specific responsibility of hospital staff. Nurses should play a pivotal role in preventing malnutrition in hospital but, in most cases, they do not.

Vague musculoskeletal complaints in these chronically ill patients may be attributed to multiple underlying disease processes rather than a deficiency in vitamin D.4 some hospital formularies continue to provide multivitamin supplements that contain less vitamin D than currently is recommended.

Hypovitaminosis C and D are highly prevalent in acutely hospitalized patients, but the clinical significance of these biochemical abnormalities is not known. Because deficiencies of vitamin C and D have been linked to psychologic abnormalities, vitamin C or D provision could improve the mood state of acutely hospitalized patients. Treatment of hypovitaminosis C improves the mood state of acutely hospitalized patients.5

Unintentional weight loss is used as a reliable indicator of malnutrition. Peripheral parenteral nutrition is an alternative when caloric intake is impossible or insufficient or refused by the patient, as it minimizes the complications of the central catheter.

Serum phosphate levels are associated with anemia in hospitalized patients. Maintaining optimal phosphate reduces the likelihood of anemia and whether ideal phosphate during acute care hospitalization influences clinical outcomes.

Nutritional support should be considered in people who are malnourished, as defined by any of the following: A body mass index (BMI) of less than 18.5 kg/m2, unintentional weight loss greater than 10% within the preceding 3-6 months, and A BMI of less than 20 kg/m2 .The most obvious medical conditions that contribute to malnutrition include those that are those that prevent oral food intake, such as oral cancer, tumors or strictures in the throat or esophagus, stroke, and degenerative neurologic disorders that result in dysphagia.

Trauma patients and others who are ventilator dependent rely on the timely initiation of nutrition support. Conditions such as chronic obstructive pulmonary disease, chronic infections, and cancer can result in increased metabolic demand and weight loss due to cachexia and poor oral intake.

Any patient identified to be at risk should have a nutrition assessment, using information on weight and weight changes, food intake, gastrointestinal symptoms, functional capacity, disease state, physical characteristics, and symptoms of micronutrient deficiencies. There is increasing awareness that chronic wound healing is very dependent on the patient's nutritional status.

The anesthesiologist's involvement in perioperative medicine has significantly changed. In order to identify patients at risks of perioperative complications, the anesthesiologist has to consider, amongst others, screening and management of undernutrition. In other words, the anesthesiologist could play an important role in undernutrition screening and its management in order to reduce perioperative morbidity.

With the move to a more integrated curriculum and problem-based learning at many medical schools, a substantial portion of the total nutrition instruction is occurring outside courses specifically dedicated to nutrition. The amount of nutrition education in medical schools remains inadequate.

The primary mission of the Nutrition in Medicine (NIM) project is to provide tools to facilitate the nutrition training of undergraduate medical students. These innovative strategies should allow a better fit of NIM within diverse medical school environments and help to promote incorporation of the curriculum into more medical schools.

A high level of malnutrition has been reported in adults in hospital and is linked to poor clinical outcome. Almost 50% of patients are malnourished on hospital admission. Many others develop malnutrition during admission. Malnutrition contributes to hospital morbidity, mortality, costs, and readmissions.

Malnutrition is an under-recognized problem in hospitalized patients. Nutrition support is recognized as an important cofactor in altering morbidity and mortality of hospitalized patients. Malnutrition in hospitals remains a serious issue. It occurs worldwide and affects patients of all ages. Almost 50% of patients are malnourished on hospital admission; many others develop malnutrition during admission.

The prevalence of malnutrition for older adults (>65 years) in hospital and rehabilitation units has been reported as being as high as

60%; some older patients with good appetites do not receive sufficient nourishment because of inadequate feeding assistance.

Malnutrition contributes to hospital morbidity, mortality, costs, and readmissions. The Joint Commission requires malnutrition risk screening on admission. Disease states and acute events predispose patients to malnutrition, the degree of which is usually determined by the severity of the illness.

The Joint Commission requires malnutrition risk screening on admission. If screening identifies malnutrition risk, a nutrition assessment is required to create a nutrition care plan. The Joint Commission has mandated universal screening and assessment of hospitalized patients for malnutrition since 1995.

The plan should be initiated early in the hospital course, as even patients with normal nutrition become malnourished quickly when acutely ill. Patients with inadequate intake over time may develop potentially fatal refeeding syndrome.

The hospitalist must be able to recognize the risk factors for malnutrition, patients at risk of refeeding syndrome, and the optimal route for nutrition support. Finally, education of patients and their caregivers about nutrition support must begin before discharge, and include coordination of care with outpatient facilities.

Malnutrition in hospitals remains a serious issue. It occurs worldwide and affects patients of all ages. Patients who are at risk for malnutrition-related complications (MRCs) must be identified. The characteristics that correlated best with malnutrition-related complications risk level assignment were occurrence of a wound, poor oral intake, malnutrition-related admission diagnosis, serum albumin value, hemoglobin value, and total lymphocyte count.

A model using four variables (malnutrition-related admission diagnosis, serum albumin value, hemoglobin value, and total lymphocyte count) was almost as good as that using six predictors. The ability of admission information to accurately reflect MRC risk is crucial to early initiation of restorative medical nutritional therapy.

For years, physicians have attempted to improve the metabolic status of patients after surgery or trauma. Currently, major emphasis is placed on perioperative nutritional status and its effect on postoperative wound healing.

It is suggested that the issue of nutrition in hospitals is of concern and that there are numerous factors which contribute to this. However, this aspect of patient care is not identified as the specific responsibility of hospital staff. Nurses should play a pivotal role in preventing malnutrition in hospital but, in most cases, they do not.

Vague musculoskeletal complaints in these chronically ill patients may be attributed to multiple underlying disease processes rather than a deficiency in vitamin D.4 some hospital formularies continue to provide multivitamin supplements that contain less vitamin D than currently is recommended.

Hypovitaminosis C and D are highly prevalent in acutely hospitalized patients, but the clinical significance of these biochemical abnormalities is not known. Because deficiencies of vitamin C and D have been linked to psychologic abnormalities, vitamin C or D provision could improve the mood state of acutely hospitalized patients. Treatment of hypovitaminosis C improves the mood state of acutely hospitalized patients.

Pain management is a crucial issue for patients, and patients' perception of care is an important quality outcome criterion for health care institutions. Pain remains a common problem in hospitals, with subsequent deleterious effects on well-being.Unintentional weight loss is used as a reliable indicator of malnutrition. Peripheral parenteral nutrition is an alternative when caloric intake is impossible or insufficient or refused by the patient, as it minimizes the complications of the central catheter.

Serum phosphate levels are associated with anemia in hospitalized patients. Maintaining optimal phosphate reduces the likelihood of anemia and whether ideal phosophate during acute care hospitalization influences clinical outcomes. Nutritional support should be considered in people who are malnourished, as defined by any of the following: A body mass index (BMI) of less than 18.5 kg/m2, unintentional weight loss greater than 10% within the preceding 3-6 months, and A BMI of less than 20 kg/m2 .

The most obvious medical conditions that contribute to malnutrition include those that are those that prevent oral food intake, such as oral cancer, tumors or strictures in the throat or esophagus, stroke, and degenerative neurologic disorders that result in dysphagia.

Trauma patients and others who are ventilator dependent rely on the timely initiation of nutrition support. Conditions such as chronic obstructive pulmonary disease, chronic infections, and cancer can result in increased metabolic demand and weight loss due to cachexia and poor oral intake.

Any patient identified to be at risk should have a nutrition assessment, using information on weight and weight changes, food intake, gastrointestinal symptoms, functional capacity, disease state, physical characteristics, and symptoms of micronutrient deficiencies. There is increasing awareness that chronic wound healing is very dependent on the patient's nutritional status.

The anesthesiologist's involvement in perioperative medicine has significantly changed. In order to identify patients at risks of perioperative complications, the anesthesiologist has to consider, amongst others, screening and management of undernutrition. In other words, the anesthesiologist could play an important role in undernutrition screening and its management in order to reduce perioperative morbidity.

With the move to a more integrated curriculum and problem-based learning at many medical schools, a substantial portion of the total nutrition instruction is occurring outside courses specifically dedicated to nutrition. The amount of nutrition education in medical schools remains inadequate.

The primary mission of the Nutrition in Medicine (NIM) project is to provide tools to facilitate the nutrition training of undergraduate medical students. These innovative strategies should allow a better fit of NIM within diverse medical school environments and help to promote incorporation of the curriculum into more medical schools.Pain was both prevalent and severe in the hospital, but patient participation in decision making was related to better outcomes. Optimal pain management, with emphasis on patient participation in decision making, should be encouraged in an effort to improve the quality of care in hospitals.

Although professional knowledge and attitudes about pain and nursing pain assessment rates have been shown to be improvable, no systematic, hospital-wide intervention has yet to be associated with improvement in pain severity. Future research on the development of new interventions, perhaps targeted specifically at physicians, is urgently needed.

Healthcare professionals must be familiar with their hospital policies and openly discuss pain control with patients and their families. Consult with patients about methods that have and have not worked well in the past. Patients also should have a chance to voice their concerns about medications and how to administer them. When appropriate, healthcare professionals should discuss their roles in managing pain and the potential limitations and side effects of treatment with patients and their families.

The American Nurses Association (ANA) differentiates between medication and non-medication pain management. Teaching patients breathing exercises and the benefits of massage, positioning, cold pack care, and relaxation can be used to decrease pain in a hospital setting as well as emphasizing proper nutrition.

38. PALATIVE CARE

Palliative Care is a relatively new medical specialty. The goal of palliative care is to improve the quality of life for patients as well as their families. Palliative care is appropriate at any point in an illness. Palliative care can be provided at the same time as conventional treatment that is meant to cure you. Palliative care is dedicated to maximizing a person's comfort, independence, and quality of life when the prolongation of life is no longer a realistic goal. More than 50% of dying patients do not receive adequate symptomatic relief. Fear of hastening death is the primary reason for physicians' reluctance to prescribe high-dose pain medication.

Hospice became a Medicare benefit in 1983 for people with terminal conditions who had less than six months to live. A surge of public support eventually led to a government benefit that allowed patients to forgo heroic lifesaving measures in return for comfort measures and the opportunity to die at home. Medicare pays hospices about $154 a day for people with terminal medical problems who receive care at home, the most popular option. For providers, there are few quality standards to meet and no minimum requirements for how often to provide care.

Palliative care and. hospice care are similar but different. Palliative care focuses on relief from physical suffering. The patient may be being treated for a disease or may be living with a chronic disease, and may or may not be terminally ill. It uses life prolonging medications. Hospice care makes the patient comfortable and prepares the patient and the patient's family for the patient's end of life when it is determined treatment for the illness will no longer be pursued. It does not use life-prolonging medications.

Hospice care is not designed to extend life, so the treatment offered is not intended to cure, but rather to provide comfort. Still, fewer patients have been dying within Medicare's six-month guideline. The principal incentive the hospice has is to keep its census high. For a hospice, death means money. From 1992 to 1998, the number of Medicare beneficiaries who used hospice care more than doubled, from 143,000 in 1992 to 360,000 in 1998. One of the areas under constant federal scrutiny is the length of time that patients stay in a hospice before they die. Hospices must be able to prove to regulators that the end was near for each patient.

No one knows how big the problem of hospice fraud is and all types of improper Medicare payments are estimated at $65 billion for 2010 but federal investigators prosecuted more than 60 cases in the last year alone, involving hundreds of millions of dollars nationwide. The system that was built to help dying patients live out their remaining days with dignity and comfort has few quality metrics to meet, no minimum requirements for how often care is provided, and low barriers to getting into the business. Critics say that can make end-of-life care seem ripe for abuse.

Palliative care is the active total care of patients whose disease is not amenable to curative treatment. Control of a patient's pain and other symptoms, and of psychological, social, and spiritual problems is mandatory. The goal is achievement of the best possible quality of life for patients and their families.

Palliative care aims to relieve symptoms such as pain, shortness of breath, fatigue, constipation, nausea, loss of appetite and difficulty sleeping. It helps patients gain the strength to carry on with daily life. It improves their ability to tolerate medical treatments. And it helps them better understand their choices for care. The goal of palliative care is to offer patients the best possible quality of life during their illness.

Palliative care is not the same as hospice care. Palliative care may be provided at any time during a person's illness, even from the time of diagnosis. And, it may be given at the same time as curative treatment. Hospice care always includes palliative care. However, it is focused on terminally ill patients-people who no longer seek treatments to cure them and who are expected to live for about six months or less. Palliative care affirms life and regards dying as a normal natural process. It neither hastens nor postpones death.

Palliative care provides relief from pain and psychological symptoms. Its goal is to integrate the psychological and spiritual aspects of a patient's care. It offers a support system to help patients live as actively as possible until their death. It offers a support system to help families cope during the patient's illness.

Palliative care is not provided by one physician but by a team of experts, including palliative care doctors, nurses and social workers. Chaplains, neuropaths, massage therapists, pharmacists, nutritionists and others are also a part of the team. Palliative care can be provided when you are at home, in an assisted living facility, nursing facility or hospital. Palliative care in contrast to hospice care is not just for patients who are very close to death.

Palliative care is therefore, more than health care just for dying persons. Palliative care is a health care philosophy aimed at improving the essence of life when cure is no longer possible. Palliative care is a health care discipline with its own research knowledge base and a specific set of skills aimed at pain and other forms of suffering which becomes the major focus of treatment.

A former hospice chief operating officer has been under indictment in federal court in Pittsburgh on charges of inflating enrollment at her company's facility by recruiting patients who often weren't really dying. In the Horizons case, prosecutors say the CEO. Stewart was pressuring her employees to recruit anyone they could find including people at bus stops in an inner-city. The goal was to keep the census high in order to bill Medicare and Medicaid for millions.

Federal prosecutors are seeking $202 million from West Allis, Wis.-based AseraCare Inc., where they allege nurses and other staff were instructed to increase hospice census "at all costs" and the mere suspicion of lung cancer was enough to enroll a patient for end of life care.

The American Board of Anesthesiology has subspecialty certification in palliative care. Palliative care is totally defined by prognosis but by what it inspires, offers, and achieves. A patient does not have to be dying to have palliative care. Palliative care is in addition to providing medical care, is also a provider of paramedical support services. Palliative care ensures informed choices be offered to patients.

The management of pain is an important aspect of palliative care. The patient must be regarded as a living person and therefore the full human experiences; physical, emotional, and spiritual, must be addressed. A patient must not die with severe pain. The patient must be comfortable.

Most important a patient must be able to live out his or hers last moment as fully and consciously as possible. In fact palliative care should make dying to be a patient's finest hour. A dying patient is unique and should be treated as someone special.

Palliative care is any form of medical care or treatment that concentrates on reducing the severity of disease symptoms rather than trying to seek a cure. he goal is to prevent and relieve suffering and to improve quality of life for people facing serious, complex illnesses. It should not be confused with hospice care which delivers palliative care to those at the end of life. In essence, palliative care provides care to those with life limiting illness at any stage of their disease.

Given that no two people are alike, if you are taking any medications and begin to take nutritional supplements you should be aware that potential drug-nutrient interactions may occur and are encouraged to consult a health care professional before using any natural product. Combining certain prescription drugs and dietary supplements can lead to undesirable effects such as: diminished prescription drug effectiveness, reduced supplement effectiveness and impaired drug and/or supplement absorption.

The foundations of good nutrition, exercise, stress reduction, and reengagement in life can contribute much to restoring the quality of life to a pain patient.1

Nutrition in palliative care and at the end of life should be one of the goals for improving quality of life. It is important to address issues of food and feeding at this time to assist in the management of troublesome symptoms as well as to enhance the remaining life. Cancer and its treatments exert a major impact upon physical and psychological reserves and at the end of life problems with appetite and the ability to eat and drink compound such impact.

Previous studies have shown that the dietary habits of cancer patients and survivors have significant implications for their recovery and quality of life. Nutrition and eating behaviors have a significant effect on cancer patients' physical and emotional adjustment. The aims of nutritional care minimize food-related discomfort and maximize food enjoyment. Ethical questions will be raised concerning the provision of food and fluids to a person nearing the end of their life. Nurses need to acknowledge that food has greater significance than the provision of nutrients.

The Office of Inspector General (OIG) has issued a special fraud alert, alerting the public to the high potential for fraud between hospices and nursing home operators.

Medicare provides palliative care in the form of hospice benefits to individuals who are terminally ill. That means the emphasis is on pain control, symptom management, and individualized counseling for not only the patient but her family too. The hospice must meet level and type of service requirements as well and have a written plan to fulfill them. Typical service requirements include physician and nursing services, speech, physical and occupational therapy, counseling and respite care as examples.

Although some of the core hospice services must be provided by the hospice directly to the beneficiary, others may be provided by other caregivers. However all must be under the management of the hospice provider. The largest area for potential abuse in this cozy relationship between hospices and nursing homes stems from the nursing home's control over whom it will allow to provide hospice services in its facilities.

A hospice can derive substantial and recurring revenue if it has an ongoing exclusive contract to serve a large nursing home's patient base. This situation is ripe for the offer or request of financial kickbacks, incentives and other lucrative means to both parties. An OIG study showed that it's sometimes the case that nursing home hospice patients receive fewer services than their home-bound counterparts. And since hospice providers are paid a flat rate, providing fewer services may positively affect their profitability and lessen their operating costs.

As in many health care fields, kickbacks are strictly prohibited by federal health care program, including Medicare and Medicaid. The ant kickback statute strictly prohibits the solicitation, receipt, offer or payment of "anything of value" to induce referrals of items or services payable by any federal health care program.

One particular area the OIG has observed as a potential source of abuse is when a hospice is paid a higher daily rate for a patient it refers to a nursing home. The law states that a hospice patient should be charged no more than if he had been enrolled as a non-hospice patient. Hospice patient referral to a nursing home as an inducement to the nursing home to its patients to the hospice is not legal.

In Metro Detroit, the arrested included six doctors, a social worker, a pharmacist and two physical therapists. According to officials, the schemes involved medical services that were unnecessary or never rendered, including hospice and home health care plus the billing, but not dispersal, of drugs. Authorities said the owners of home health care and hospice companies in Metro Detroit, two of whom are physical therapists, allegedly paid kickbacks to doctors and recruiters for referring patients to them, then billed Medicare for unnecessary services.

In another case, the administrator and part owner of a hospice orchestrated an extensive scheme to fraudulently bill Medicare and Medicaid for millions of dollars by falsifying the level of hospice care provided for patients at nursing homes which he controlled.

According to the charges, this administrator trained nurses to look for signs that allegedly would qualify a hospice patient for general inpatient care, resulting in payments per day more than four times higher than routine care rates. In many instances, patients were not terminally ill and wound up enrolled in hospice care far longer than the required life expectancy of six months or less.

In another case, the government contends that since at least 2007, a Texas-based hospice has fraudulently certified patients as terminally ill to illegally collect Medicare payments. The United States alleges that the hospice through its reckless business practices, admitted and retained individuals who were not eligible to receive Medicare hospice benefits, because it was financially lucrative and this hospice misspent millions of Medicare dollars intended for Medicare recipients."

In some instances, patients were admitted to hospice care, then discharged just before the date at which the patient would reach the Medicare payment cap. That individual is then placed in the company's nursing home facilities until that Medicare cap is reached, before being admitted once again to its hospice care.

The government is increasing scrutiny on these fraudulent institutions and increasing the incidence of prosecution.

39. RSD

According to the National Institute of Neurological Disorders and Stroke (NINDS), RSD is "a chronic pain condition that is believed to be the result of dysfunction in the central or peripheral nervous systems. RSD usually affects one of the extremities (arm, leg, hand, or foot). The primary symptom of RSD is intense, continuous pain. Reflex sympathetic dystrophy (RSD) affects one or more of your arms or legs but also can affect your face following a tooth extraction. Reflex sympathetic dystrophy is now called the Complex Regional Pain Syndrome (CRPS). Reflex sympathetic dystrophy is serious, painful, and potentially disabling. Pain associated with this entity is throbbing, burning, or aching.

A patient's clinical history (signs and symptoms) are the major factor in diagnosing RSD. The diagnosis is made difficult because many of the symptoms overlap with other conditions. There is no specific blood test or other diagnostic tests for RSD. X-rays may show thinning of bones (osteoporosis) and nuclear bone scans may show characteristic uptake patterns which help diagnose RSD.

You can have pain just to light touch (allodynia). You can have swelling of one or more of your extremities as well as either warmth or coldness depending on the phase of your RSD and sweating also occurs on the palms of your hands or the soles of your feet. Your hair may grow faster on the extremity with RSD at first, only to progress to loss of hair on your arm or leg. Your extremity will sweat if you have RSD. It can turn color. The nails in your affected limb can grow faster on the extremity that suffers from reflex sympathetic dystrophy.

Reflex sympathetic dystrophy usually occurs following an injury. However, a heart attack or stroke can also trigger reflex sympathetic dystrophy. It can be seen in the knee as well as in the shoulder. Reflex sympathetic dystrophy occurs in 40 percent of the cases followed an injury to a muscle or a nerve. Simple bruises or sprains can also trigger reflex sympathetic dystrophy.

Fractures accounted for 25 percent of reflex sympathetic dystrophy cases. Twenty percent of the RSD patients were postoperative on an arm or leg, whereas 12 percent occurred after a heart attack. Three percent occurred after a stroke. Approximately 37 percent of patients in the study had emotional disturbances at the time of the onset of the reflex sympathetic dystrophy.

It was once thought that reflex sympathetic dystrophy was caused by an emotional problem. Many people do not suffer from emotional problems at the time of the onset of reflex sympathetic dystrophy. Treatment usually consists of oral medications as well as injection therapy by an anesthesiologist using local anesthetics. Steroids may also be used effectively to treat RSD. If you sustained actual nerve damage, your reflex sympathetic dystrophy is called causalgia or complex regional pain syndrome II. Complex regional pain syndrome I does not have a nerve injury associated with it.

Reflex sympathetic dystrophy is a syndrome that consists of burning pain, pain to touch over the skin of the injured extremity, shiny skin, and skin that has different colors consisting of either redness or a blue cyanotic color. Blue or cyanotic discoloration usually occurs when skin or other tissues do not get enough blood and oxygen. With this disease, the pain in your extremity is out of proportion to your injury.

It was originally hypothesized that if your sympathetic nervous sys-tem became hyperactive, this hyperactivity caused of reflex sympathetic dystrophy. Your sympathetic nervous system is one component of your autonomic nervous system. The other component is called the para-sympathetic nervous system. Your autonomic nervous system regulates your circulation and your breathing as well as your stomach and bladder functions. You have no control over your autonomic nervous system.

Your sympathetic nervous system sends sympathetic nerve fibers to the blood vessels in your head and neck as well as to your skin, muscles and sweat glands in your arms and legs. Your hands and feet can sweat profusely if you have reflex sympathetic dystrophy and the hair on your arms and legs can grow faster or fall out. Your sympathetic nerve fibers can also restrict circulation in certain areas of your body. Sometimes if your doctor blocks your sympathetic nerve pathways with a numbing medicine, you can have some relief of your reflex sympathetic dystrophy.

The treatment of reflex sympathetic dystrophy includes weekly repetitive sympathetic blocks up to 5 or 6 or removal of the sympathetic nerves, either surgically or by chemicals such as phenol or by intense heat. Sympathetic blocks involve placing a local anesthetic about the bundles of nerves that exist outside of your central nervous system.

These nerve bundles that are called ganglia are in your neck as well as your lower back. The ganglion in your neck influences your arm pain- while your ganglion in your lower back influences RSD pain in your leg.

For you to be diagnosed with RSD, you should have the following: An initiating traumatic event to your body (e.g. bone fracture), an onset of spontaneous pain, excruciating pain to light touch (allodynia) as well as pain from a noxious stimulus that lasts longer than expected. Your pain must be global and not just confined to a specific area.

For example, if you have injured your hand, you may have an injury to one of the nerves in your hand. Your ulnar nerve will give you pain or numbness in your last two fingers of your hand if this nerve is affected. This is the definition of a neuritis that means inflammation of a nerve. This is not RSD. This is an example of neuralgia. RSD means that the whole hand (global) is painful and not just in the distribution of one nerve.

Other signs of reflex sympathetic dystrophy include evidence of swelling of your extremity, an increase or a decrease in your skin blood flow noted by imaging as well as alterations in the color of your skin and sweating. Cold applications to your skin can worsen your pain. Movement of your joints can also cause pain if you have RSD. You skin may be shiny. Your nails should grow faster on the side of the reflex sympathetic dystrophy. At first your hair will grow faster on the side of your reflex sympathetic dystrophy but eventually your hair pattern will decrease and you may even lose hair in this area.

Tremors or spasms may be noted on the side of your reflex sympathetic dystrophy. If you have complex regional pain syndrome, you should also have complaints of stiffness at the joints where your fingers meet your hand or where your toes meet your foot. Some physicians can over diagnose complex regional pain syndrome.

Unfortunately, some surgeons call botched surgery that they did that had a bad outcome RSD. They will make a presumptive diagnosis of RSD rather than admit that he or she caused a problem. This situation however, is rare.

RSD must be treated immediately once it has been diagnosed. If you have any of these symptoms mentioned in this chapter, notify your doctor. A three-phase bone scan can be useful in diagnosing reflex sympathetic dystrophy (figure 1). This imagery is related to the distribution of a radioactive isotope throughout the body, and a nuclear medicine doctor will examine the distribution of the radioactive isotope in the affected extremity.

The distribution of the radioactive isotope is dependent upon blood flow as well as the activity of the bone. In early RSD, you will have increased blood flow and after 3 months your blood flow will be decreased. If your three-phase bone scan is negative, this does not mean that you do not have reflex sympathetic dystrophy. A three-phase bone scan may be effective for staging the early or late forms of RSD. Magnetic resonance imaging (MRI) can also aid in the diagnosis of RSD by identifying swelling in the center of your bone. This bone marrow edema is characteristic of complex regional pain syndrome. This study is more reliable than a three-phase bone scanning or plain X-ray exams.

Contact and infrared thermography have both been used for the diagnosis of reflex sympathetic dystrophy, but the problem with thermography is that it can be influenced not only by skin blood flow but also by the temperature of the room environment as well as by your muscle and your deep tissue metabolism. A new method called laser Doppler imaging has been shown to be effective for the diagnosis of complex regional pain syndrome. The laser Doppler is important because the results of this study are influenced by your skin blood flow. Your skin blood flow is under the control of your autonomic nervous system.

After you have sustained an injury to your extremity, the blood vessels to your extremity initially increase in caliber. This allows more blood flow to go to your extremity. Your hand or foot will therefore, feel warm and may appear to be red. This phase usually occurs within the first month of your injury. A three-phase bone scan at this time will demonstrate increased isotope activity in your extremity, which indicates phase 1 reflex sympathetic dystrophy.

As your RSD progresses, the blood vessels to your extremity will de-crease in caliber. They go from their enlarged diameter to a normal appearing diameter. This is phase II. You will have some swelling as well at this time and global pain about your extremity and sweating of your extremity as your sympathetic nervous system becomes overactive. This phase can progress on to phase III.

During phase III, your blood vessels become extremely small and you have decreased blood flow to your hand, foot, or your affected extremity. This will cause your skin to become cold. By this time, you will notice that your skin has become shiny and that the sweating in your hand or foot may have increased. A three-phase bone scan at this time can detect a significant decrease in your blood flow to your extremity. Your treating doctor should try and prevent you from progressing through these phases by being aggressive in his or her treatment.

Be aware that on rare occasions RSD can spread into more than one extremity. If you have chronic RSD, you can have skin infections associated with persistent swelling of your skin as well as blood vessels that can spontaneously rupture. You may have a change in skin pigmentation and your fingernails or pump, which sends a narcotic into your spinal fluid, needs to be implanted to control your RSD pain.

Clonidine, which is frequently prescribed as a patch over your skin, can also be administered into your epidural space for the control of your pain as well. Baclofen or a snail toxin toenails on the affected extremity can become thick and clubbed.

The frequency of reflex sympathetic dystrophy shows a peak incidence of this entity around 50 years of age. However, you must be aware that both children and elderly individuals can develop RSD. RSD can be refractive to treatment with sympathetic blockade. This type of RSD is called sympathetically independent pain. RSD related pain that responds to sympathetic blockade is classified as sympathetically maintained pain. Sympathetically maintained pain usually has a decrease in your pain component following a sympathetic block. The onset of reflex sympathetic dystrophy can occur at any time following a traumatic event ranging from days to months.

The exact cause of reflex sympathetic dystrophy is unknown. If you have had a nerve injury where your nerve was cut, your nerve endings will attempt to grow together. The nerve endings will sprout small nerve fibers. Sometimes as your nerves attempt to grow together, the area where they come together can be extremely painful. Where the nerve endings come together can cause an extremely painful area called a neuroma. This neuroma is sensitive to the chemicals released by your sympathetic nervous system.

Females are more vulnerable to sympathetically mediated pain than males. The chemicals that are involved that cause you to have reflex sympathetic dystrophy are potentially affected by your sex hormones. It is believed that your hormone status at the time of your trauma is important for the development of the pain associated with reflex sympathetic dystrophy.

The effects of reflex sympathetic dystrophy on the central processing in your central nervous system may be the basis for the spread of reflex sympathetic dystrophy to your other extremities. Many recommendations for the treatment of reflex sympathetic dystrophy exist. Because there are so many different treatments proposed, you should be aware that no single treatment is superior to the others. Remember that no treatment for complex regional pain syndrome is consistently successful.

It is known that early recognition and active treatment of the complex regional pain syndrome improves your outcome. For example, injections of local anesthetics about your sympathetic nervous system can alleviate your symptoms of reflex sympathetic dystrophy for weeks to months.

In some instances the relief may be permanent. These types of injections must be done early following the onset of your symptoms of reflex sympathetic dystrophy. The injections can be done in your stellate ganglion, which provides sympathetic fibers to your arms, or the injections can be done in the lumbar sympathetic ganglion, which supplies sympathetic fibers to your legs and feet.

A clonidine patch can be used to decrease your pain. This patch is usually used to treat high blood pressure. However, the patch does decrease the sympathetic nervous system chemicals that can be released if you have reflex sympathetic dystrophy. The patch is usually worn for one week before it is changed.

Steroids administered by mouth are effective for the treatment of re-flex sympathetic dystrophy. Steroids will decrease inflammation caused by prostaglandins. If your pain is severe, your doctor will probably prescribe a narcotic drug for you. Depending on the severity of your pain, your doctor will prescribe a mild narcotic such as Darvocet (propoxyphene) or a stronger narcotic such as methadone.

Anticonvulsive medications can be helpful in decreasing your pain. Gabapentin (Neurontin) is frequently used now for the treatment of pain associated with your complex regional pain syndrome.

Narcotic medications administered into your spinal fluid can help decrease your pain. Sometimes a morphine (Prialt) placed in the pump may also decrease your pain. Antidepressant medications such as amitriptyline have also been shown to be effective. Amitriptyline increases certain chemicals in your central nervous system that are helpful in decreasing the amount of pain that reaches your brain. Implantation of an electrical spinal wire attached to a battery into your epidural space can also provide you with significant pain relief. This apparatus is called a dorsal column stimulator.

Psychological intervention is also helpful; because of the severity of the pain associated with reflex sympathetic dystrophy, you can develop fear, anxiety, and depression. Psychological intervention including the use of biofeedback and sometimes hypnosis can successfully be used to treat your pain.

A technologically advanced solution for chronic pain management. It is reported to be effective in the treatment of CRPS/RSD. This device has been shown to be highly effective in the treatment of chemotherapy induced peripheral neuropathy (CIPN), drug-resistant chronic neuropathic and cancer pain, having long-lasting effects. The Calmare® device is a U.S. FDA cleared and European CE mark-certified pain therapy medical device for the non-invasive treatment of chronic neuropathic.

Scrambler therapy does not present toxicity and allows opioids dosage reduction, and it is also a repeatable treatment. Present novel data support that scrambler therapy seems to be effective for the treatment of cancer pain.

The Calmare device uses a biophysical rather than a biochemical approach. A 'no-pain' message is transmitted to the nerve via disposable surface electrodes applied to the skin in the region of the patient's pain. The perception of pain is cancelled when the no-pain message replaces that of pain, by using the same pathway through the surface electrodes in a non-invasive way. Regardless of pain intensity, a patient's pain can be completely removed for immediate relief.

Maximum benefit is achieved through follow-up treatments. A patient may be able to go for extended periods of time between subsequent treatments while experiencing significant pain control and relief. The period of time between treatments depends on the underlying cause and severity of the pain in addition to other factors. A neuropathic or mixed neuropathic-nociceptive pain condition was associated with a positive treatment outcome in one study.

Treatment for CRPS/RSD must be individualized. No one treatment will work for everyone. Most treatments and medications were developed to treat other chronic pain syndromes and may not be covered by your insurance Treatment for CRPS may be difficult. The goal is to seek pain relief and to restore function. There are 20 percent of people who don't respond to anything, but it seems like the other 80 percent get at least minimal, if not substantial relief.

the AMA guides does not recognize (rate) chronic pain and how does this impact injured workers who, for example suffer from really extremely painful, debilitating complex regional pain syndrome (CRPS), aka as Reflex Sympathetic Dystrophy (RSD). physical injuries must be assessed in accordance with The American Medical Association Guides For The Evaluation Of Permanent Impairment.

In 2003, a member of the AMA and Chairman of the Scientific Advisory Committee of the International Research Foundation for RSD/CRPS (Dr. Anthony Kirkpatrick) filed a complaint with the AMA putting the AMA on notice that it was causing ongoing injury to patients by disseminating false and misleading information about the diagnosis of reflex sympathetic dystrophy (RSD) also referred to as complex regional pain syndrome (CRPS Type I).

Dr Kirkpatrick wrote: "The false assertions by the AMA are particularly egregious because RSD/CRPS is a syndrome that must be treated in a timely manner in order to avert exacerbation of symptoms leading to irreversible impairment and suffering.

There are countless injured workers who suffer from this debilitating, chronic, neurological syndrome. The syndrome can start after minor trauma, such as one caused for example by a sprained finger, or following minor trauma. But it can also be triggered by surgery or repetitive vibration motion such as the kind that comes from a jackhammer or weed-cutting tool.

As RSD progresses over time, especially without treatment, the syndrome tends to become more unresponsive to treatment. Hence, early diagnosis and treatment are imperative. RSD can remain localized to one region of the body indefinitely. In other cases, it spreads to large segments of the body spontaneously or by trauma leading to permanent deformities and widespread immobility of limbs. At an advanced stage of the illness, all patients develop significant psychiatric problems and narcotic dependency, and are left completely incapacitated.

Treatment cons include multiple sympathetic injections by anesthesiologists. If one does not provide relief subsequent injections will not be effective. Needle jockeys believe that more is better.

However, the most horrific "con" or "fraud" is an insurance company's denial that the entity of RSD/CRPS even exists. This may be seen in more frequently in Workman's Compensation injuries. RSD treatment can be costly and enduring. It saves insurance companies money by denying that RSD/CRPS even exists.

For example, the harm caused by the AMA's (5th edition) error has been devastating to injured workers with RSD. There "must" be at least eight (8) concurrent, objective signs for RSD in order to make the diagnosis. The AMA clinical guidelines refer to objective diagnostic criteria such as changes in skin temperature, color, sweating, swelling, etc. Under Workman's Compensation laws injured workers with RSD may never be able to work again and yet they will not ever qualify for even a meager "lump sum", let alone a common law damages claim.

An early diagnosis and treatment can help reduce or prevent permanent damage. Treatments may include: Biofeedback, Exercise, Medications: alpha-blocking drugs, calcium channel blockers, Local anesthetic blockers, Bier blocks, Physical therapy, Surgery, spinal pumps and transcutaneous electrical nerve stimulation.

Whatever treatment is chosen to treat RSD, the most important consideration is the rapid diagnosis and institution of treatment to prevent this disease from becoming disabling.

40. ELDERLY PAIN MANAGEMENT

Between the years 2010 and 2030, the population of the United States over 65 years of age will increase by 73%. One out of every five Americans will be over 65 at that time. Between 1900 and 2000, the total US population increased 3 times but the population of people 65 years or older increased more than 10 times. The growth rate for the population 65 years or older is expected to outpace that for the total population during the next several decades. By 2040, the percentage of elderly patients will increase 20%. Elderly patients in the United States are estimated to be 55 million by 2020 and 80 million by 2040.

The treatment of older adults with pain is complex and affected by age-related changes in pharmacokinetics and pharmacodynamics. Improved management of chronic pain can significantly reduce disability in older adults but pain management in elderly patients can be a challenge. Elderly patients can be taking many different medications. Some of these drugs can adversely interact with some pain medications. Senile patients may forget to take their medications as prescribed. Their kidneys do not function as well as in younger patients. An estimated 50% of older adults living at home and up to 80% of elderly patients in long term care facilities suffer from persistent pain. Data suggest pain in the elderly is widely under recognized and undertreated

The use of nonsteroidal anti-inflammatory agents is suggested as a treatment for pain in elderly individuals. These types of agents are helpful only for short-term therapy. Gastrointestinal toxicity, platelet dysfunction, renal dysfunction, and sodium retention limit their usefulness in some patients. Untreated pain in the elderly can result in depression, decreased activity or decreased food and fluid intake. It can cause pain in other areas from guarding arms, legs or back, putting pressure on other areas of the body.

Your kidneys are responsible for eliminating drugs. As a result, drugs like morphine can accumulate within an elderly patient's body which could cause an overdose. Your liver metabolizes (breaks down drugs). Some elderly patients cannot afford some medications and therefore do not take them. Liver function can also be compromised in elderly patients. This decreased function can affect the breakdown of many drugs. An elderly patient's body mass may be decreased as well. As a result, there is less body volume where a drug can go. A dose of drug will be distributed through various body tissues. If you are emaciated, a dose of drug will remain in your blood stream instead of being distributed throughout your body. As a result, the concentration of drug in your blood stream may be higher than expected.

Your kidneys become smaller with age. As a result, there is decreased blood flow to the kidney and less effective filtration with removal of a drug from the kidney. As one ages, the liver undergoes a decrease in mass and blood flow. Decreased saliva noted in some older patients may interfere with swallowing. Drugs prescribed by mouth may be absorbed differently because of changes in stomach acid levels in older patients. The changes in physiology with aging may alter the side effect profile of many drugs.

One other important consideration is that of elderly persons being able to adequately monitor and adhere to their own scheduled pharmacological administration. Elderly patients may skip medication doses or cut them in half. Because pain is very common among the elderly, all elderly patients should be asked about their pain. Chronic pain can lead to depression, and polypharmacy. The cause of an elderly patient's pain may be difficult to identify and may be multifactorial. Inadequate treatment of pain is common among elderly patients. Thus, psychosocial support and nondrug treatments that reduce pain are particularly important. Patient and caregiver education and active caregiver involvement can help reduce pain and improve quality of life.

The prevalence of pain in elderly patients is higher among nursing home residents. In elderly patients, the most common sites of pain are joints, and the most common causes of pain are musculoskeletal disorders. Cancer related pain is not infrequent. Psychological factors such as depression and anxiety can prolong or amplify pain. The effect of age on pain perception is unknown. Perception may be influenced by many sociologic factors.

Chronic pain is characterized by a vague onset. The cause is often a chronic disorder. Sometimes the cause is clear, but the pain lasts longer than the expected time for healing. Neuropathic pain often manifests as spontaneous burning pain with superimposed lancinating pain. Neuropathic pain tends to follow the distribution of a neural pathway. Chronic pain in elderly patients may gradually lead to insomnia, decreased appetite, weight loss and constipation. Patients may become preoccupied with physical symptoms, become inactive, and withdraw socially.

Depression is common in older patients. Inactivity can lead to deconditioning. Many elderly patients take pain for granted and do not mention it unless they are asked. The assessment of patients with impaired cognition may be challenging. Patients with dementia may be able to describe their current symptoms but unable to reliably report their previous symptoms. Depression, secondary gain, personality disorders, and psychological stress should be evaluated in all elderly patients.

The patient's physical examination should focus on the musculoskeletal system and include palpation for trigger points, evaluation for joint swelling and inflammation, and evaluation for pain with passive range of motion. Pain is suggested by facial grimacing, frowning, or repetitive eye blinking. In the elderly, pain often has multiple causes, and no single pre-dominant cause can be identified.

Poor pain management decreases the patient's quality of life and may contribute to suicide. The elderly are more likely than younger patients to experience adverse effects of analgesics. Drug dosing starting low and going upward slowly. Oral analgesic administration is usually preferred because it is convenient and results in relatively steady blood levels.

Acetaminophen is the analgesic of choice for most elderly people with mild to moderate pain. Despite its relative lack of anti-inflammatory activity, acetaminophen is usually the best drug for initial treatment of osteoarthritis. NSAIDs are indicated when inflammation contributes significantly to pain. Adverse effects vary, and a patient may tolerate one NSAID better than another. NSAIDs tend to have a ceiling analgesic dose.

The most common adverse effect of all NSAIDs is gastrointestinal upset, which may require stopping the drug. Ulceration and GI bleeding can occur. Ulceration with or without bleeding can occur simultaneously or independently of each other. Risk of ulcers and GI bleeding for people 65 years or over is 3 to 4 times higher than that for middle-aged people.

NSAIDs can impair renal function and cause sodium and water retention; they should be used cautiously in the elderly, particularly in those who have a renal disorder. Nonacetylated salicylates may have less renal toxicity and fewer antiplatelet effects than other NSAIDs. Opioids are the most potent analgesics. Opioids act by blocking receptors in the brain and spinal cord. In the elderly, opioids have an increased half-life and possibly a greater analgesic effect than in younger patients. Nonetheless, the most common error in prescribing these drugs is to give them too infrequently, allowing breakthrough pain.

A few opioids have specific advantages and disadvantages in elderly patients. Fentanyl causes less histamine release and thus less vasodilation and hypotension. Meperidine should be avoided in elderly patients. Meperidine is less effective when given orally and can cause confusion; also, it is metabolized to an active form that tends to accumulate and thus may lead to central nervous system excitement and seizures.

Opioid agonist-antagonists, which have both agonist and antagonist effects on opiate receptors, often have psychotomimetic effects in the elderly. For this reason, pentazocine (Talwin) and butorphanol (Stadol) are rarely appropriate for the elderly patient. The analgesic effect of propoxy-phene (Darvon) which is no longer available is similar to that of aspirin or acetaminophen, but dependency and renal impairment may occur.

As a result, propoxyphene should not be used in the elderly. In patients with renal insufficiency, excretion of morphine and codeine may be delayed, resulting in undesirably long therapeutic or adverse effects, particularly with sustained-release formulations. In these patients, hydromorphone or oxycodone is less likely to accumulate and may be preferred.

Opioids can be given transdermally (on your skin). However, trans-dermal fentanyl should be used only in patients who have already been stabilized on opioids. Transdermal fentanyl is long-lasting. The peak analgesic effect of transdermal fentanyl occurs 18 to 24 h after application.

If this drug is used, a rapid-onset analgesic is required in the meantime. It is important to know that the reservoir for this system is the skin and not in the patch. If an overdose occurs, removing the patch does little to stop drug delivery within the first 18 h after removal. Patients must be closely observed if they have a fever. A fever can cause an increased uptake of the drug into the elderly patient's body. As a result an overdose could occur.

A heating pad can also cause a fentanyl overdose. Continuous opioid infusion provides steady-state analgesic drug levels. This means that there are no peaks and valleys in the elderly patient's bloodstream. Continuous infusion in palliative care patients may also be useful if regional techniques and NSAIDs are ineffective or inappropriate in patients near the end of life.

Patient-controlled analgesia enables a patient to increase drug delivery as needed. This technique results in a more stable blood drug level, thus avoiding the roller-coaster effects of intramuscular dosing. Patient-controlled analgesia reduces overall drug use and has fewer adverse side effects. However, patients with confusion or dementia cannot effectively use patient-controlled analgesia. Opioid muscle injection is rarely used. Initially, drug blood levels are high, resulting in more frequent adverse effects. The blood drug levels decrease rapidly, resulting in pain recurrence.

Unlike NSAIDS, opioids have no ceiling analgesic effect as dosage is increased. The maximum dose is whatever is needed to relieve pain. However, adverse effects may limit the maximum dose that is used. Opioids cause dose-related sedation and respiratory depression.

Most elderly patients taking opioids should not drive and should take precautions to prevent falls. Opioids may cause confusion. If confusion is due to an opioid, pupils are usually very constricted. Sometimes decreasing the dose may relieve confusion without significantly decreasing analgesia. If this approach is ineffective, a different analgesic may be necessary.

Opioids almost always cause constipation or urinary retention. Patients do not develop tolerance to these adverse effects. When an opioid is started, the patient's intake of fluid and fiber should be increased to try to prevent constipation. If a laxative is needed, a fiber laxative may be used.

Gabapentin (Neurontin) is frequently prescribed in elderly patients. Dose reductions of gabapentin are recommended in patients with renal insufficiency. Dizziness and drowsiness are common adverse effects. Pregabilin (Lyrica) is frequently in elderly patients with post herpetic neuralgia.

Antidepressant medications are also prescribed as adjunct medications for elderly patients who suffer from pain. For tricyclic antidepressants, amitriptyline, which is highly sedating and anticholinergic, should be avoided in the elderly. Local anesthetics injected into painful muscle areas are sometimes effective.

Local anesthetics injected into joints can relieve joint pain as well. Topical drugs are frequently used for pain originating in peripheral nerves. Capsaicin cream, NSAID creams, or a Lidoderm (lidocaine 5%) patch should be considered as well. Physical therapy can reduce pain due to musculoskeletal disorders in elderly patients. Aquatic therapy can help muscle and joint pain. Pain due to muscle spasm may be reduced by stretching, muscle massages, cold therapy or heat therapy. Ultrasound therapy may relieve musculoskeletal pain originating in your deep tissues.

Transcutaneous electrical nerve stimulation (TENS) can relieve many types of pain as well. Alternative therapies are also used by many patients to control their pain. Occupational therapy can be helpful as well. There are not specific recommendations about the long-term use of complementary and alternative therapies and although their effectiveness remains unproven they should not be discouraged. Palliative sedation may be a valid palliative care option to relieve suffering in the imminently dying patient. Polypharmacy, defined as either the use of multiple medications or the use of unnecessary medications, is common in older people and increases the risk of adverse drug reactions, nonadherence, and increased cost

While low back pain is related to the functional deterioration of lumbar spine structures, paying attention to posture and continuing physical exercise in daily living can improve the health of the lumbar region. Furthermore, therapeutic exercise should be prescribed based on specialist evaluation of the pain reduction achieved by medication.

For all opioids half-life of the active drug and metabolites is increased in the elderly. It is, therefore, recommended that doses be reduced, a longer time interval be used between doses, and creatinine clearance be monitored because the kidneys excrete the opioids from the body. Therefore, decreased kidney function could possibly result in a drug overdose.

One should be aware of the under treatment of pain in elderly patients with dementia. A myth exists is that people with dementia have less sensitivity or awareness of pain. Lab tests can be helpful to determine if the pain is from a urinary tract infection or a systemic infection. A physical exam can help the physician determine if something is swollen or an internal organ is enlarged. If the doctor can determine the cause of the pain, he/she can then consider treatments.

If the physician cannot determine the cause of the pain, it might be necessary to work proactively with the physician to treat the pain even without a cause. Often people do not get good pain management for fear of addiction to opioid medications, such as the Fentanyl patch or OxyContin but there is little incidence of addiction when the medication is taken properly for pain. Massage, soft touch, and warm applications are relaxation techniques that are beneficial for patients who are open to these practices.

The FBI has identified elder fraud and fraud against those suffering from serious illness as two of the most insidious of all white collar crimes. Memory loss and forgetfulness are often associated with aging and unfortunately, con artists try to take advantage of this by trying to pull scams on seniors. Seniors are an attractive population to run scams on because they are more likely to own their own homes and have good credit scores and they are often polite and trusting which make them easy targets for con artists.

There are a number of scams that seniors are the target of, including:. Healthcare fraud, including Medicare fraud. This includes insurers getting charged for medical equipment that wasn't delivered to seniors, unnecessary and fake tests being performed on seniors, customers or providers billing for services that weren't performed on seniors, counterfeit prescription drugs being given to seniors and/or companies offering free products in exchange for a seniors Medicare number.

Older Americans are less likely to report a fraud because they either don't know who to report it to or are too ashamed at having been scammed. Pain specialists order costly tests for illegal drugs such as cocaine and angel dust, which few seniors ever use.

Although the FBI has identified several instances where dietary and nutritional supplements promise anti-aging effects have been utilized to defraud American citizens, the number of complaints and related dollar losses have not indicated a substantial crime problem falling within the jurisdiction of the FBI.

Though a growing number of experts believe the drugs may do more harm than good, the country's aging population has become a prime market for the multibillion-dollar-a-year industry. Since 2007, top-selling opioids dispensed to people 60 years and older have increased 32%. That's double the growth for prescriptions dispensed in the 40- to 59-year-old age group.

The increase has been fueled in part by doctors and pain advocacy organizations that allegedly receive money from drug companies and make misleading claims about the safety and effectiveness of opioids, including a reassuring statement that that the addiction rate is rare in elderly populations. However, many pain specialists feel that the majority of older patients should not stay on the drugs because of side effects, because they do not frequently get adequate pain relief, or because they exhibit signs of abuse.

Pain medicine scams for natural substance pain relieving substances can be found on the internet. The internet is often just a new method of perpetrating some of the oldest scams, but allows it to be done more easily with automation and from anywhere in the world. There are also new areas of vulnerability via spyware and viruses.

The FBI previously arrested a pain management doctor in Texas who caused fraudulent claims to be submitted to Medicare, Medicaid, and TRICARE for procedures which he did not perform or were non-reimbursable. These kinds of criminals hurt the very nature of our health care system by falsely inflating the cost of health care for all of us.

41. VASCULAR PAIN

Vascular diseases have tendencies to obstruct blood flow to areas throughout your body. For example, patients with Raynaud's disease have complaints of burning pain, numbness and swelling in their fingers, toes or hands or feet on both arms. Raynaud's phenomenon usually involves one hand and is related to some lesion that compresses arteries to your hands. Raynaud's disease affects both hands while Raynaud's phenomenon can affect one hand.

Diseases that contribute to Raynaud's disease or phenomena include obstructive arterial disorders, vascular disorders, and scleroderma. Drug intoxications as well as some cancers and neurological entities can cause Raynaud's disease. Raynaud's disease is a vascular pain. Raynaud's disease pain can last a few minutes to hours. The average length of attack is 5 minutes to 60 minutes.

Raynaud's disease is a disorder of blood flow to your fingers, toes, nose, ears, and sometimes your tongue. When you have symptoms, you will suddenly experience a decrease in your blood flow to these areas. You will have color changes of your skin, especially on your fingers and toes, with exposure to cold or emotional stress. Cold exposure to your face can also cause changes in your fingers and toes. Many people use the term Raynaud's disease to include Raynaud's phenomena. This disease is classified as one of two types: primary and secondary. Secondary Raynaud's disease is also called Raynaud's phenomena.

Primary Raynaud's disease has no underlying medical problem and is mild and causes fewer complications than secondary Raynaud's disease. Approximately 50 percent of people diagnosed with Raynaud's disease are primary Raynaud's disease and 50 percent are Raynaud's phenomena. Women are five times more likely than men to develop primary Raynaud's disease. Most patients develop Raynaud's disease before age 40.

Be aware that 30 percent of individuals with primary Raynaud's disease progress to secondary Raynaud's disease. Approximately 15 percent of individuals with primary Raynaud's disease do improve. The secondary Raynaud's disease or Raynaud's phenomena is essentially the same as primary Raynaud's disease but secondary Raynaud's disease occurs in individuals who have predisposing factors.

You need to know that there are three phases of Raynaud's disease. When you are first exposed to cold, your small arteries contract and your fingers, toes, ears, or the tip of your nose and tongue become pale and white. This observation occurs because you are deprived of blood. Remember if you have an increased blood flow to your tissues, the tissue will appear red. After your oxygen is deprived, your blood vessels will expand. It is the veins that expand most. The veins carry blood that has minimal or no oxygen. This will give your blood a bluish tint. The area of the low-oxygen-carrying blood will appear blue. The area also feels cold to touch. When your arteries begin to dilate, the blood flow is increased. Oxygen is increased and your tissue color will appear normal.

I have mentioned the associated diseases that you might have if you have secondary Raynaud's disease. Primary Raynaud's disease can be later classified as a secondary Raynaud's disease after a predisposing underlying disease has been diagnosed. This observation is seen in 30 percent of patients. A secondary type of Raynaud's disease is more complicated and severe. This type of Raynaud's disease is more likely to worsen. Diseases that can predispose you to secondary Raynaud's disease include scleroderma, SLE, rheumatoid arthritis, and polio.

For some reason, herniated discs and spinal cord tumors as well as cerebrovascular accidents and polio can also cause Raynaud's disease. Vascular pain in general can be divided into three categories: Arterial pain, pain due to dysfunction of the capillaries in your tissue and pain related to pathology of your veins. You can have obstruction of both your arteries and veins of your limbs. When this happens you have what is called Burger's disease. Swelling of the small arteries and veins in your extremities causes this disease. The painful symptoms that you note are a result again of decreased oxygen flow to your tissues.

When your blood supply to a part of your body is decreased, which happens in Burger's disease, your oxygen to your tissue is significantly decreased. You will develop pain in the calves of your legs. If the oxygen deficit is extremely low, your nerves to your legs will suffer injury. This nerve injury will cause you pain as well as lack of oxygen to your extremity muscles. If your pain is severe, you may not experience relief with rest. If your tissues are deprived of oxygen for a long time, you can develop ulcerations in your skin and also develop gangrene.

Another problem with your blood vessels that can cause you to have pain is Takayasu's syndrome. This syndrome is due to inflammation or swelling of your small arteries of the upper part of your body, including your eyes. It occurs more in young girls as well as young women. More than 60 percent of individuals complain of weakness and fever as well as joint pain and pain in the upper extremities. When this pain occurs, you will soon develop the pain about the arteries that are inflamed. This disease can progress to even cause you to have angina pectoris. If this angina pectoris progresses, you may have a heart attack as well.

Temporal arteritis is another inflammation of the large arteries, especially around your temples. Inflammation of one or both of these arteries can cause you to have significant headaches. It can also involve other branches of your carotid artery. Temporal arteritis occurs usually if you are over 55 years of age. Temporal arteritis is more common in women than in men. Occasionally if you have temporal arteritis you will have headaches that are occasionally unbearable. Your headache will begin over your involved arteries. As stated, the pain mostly begins about your temples. However, this disease can also affect your occipital arteries. These are the arteries that are toward the back of your head and approximate an area where the back of your skull meets your neck.

You may have tenderness to touch over the swollen and inflamed arteries. The areas around your inflamed arteries are extremely sensitive to firm touch. You may even have decreased blood flow to your jaw muscles. Therefore, when you chew you may have significant pain in your jaw muscles. Temporal arteritis can affect arteries in multiple locations throughout your body. You may develop a flulike syndrome with generalized muscle pain as well as fever and weakness. The muscle pain can progress and involve your neck, shoulders, and pelvis as well as your legs. The arteries are usually affected on both sides of your body.

Erythemalgia is a syndrome that can affect both your arms and your legs. The temperature in your extremities will be elevated and you will have redness in either your arms or legs. Along with the change in color, you will have burning pain as well as tingling in your extremities. Sometimes you will experience swelling in your hands and feet. Usually this disease affects your legs. However, it can also affect your arms. This entity is usually seen if you are exposed to an increased temperature. When you experience the pain, it can last for a few minutes up to hours. This type of pain in this syndrome can be associated with diabetes.

Sickle cell disease affects the arteries throughout your body. This pain can be severe. The sickling cells can stop blood flow to your blood vessels. As a result, you have generalized lack of oxygen to all of your tissues and have severe pain. Sickle cell disease is inherited. Sickle cell disease is more prevalent in African Americans or individuals of Mediterrean decent. In Africa, the sickle cell gene gave advantage to individuals because it would resist infection caused by malaria. This is the reason why the disease is prevalent in populations of African descent. The deposition of sickled cells within your arteries decreases blood flow to your tissues. This causes a painful crisis to the majority of your organs.

If you have sickle cell disease and if you have a painful crisis, you will note the development of severe pain. The frequency of the pain occurs most in the third and fourth decades. Cold and infection can induce you to have a sickle cell crisis. Furthermore, dehydration and alcohol consumption can cause you to have a crisis as well as exposure to low-oxygen tension. You can have pain in different parts of your body. Chest pain can occur. This is usually accompanied by a fever.

You back, legs, and stomach may also develop significant pain. If you have pain in your abdomen, this pain can mimic appendicitis. The sickle cell related pain can last from hours to even weeks. You can have a gradual or sudden onset of pain. You can have decreased blood flow to your bone. This will cause some tissue death in your bone. You can have pain in your joints as well as swelling. This pain is severe enough to cause you to experience depression.

The initial treatment of this disease is usually the administration of either steroids or nonsteroidal anti-inflammatory drugs. If your pain is severe, your doctor may prescribe narcotic medications until your crisis subsides. If you have infection as a cause of your sickle cell crisis, you may require antibiotics. Because of the depression associated with this entity, you may need to have a psychological evaluation as well as the administration of antidepressant drugs. Sometimes narcotic medications are necessary for pain control.

Scleroderma also affects your skin. By definition, it is called "hard skin." It is uncommon. Scleroderma is classified according to the degree of your skin thickening. Scleroderma is most common in adults. However, it can be seen in children. The hallmarks of scleroderma are light skin and Raynaud's phenomena. Scleroderma is a generalized disorder of the small arteries as well as the connective tissue around your arteries.

Not only can your gastrointestinal tract be affected but also your lungs, your heart, and your kidneys. Most all patients who have scleroderma have Raynaud's disease. Patients with scleroderma can have pallor of the digits following cold exposure or emotional stress. Your fingers and toes can turn blue followed by redness in addition to burning pain and tingling.

This disease can be severe and devastating. You can get gangrene in your fingers and toes and end up with an amputation. Swelling can be seen over your hands and feet. Over time, thinning of your skin can occur. The thinning of your skin is easily noted over joints. Usually scleroderma begins before age 40 and is more common in females. Approximately 80 percent of scleroderma patients are females.

Scleroderma can affect your kidneys and may cause you to have kidney failure. Scleroderma can also affect your heart and cause heart arrhythmias and palpations.. You may need an echocardiograph if you have chest pain. This test can reveal some thickening around the outer wall of your heart. You will have muscle pain as well as joint pain if you have scleroderma. You will have stiffness in the morning. Systemic lupus erythematosus is a disease of unknown cause. It can also be associated with Raynaud's disease.

Systemic lupus erythematosus (SLE) is caused by your body's production of antibodies that injure the tissues of some of your organs in your body. The symptoms can come and go. You may have a rash develop on your face. However, SLE can be life threatening if it involves your internal organs. SLE can cause you to have failure of your kidneys or hemorrhage as well as a pulmonary disease.

Dermatomyositis is an inflammatory disease that can affect your muscles. You will have muscle pain and tenderness. A rash usually accompanies this disease. The rash occurs on your upper eyelids. You may have some swelling around your eyes as well. You can have redness about the knuckles of your fingers. This disease can affect almost any organ system in your body. You can have involvement of the muscles of your fingers and toes. The muscles in your legs can become weak. This disease can be caused by an abnormality in your immune system. The diagnosis of this disease can be done by taking samples of your muscle.

Polyarteritis nodosa is caused by inflammation or swelling of the walls of your blood vessels. This disease can affect blood vessels of any size as well as in any location. It usually occurs between ages 40 and 50. Men are affected more than women. Your kidneys can be affected. If the disease progresses, you can develop kidney failure. This disease can affect your arteries going to your heart and can cause you to have a heart attack. It may cause abdominal pain and bleeding. This disease can affect your nervous system as well. It can cause you to have weakness as well as loss of sensation. As stated previously, it can be associated with rheumatoid arthritis.

Supplements haven't been tested for safety and due to the fact that dietary supplements are largely unregulated, the content of some products may differ from what is specified on the product label. Also keep in mind that the safety of supplements in pregnant women, nursing mothers, children, and those with medical conditions or who are taking medications has not been established.

Due to a lack of supporting research, it's too soon to recommend any alternative medicine for Raynaud's disease. If you're considering using it, talk to your doctor to weigh the potential risks and benefits. Keep in mind that alternative medicine should not be used as a substitute for standard care. Self-treating a condition and avoiding or delaying standard care may have serious consequences.

DigestaCure, is a 100% natural product by Pristine Nutraceuticals which is made by the base ingredient of Aloe for curing autoimmune disorders. DigestaCure promotes healthy healing of autoimmune disorders. To be on the safer side, Pristine Nutraceuticals do come with a statutory message that DigestaCure does not heal any "symptoms" or "conditions" of autoimmunity but reaches to the root cause and heals the said issue. There are no adverse reports on this product that would suggest fraud.

42. CANCER PAIN

Cancer pain is usually not evident until the cancer growth has become far advanced. Most non-solid tumors cause minimal pain while solid tumors like prostate cancer can cause significant pain. If you have myeloma, you will have a malignant formation of your plasma cells. Plasma cells are antibody-producing cells found in bone forming tissue as well as in your lungs and your abdomen. This increase in your plasma cells can affect your organs and cause you to have painful symptoms. Usually bone pain is the most common pain noted involving multiple myeloma.

Multiple myeloma can be an extremely painful entity affecting your bones and is usually treated by a medical specialist who treats cancer called an oncologist. Lung cancer is common in the United States. Lung Cancer is a disease that begins in the tissue of the lungs. Oxygen is taken up by your body and carbon dioxide is removed. The vast majority of lung cancer cases fall into one of two different categories: Non-Small Cell Lung Cancer is the most common type of lung cancer, making up nearly 80% of all cases. This type of lung cancer grows and spreads more slowly than small cell lung cancer. Small Cell Lung Cancer makes up nearly 20% of all lung cancer cases.

It is associated with cancer cells smaller than most other cancer cells. These cells may be small, but they can rapidly reproduce to form large tumors. Their size and quick rate of reproduction allows them to spread to the lymph nodes and to other organs of the body. Cigarette smoking causes this type of cancer.

Symptoms of lung cancer include the following: coughing, shortness of breath, wheezing, pain in your chest, shoulder, upper back, or arm, coughing up blood, frequent pneumonia, generalized pain and hoarseness. Lung cancer can spread to your brain liver or bone.

As a result, you may experience headaches, seizures, abdominal pain or bone pain. Non-small cell lung cancer can be treated with surgery while small cell cancer is treated with chemotherapy. Sometimes, a small segment of the lung can be removed while in other cases, the whole lobe must be removed.

Colon cancer is another common cancer that you need to be aware of. The colon is the part of your body where the waste material is stored. The rectum is the end of the colon adjacent to the anus. Together, they form a long, muscular tube called the large intestine (also known as the large bowel). Tumors of the colon and rectum are growths arising from the inner wall of the large intestine. Benign tumors of the large intestine are called polyps. Malignant tumors of the large intestine are called cancers. Cancer of the colon and rectum (also referred to as colorectal cancer) can invade and damage adjacent tissues and organs. Cancer cells can also break away and spread to other parts of the body (such as your liver and lung).

Factors that increase a person's risk of colorectal cancer include high fat intake, a family history of colorectal cancer and polyps, the presence of polyps in the large intestine, and chronic ulcerative colitis.

Symptoms of colon cancer are usually nonspecific. They include: fatigue, weakness, and shortness of breath, change in bowel habits, bloody stools, diarrhea and/ or constipation, blood in your stool, weight loss, abdominal pain or cramps. If colon cancer is suspected a barium enema X ray or a colonoscopy will be done. Surgery is the most common treatment for cancer of the rectum and colon. If the cancer has spread you may also require chemotherapy. If your cancer is limited to your rectum, you may be treated with radiation therapy.

Some cancers can be gender specific. For example, if you are a female, you can develop cancer of your breasts, cervix, uterus, or ovary. If you are male, you can develop cancer of your testicles, prostate gland or breast. Cancer-related pain can be excruciating in some cases. Various treatment methods and therapies are available to help relieve your pain if it is caused by a cancer. Breast cancer is the most common malignancy in women in the United States. Approximately 182,000 women develop breast cancer and more than 46,000 die with it. It occurs in one in eight women. Approximate-ly two thirds of cases occur after menopause. Fifteen percent of cases occur before the age of 40. Screening for female cancers is very important.

The actual cause of breast cancer is not known. There are different types of breast cancer. Some breast cancers can affect the ducts of the breasts, whereas other types affect the lobules of the breasts. Cancer of the ducts usually occurs on one side of the body, whereas lobular cancer is bilateral. You must be taught how to do self-examination of your breasts. The majority of women detect their own breast cancer. You should have a breast examination by your doctor at the time of your regular physical examination if you are over age 40. Mammography is recommended every 1 to 2 years if you are older than 40 years of age.

If you have a history of breast cancer, you should have a mammogram yearly. If you are over 40 and have a family history of breast cancer, you should also have a mammogram every year. The survival rate is lower if your cancer is detected by a mammogram as opposed to palpation. Breast cancer is usually painless and presents with a palpable mass in a postmenopausal woman. If it had associated pain, the diagnosis would be earlier diagnosed. You should perform routine self-examinations as your cancer can be diagnosed early as opposed to waiting for your doctor or mammogram to make the diagnosis.

An accurate diagnosis of breast cancer requires a needle aspiration, a percutaneous needle biopsy, or an incisional (surgical) biopsy. A biopsy should be done on every suspicious breast mass. You must have a chest x-ray to see if your breast cancer may have spread to your lungs, ribs, or spine. A bone scan may also be required to see if your breast cancer has spread to your bones. If you have breast cancer, your doctor will want to get a CAT scan of your abdomen to see if the cancer has affected your liver as well.

Your doctor will also obtain a liver function test from you because your cancer can spread to your liver. Risks for breast cancer include increasing age, a family history of breast cancer, previous cancer in one breast, early menstruation (meaning before age 12), late menopause (meaning after age 52), a history of having no children, obesity, a high fat diet, alcohol use, and a family history of cancer of the ovary, uterus, or colon.

A pathologist will stage your cancer. Staging determines the severity of your cancer. A 0 stage cancer is confined to an area of your organ. A stage greater than III usually means that the cancer has spread beyond your affected organ. Your survival rate depends on the stage of the cancer. The stages are based on the severity of the cancer. The higher the stage correlates with a lower survival rate. If you have cancer in your breast that has not spread to your bones or other organs, your 5-year survival rate is greater than 95 percent. However, if your cancer has spread to other areas of your body, your 5-year survival rate is only 10 percent. If your cancer is only in your tissue, you may only need removal of that part of the tissue from your breast.

Cancer treatment is complex and new methods are frequently being developed to treat advanced metastatic cancer. However, you are encouraged to do your own breast exams. This may help you to discover the cancer much earlier than if you wait to have an exam at your yearly physical examination or during a mammogram.

If your breast cancer has spread to other areas of your body, you will most likely require a mastectomy (removal of your breast, radiation therapy, chemotherapy, as well as hormone therapy). Your oncologist will discuss with you the best options for your treatment. Breast cancer can also occur in males. Males can have an enlargement of their breast tissue. Estrogens stimulate breast development. Androgens such as testosterone inhibit breast development. Male breast cancer is usually on one side and presents as a firm mass that appears to be fixed to the male's underlying muscle. There may even be a nipple discharge. There may also be retraction of the skin around the male breast.

With respect to female cancer, cervical cancer accounts for approximately 2 to 3 percent of all cancers involving women in the United States. More than 15,000 cases of cervical cancer are diagnosed each year, and approximately 5,000 women die from this disease. Risk factors for develop-ing carcinoma of the cervix include suppression of the immune system, a history of genital herpes or genital warts, multiple sexual partners, partners with penile warts or cancer, low economic status, intercourse before age 17, and cigarette smoking. Usually cancer of the cervix is painless. A Pap smear detects many cases of cervical cancer.

Cancer from your cervix can spread and can cause you to experience lower back pain, leg pain, weight loss, or swelling in your legs. If you have an abnormal Pap smear, you will have a biopsy of your cervix. If the biopsy is unable to determine whether a suspicious-looking tissue is cancerous, you will have a greater portion of your cervix removed, which is called a cervical conization.

Your doctor will obtain liver function tests from you, a creatinine level, and a squamous cell carcinoma antigen level. A chest x-ray will be obtained to see whether the cancer has spread to your ribs or lungs. An MRI of your pelvis and abdomen will be obtained to see whether the cancer has spread to other organs. Your gynecologist may place a scope in your bladder and one in your sigmoid colon to see whether the cancer has advanced to your gastrointestinal tract or urinary tract.

As with most cancers, a pathologist will assign a numeric stage to your cancer. A high number means that your cancer has spread beyond the organ where it began. If your cancer is only confined to your cervix, you have a 5-year survival rate of 100 percent. If your cancer has spread throughout your pelvis and involved your bladder or rectum, your 5-year survival rate is 20 percent.

If your cancer is in an advanced stage and has spread outside of the cervix to other areas of your body; your oncologist will probably prescribe radiation therapy and possibly chemotherapy. If your cancer has spread to your upper vagina, your gynecological oncologist may elect to do abdominal hysterectomy as well as removal of your lymph nodes. On the other hand, this doctor may elect to do radiation therapy.

Many times the treatment chosen by your doctor depends on your overall health status. After your treatment, your gynecological oncologist will perform a comprehensive pelvic examination as well as a Pap smear every three months for the first two years following your initial treatment. After that, the examination and Pap smear should be every six months from years three to five. If you develop a recurrent cancer of your cervix, you will then probably experience vaginal bleeding or discharge. You can develop pain in your back and legs as well. Again you may experience weight loss. If this happens, you may be treated with radiation therapy or with an extensive removal of the organs in your pelvis.

If you are taking estrogen replacement and are over age 52, you have an increased risk of developing uterine cancer. As with the other cancers mentioned in this chapter, there are stages. Stage 0, which is the cancer in your uterus, has a 100 percent success rate. If your cancer involves your bladder or your rectum, your survival rate decreases to 20 percent.

If you have stage 0 uterine cancer, a simple procedure that removes the area of the cancer can be done. If you have the fourth stage, which involves your bladder, pelvis, or rectum, you will have radiation therapy. If you have stage 2A, you will have a radical hysterectomy with removal of your lymph nodes followed by radiation therapy. The clinical presentation of this cancer is abnormal uterine bleeding. If you are in menopause and begin bleeding, your gynecologist or primary care doctor should evaluate you immediately.

Standard therapy for uterine cancer is an abdominal hysterectomy with removal of both your ovaries. As with other cancers mentioned in this chapter, you should have a pelvic exam and Pap smear every three months for the first two years after treatment. Other tests should be done only if you have a recurrence of symptoms. If you do have recurrence of the cancer, a major surgical procedure will need to be done. Ovarian cancer develops in 1 in every 70 women. Approximately 1 percent of women die from this cancer. Approximately 24,000 cases of ovarian cancer are diagnosed in the United States each year. More than 13,000 women will die with ovarian cancer each year.

You can have abnormal uterine bleeding. If you are a postmenopausal female and if your doctor can palpate your ovary on a routine pelvic exam, this suggests that you may have an ovarian tumor. Usually, normal ovaries cannot be palpated. If you have an enlarged ovary, an ultrasound of your pelvis may be helpful in diagnosing cancer of your ovary. Your pelvis, abdomen, and chest will be carefully examined as well. Liver-function tests will be done as well as a CAT scan of your abdomen. Occasionally a further gastrointestinal workup is indicated.

Males suffer from gender specific tumors as well. The testes secrete testosterone and estradiol, which are two hormones. Testicular cancer represents approximately 2 percent of all cancers in men. It is the second most common cancer in men between the ages of 20 and 34 years of age. These tumors usually manifest as an enlargement of the testicle. You may have pain and tenderness in your testicle. A male with a testicular tumor can have breast enlargement. Approximately 10 percent of these tumors will have distant spread of the cancer at the time of the diagnosis.

Prostate cancer is the second most common tumor in men. Lung cancer is the most common. Approximately 200,000 new cases are diagnosed each year in the United States. Prostate cancer is more common among African Americans and men who have a family history of prostate cancer. The problem with prostate cancer is that it is usually painless and has no other symptoms that are seen with prostatism. Prostate cancer can be detected by routine digital examination or elevation of your prostate specific antigen (PSA). Sometimes if you have surgery to remove an enlarged prostate gland, cancer tissue can be found in your prostate gland.

When the cancer travels from your prostate gland and goes to your bone, you can have severe back pain or other bone pain. In many instances, an MRI will be done to see whether your tumor has spread to other organs. Other chemical body markers can be measured as well if cancer is suspected to be present in another organ. A bone scan may be necessary to detect a cancer that has gone to your bones. If you have prostate cancer, your surgeon may do a prostatectomy (removal of your prostate gland), radiation therapy, hormone therapy, or chemotherapy.

Prostate cancer can be detected early; if it is detected early, your prognosis for survival is excellent. This means that you need to follow up with your primary care doctor regularly and have a regular rectal examination so that your doctor can feel your prostate to see if it is enlarged or if it has possible cancer masses in it. You will also need to have your PSA done on a regular basis.

There is no reason why cancer pain cannot be controlled. There are multiple modalities now available to adequately control cancer pain. If you have been diagnosed with cancer, you face a wide range of psychological and physical problems throughout your cancer. You may have a fear of a painful death or disfigurement. One of the most feared consequences of cancer is pain. To treat your pain appropriately, a multidisciplinary approach may be necessary, including your oncologist, your psychologist or psychiatrist, and your pain-management doctor.

Neuropathic pain causes you to experience symptoms that are sharp and electrical shock like. This type of pain can be controlled by antiseizure medications such as Neurontin or Lyrica. You can have pain that is severe and excessive for the extent of tissue damage that has occurred. This type of pain is called idiopathic and usually has a psychological pathology associated with it.

Anticonvulsant medications can relieve severe lancinating pain when your tumor affects one of your nerves. In case you are wondering why a seizure medication would be prescribed, it's because these medications are also pain medications. In the United States, about 5 percent of all anticonvulsant medications are prescribed for pain management.

Narcotics can relieve your cancer pain. Morphine is the standard of comparison for the rest of the narcotic analgesics. A sustained-release preparation is available called MS Contin releases the drug over 8 to 12 hours. Oxycontin also provides a release of oxycodone over 8-12 hours. There is also a drug that you can take once a day that will give a sustained release over 24 hours called Kadian.

Dilaudid is stronger than morphine, but it has a shorter duration of action than morphine. Methadone is another drug that can be prescribed for cancer pain. It is very effective when given in a pill form. Another drug more potent than morphine is Levo-Dromoran. It is stronger than morphine and can last up to 16 hours per dose. Opana, a long acting oxymorphone is also available. Fentanyl is a potent drug that is more potent than the drugs men-tioned. A transdermal fentanyl patch gives you a continuous dose of drug. There is also an oral fentanyl lozenge that is available for treatment of your breakthrough pain when you are taking around-the-clock opioids.

Demerol (meperidine) is another drug that is available for pain management. It is not recommended for chronic pain because the breakdown products of this drug can cause seizures and also because of its relatively short duration of pain-relieving action, one and a half to two hours, as compared to other opioid preparations. Narcotic medications can be placed into your epidural space or actually even placed into the fluid that surrounds your spinal cord through an implanted pump. A snail toxin called Prialt can also be placed in a pump to control your pain. This pump deposits the drug in the spinal fluid. Other routes of drug administration are the oral routes, but you do not have to swallow a pill.

Sublingual (under the tongue) morphine when it is in a high concen-tration (Roxanol 20 mg/ml) can provide you with pain relief if you cannot swallow pills. Actiq is a fentanyl preparation on a stick that resembles a lollipop. Rectal suppositories are another way of providing you with narcotic medications. Rectal suppositories are available for hydromorphone, oxymorphone, and morphine. The rectal administration of morphine, for example, can provide pain relief within 10 minutes.

Cancer pain can be successfully treated. In order to do so, a timely and accurate diagnosis must be done. This is one of many reasons why you should have a routine physical examination by your doctor. Given that no two people are alike, if you are taking any medications and begin to take nutritional supplements you should be aware that potential drug-nutrient interactions may occur and are encouraged to consult a health care professional before using any natural product.

Fraud involving cancer treatments can be particularly heartless. There can be a great temptation to jump at anything that appears to offer a chance for a cure. Advertisements and other promotional materials touting bogus cancer 'cures' have probably been around as long as the printing press. However, the Internet has compounded the problem by providing the peddlers of these often dangerous products a whole new outlet. Another unproven "remedy" that has been sold for decades is an herbal regimen known as the Hoxsey Cancer Treatment. The FDA has taken regulatory and enforcement action against this discredited course of therapy beginning in the 1950s.

There is no scientific evidence that it has any value to treat cancer. Yet consumers can go online and find all sorts of false claims that Hoxsey treatment is effective against the disease. Fraudulent products, on the other hand, are unapproved and typically have never been clinically tested or reviewed by FDA for safety and effectiveness.

Recently a man was arrested on charges of doctor and prescribing phony cancer medication. The arrest is not an isolated incident. Last year, a Northern California man was arrested on charges of practicing medicine without a license and prescribing patients "natural" cures that investigators say included bags of dirt. In 2013, an evangelical minister was sentenced to 14 years in prison for pushing phony herbal supplements on parishioners dying of cancer. Experts testified that the supplements actually contained sunscreen preservative and beef flavoring.

A Michigan doctor was arrested on allegations of trying to make money from chemotherapy treatments to the point of intentionally misdiagnosing people with cancer. He was charged for allegedly submitting false claims to Medicare for services that were medically unnecessary, including chemotherapy treatments, Positron Emission Tomographic (PET) scans and a variety of cancer and hematology treatments for patients who did not need them. Some of the medications contained nothing more exotic than sunscreen preservatives and beef extract.

Another doctor charged patients $4,270 for a week's worth of a cancer remedy while a six-month cancer treatment program retailed for $120,000 to $150,000. The high price for the cancer remedy product was justified because the doctor alleged that it was "made with herbs from around the world and was manufactured in a laboratory according to the needs of each patient."

According to federal prosecutors, this doctor fraudulently marketed and sold a medical treatment that she claimed had a 60% to 100% rate in curing Stage 4 "metastatic or terminal cancers." A chemical analysis showed most of the products would have been ineffective against cancer or other ailments.

One victim who was diagnosed with breast cancer that was spreading through her body and the woman traveled to Southern California and was told that the herbal treatment program would shrink her tumors and kill her cancer cells. The victim and her husband paid thousands of dollars for the herbal product. The victim took the cure and at one point the doctor pronounced her "cancer-free" at a party held for patients. In fact however, the cancer continued to spread and the woman died in four months.

43. ABDOMINAL PAIN

Pain in your abdomen bladder and kidney can be disabling and severe. Abdominal pain is an indication of an array of ailments: bacterial infection in your stomach, spasms due to menstruation, digestive disorders, upset stomach, or fragility and can't stomach some foods. Abdominal pain is characteristically minor, and is often curable through self-treatment.

Identifying what instigated the persistent abdominal pain is incalculable and the expertise of a medical physician is necessary and highly recommended. You can't just personally formulate a diagnosis and do self-medication. The origin may be a digestive condition like Celiac or Crohn's disease; or a gynecological malady like ovarian cysts or endometriosis. These conditions need properly prescribed medications.

Once an initial evaluation has been completed, your health care provider may have you undergo some tests to help find the cause of your pain. These may include stool or urine tests, blood tests, barium swallows or enemas, an endoscopy, X-ray, ultrasound, or CT scan. Abdominal pain in general occurs more often in women than in men. Stress, diet, and the work environment may be causes of abdominal pain in general. Various abdominal pains can occur in your upper, mid, or lower abdomen. Cramping and intermittent pain is easily caused by disorders of your bowel, gallbladder, and ureter of your kidney or your fallopian tubes from your uterus. Pain in your abdomen and pelvis is called visceral pain and is non-specific with respect to the exact location of your pain. Many nerves from many organs can send pain signals to your spinal cord and brain.

A common syndrome in adults is the irritable bowel syndrome (IBS), which is frequently diagnosed in the general population. Approximately 30 percent of patients seen by gastroenterologists suffer from IBS. It is more common in women and may even be seen in adolescents. If you have IBS, this disease can impair your quality of life. The exact cause of IBS remains to be discovered. IBS can be caused by physiological, psychological, and behavioral factors. Sometimes you may have severe symptoms without any physical findings. This pain is not confined to one area of your gut but it is global over your stomach. Sometimes IBS is diagnosed in patients who suffer from fibromyalgia.

Usually this abdominal pain associated with IBS is relieved followed a bowel movement. You may suffer diarrhea alternating with constipation. You may have bloating or the feeling of incomplete evacuation of your stool following a bowel movement. Some physicians believe that your colon is the cause of IBS. You can have symptoms daily or you may have symptoms once a week or once a month. If you have IBS, you may also have heartburn and nausea. IBS is sometimes associated with fibromyalgia. You may also suffer from chronic fatigue and significant depression.

Pain associated with IBS can be caused by depression or other behavioral illnesses. If you have psychosocial factors, these factors can influence the frequency of your symptoms as well as the severity of your symptoms. If you suffer from IBS, you may have a previous history of physical, sexual, or emotional abuse. Usually extensive diagnostic tests are not utilized for your doctor to diagnose your IBS because there are no definitive tests for this disease. The criterion for the diagnosis of IBS is difficult because of the variety of physical complaints associated with IBS.

To be diagnosed with IBS, you need to have abdominal pain first of all. Your pain must be relieved with a bowel movement. The onset of your pain must be associated with a change in the frequency of your stool habits. The onset of your pain must be associated with a change in the appearance of your stool. You may possibly have IBS if you have an abnormal stool (in which it differs in appearance from usual stool appearance) one out of every four defecations.

If you have bloating or abdominal distention in one out of four days or passage of mucus in one out of four defecations, there is a high probability that you have IBS. You should have symptoms for at least 12 weeks or more over the previous 12 months. Your symptoms do not have to be consecutive. At one time, doctors thought that IBS was primarily a psychosomatic (mental) entity. However, it is now accepted that if you suffer from IBS, you are not "crazy." It is known through recent research that nerves in your gastrointestinal system can become oversensitive, causing them to overreact to both gas as well as food passing by these nerves. The stimulation of your nerves in your gastrointestinal tract will cause you to have pain as well as cramping.

If you have moderate symptoms, you may require psychological treatment and occasionally pharmacologic management. If you have severe and constant symptoms, you may require antidepressants as well as psychological testing and treatment and you may need to be referred to a specialist in abdominal diseases (gastroenterologist). The possibility of developing IBS is extremely high in individuals who suffer panic disorders. If you have moderate to severe depression, you are also prone to IBS. The reason for this association remains unknown.

Your brain can affect the nerves in your stomach and cause you to have an upset stomach. For example, if you are anxious or have to give a speech in front of a large crowd, you may develop "butterflies" in your stomach. You might feel the effect of your stress within your gastrointestinal system. If you are facing a stressful situation, your brain can influence specialized cells in your gastrointestinal system called mast cells to release histamine. Histamine makes the nerves in your gastrointestinal system contract the smooth muscle in your gut. This will cause you to have cramps. It can also cause you to have diarrhea is some instances.

The new drug Lotronex (alosetron) is used to treat abdominal pain and discomfort as well as any symptoms of diarrhea. Lotronex is the first drug approved by the FDA to be used for IBS treatment. Another new drug designed to treat IBS that is now unavailable is called Zelnorm (tegaserod). It is a drug that is in a class of medications called gastrointestinal serotonin agonists. This drug is used for the treatment of constipation, bloating, and abdominal pain. Because of serious side effects this drug was withdrawn from the market in March 2007. If you suffer from IBS, you may want to minimize your fat intake. Many foods inhibit your intestinal gas transit. By decreasing the passage of gas through your gastrointestinal system, bloating and the expansion of your bowel can cause you to have pain. Fructose is another food substance that can worsen your IBS symptoms. Fructose is found in honey, fruit, and in some soft drinks. Fructose can cause you to have bloating, cramps, and diarrhea. Bacteria normally live in your digestive system. The bacteria in your colon may use fructose as their food source. In the process of utilizing fructose, hydrogen gas is liberated in your colon from the breakdown of sugars.

Gastro esophageal reflux disease (GERD) can cause burning pain in your lower thorax or your upper abdomen. It is caused by relaxation of the lower esophageal sphincter that allow stomach acid to go into your esophagus. This condition can be treated with ant acids. Upper abdominal pain can come from a hiatal hernia. You may have vomiting as well as generalized abdominal pain. In this condition, your stomach herniates into your chest cavity. You may require surgery to correct this deformity.

Abdominal pain can come from ulcers where the lining of your stomach or duodenum is injured or you may have gastritis where the lining of your stomach is inflamed. Treatment for ulcers and gastritis include antacids, H2 blockers like cimetidine and if no relief occurs with these medications the use of protein pump inhibitors like omeprazole (Zegerid) may be therapeutic.

Your pancreas can also be a source of severe pain. The pain in acute situations can radiate from your mid abdomen to your back. Alcohol or a gallstone can injure your pancreas. A lab test that measures your blood amylase level will be abnormal if you have acute pancreatitis. An ultra sound will help in the diagnosis of pancreatic disease. You will need fluid replacement and analgesic medications such as narcotics if you have an acute attack of pancreatitis.

Chronic pancreatitis is an inflammation seen usually in chronic alcoholics. The diagnosis is made with a CAT scan or ultrasound or an endoscopic retrograde cholangio pancrea tography (ERCP). To help with chronic pain you may need destruction of the nerves going to your pancreas called the celiac plexus. This injection can be done with alcohol or phenol. You may need insulin replacement if you have severe damage to your pancreas. A pseudocyst may form on your pancreas that may need to be drained surgically. Both acute and chronic pancreatic disease may require admission to an intensive care unit.

An appendix or gallbladder inflammation can also be very painful. Your gallbladder is in the upper right side of your abdomen while your appendix is located in the right lower aspect of your abdomen. If either of these organs becomes diseased, you can develop nausea, vomiting and a fever. Surgery may be necessary to remove one of these diseased organs. Laboratory tests, antibiotics and analgesics are necessary. A CAT scan or a HIDA study can be used to diagnose gallbladder disease. Approximately 20 % of patients continue to experience pain post gallbladder surgery. The reason is usually related to a gallstone in the common bile duct. Appendicitis can be diagnosed with an abdominal ultrasound in most cases.

Your immune system can be a cause of abdominal pain. Inflammatory bowel disease is believed to be a disease of your immune system. IBS can respond to diet. However, the inflammatory bowel disease rarely responds to changes in diet. Inflammatory bowel disease includes ulcerative colitis and Crohn's disease. Ulcerative colitis is a chronic disease and a recurrent disease. It involves inflammation of the lining of the colon. It can also involve your rectum.

Crohn's disease can involve any part of your gastrointestinal tract, including your mouth all the way to your anus. The causes of Crohn's disease and ulcerative colitis are unknown. Usually inflammatory bowel disease begins in early adult life. However, there are cases reported in the elderly. Genetic factors can make you prone to inflammatory bowel disease. If you have a disorder of your immune system, you are again prone to develop irritable bowel disease. It is possible that your immune system may attack the lining of your gastrointestinal system. Crohn's disease involves the lower ileum (the lowest part of the small intestine). Your rectum can be involved as well. Approximately one third of Crohn's disease patients have their pathology in their colon, whereas one third of patients have their pathology in their ileum and one third have their pathology in both their ileum and colon. The inflammation of your gastrointestinal system can go from the inside of your bowel to the outside.

The inner lining of your gastrointestinal tract can develop ulcers in some cases of Crohn's disease. An ulcer is a break in the lining of the wall of your stomach or small intestine. This break in your gut lining can fail to heal and can be accompanied by inflammation. A fistula from the inside of your bowel to the outside can develop. A fistula is an abnormal communication between a hollow organ and the exterior.

With Crohn's disease, you can have fever, diarrhea, pain, and tenderness in the right lower part of your abdomen. You can also develop an abscess around your anus. The inner aspect of your intestine or colon can decrease in diameter, which is called a stricture. If you have Crohn's disease, you can have an increased incidence of gallstones. With Crohn's disease, your bile salts may not be absorbed properly through your ileum. You can also develop kidney stones. You can have a history of frequent liquid bowel movements.

Because of absorption problems of nutrients, you may have a poor nutritional status. You can feel fatigued and suffer from a loss of energy. If your bowel becomes swollen, you can perceive the inflamed bowel, which may feel like a mass or sense of fullness. This thickened loop of inflamed bowel can be tender to deep palpation. If you develop a tract from the inside of your bowel to the outside, this fistula can cause you to develop an abscess behind the lining of your bowel. You will have fever, chills, and tenderness to deep palpation about your abdomen.

A barium enema is an enema with opaque contrast liquid that outlines your intestines on x-ray images. This test helps your doctor look for abnormalities in your bowel. To examine your lower bowel, your doctor may also use air with the barium to distend your bowel. Through the colonoscope (a flexible fiberoptic instrument), your physician can obtain biopsies of your colon and ilium. If your gastrointestinal system develops an obstruction somewhere in your system, your food cannot pass through this obstruction. You will be treated with fluids through your veins, and a tube will be placed through your nose to suction out substances that are unable to pass through your bowel. Steroids can be necessary to treat the inflammation caused by Crohn's disease. Be aware that chronic cramping, abdominal pain, and diarrhea are noted in both IBS and Crohn's disease.

Antibiotics may be used for the treatment of an inflammatory disease. Sulfasalazine is effective in reducing the symptoms of your disease. Drugs that can affect your immune system such as azathioprine and mercaptopurine are also useful in the treatment of your disease if it is unresponsive to the other methods that we mentioned. If you smoke, stop smoking; smoking can cause you to have a recurrence of Crohn's symptoms. If conservative treatments fail, you may require surgery.

Ulcerative colitis is another form of inflammatory bowel disease. Ulcerative colitis involves an inflammation of the inner lining of your colon. You will have bloody diarrhea if you have ulcerative colitis. You will have pain in your abdomen. You can develop anemia and the protein in your bloodstream, albumin, will be decreased. A scope in your colon is the key to the diagnosis of your disease.

A hernia can cause abdominal pain. A hernia is an abnormal protrusion, or bulging out, of part of an organ such as a portion of your intestine through the tissues that normally contain it. In this condition, a weak spot or opening in a body wall, often due to laxity of the muscles, allows part of the organ to protrude causing a hernia to occur. A hernia may develop in almost any part of the body; but the muscles of the abdominal wall are most commonly affected.

Hernias cause pain and reduce general mobility. They never cure themselves, even though some can be cured (at least temporarily) by external manual manipulation. Depending on the nature of the protruding organ and the solidity of the structure through which it is protruding, a hernia may cause complications that are medically dangerous such as strangulation. One major danger of a hernia is that if bowel is contained within the protruding loop it may hinder or stop the blood flow through the intestine (occlusion). More serious still, if the loop itself becomes twisted outside its containing structure, or compressed at the point where it breaks through that structure (a strangulated hernia), the blood supply to the loop will also cease and the entire hernia will undergo tissue death (necrosis). This requires immediate emergency surgery.

Although there are many types of hernias, the following are the most common: An abdominal hernia is also called an epigastric or ventral hernia. This type of hernia affects one person in 100. This group of hernias also includes inguinal hernias and umbilical hernias. Indirect inguinal hernias affect men only. A loop of intestine passes down the canal from where a testis descends early in childhood into the scrotum. If neglected, this type of hernia tends to increase progressively in size causing the scrotum to expand.

On the other hand a direct inguinal hernia affects both sexes. The intestinal loop forms a swelling in the inner part of the fold of the groin. A femoral hernia also affects both sexes although most often women. An intestinal loop passes down the canal containing the major blood vessels to and from the leg, between the abdomen and the thigh, causing a bulge in the groin and another at the top of the inner thigh.

An umbilical hernia affects both sexes as well. An intestinal loop protrudes through a weakness in the abdominal wall at the navel. A hiatal hernia also affects both sexes. A loop of the stomach when particularly full protrudes upward through the small opening in the diaphragm through which the esophagus passes, thus leaving the abdominal cavity and entering the chest. An incisional hernia is a hernia that occurs at the site of a surgical incision. This is due to strain on the healing tissues due to excessive muscular effort, lifting, coughing, or extreme pressure.

An obturator hernia is a rare type of hernia, but it is a significant cause of intestinal obstruction due to the associated anatomy. This hernia can occur in your upper thigh. A correct diagnosis and treatment of an obturator hernia is important, because delay can lead to high mortality. Umbilical hernias can be present from birth, but most happen later due to pressure on openings or weaknesses in the abdominal cavity or wall from heavy lifting etc. Hernias tend to run in families, and can be caused by such things as coughing, straining during a bowel movement, lifting heavy objects, accumulation of fluid in the abdominal cavity, and obesity.

The symptoms of hernias vary, depending on the cause and the structures involved. Most begin as small, hardly noticeable breakthroughs. At first, they may be soft lumps under the skin, a little larger than a marble; there usually is no pain. Gradually, the pressure of the internal contents against the weak wall increases, and the size of the lump increases.

Early on, the hernia may be reduced which means that the protruding structures can be pushed back into their normal places. If those structures, however, cannot be returned to their normal locations through manipulation, the hernia is said to be irreducible, or incarcerated. The treatment of an incarcerated abdominal hernia is a serious surgical problem. Operations may be marked by high mortality due to the late diagnosis of incarceration and further postoperative complications.

For small, non-strangulated and non-incarcerated hernias, various supports and trusses may offer temporary, symptomatic relief. However, the best treatment is surgical closure or repair of the muscle wall through which the hernia protrudes. When the weakened area is very large, some strong synthetic material may be sewn over the defect to reinforce the weak area. Postoperative care involves protecting the patient from respiratory infections that might cause coughing or sneezing, which would strain the suture line. Recovery is usually quick and complete.

Be aware that pilonidal sinus disease is a common problem of the sacrococcygeal region. However, it is also observed in the periumbilical area. It is recommend that conservative treatment be done in patients an with umbilical pilonidal sinus. Surgery should be performed in recurrent cases resistant to conservative treatment. The importance of differential diagnosis of umbilical pilonidal sinus from other umbilical pathologies is emphasized.

Laparoscopic onlay patch hernioplasty is a safe and efficacious technique for the repair of umbilical hernia. Compared to the Mayo repair, the Laparoscopic approach confers the advantages of reduced postoperative pain, shorter hospital stay, and a diminished morbidity rate. It has been recommended that a surgeon use alloplastic material for umbilical hernia repair for patients with a BMI greater than 30.0 and hernia orifice larger than 3 cm. The decision for use of a mesh in hernial gaps from 2 to 3 cm should depend on individual factors. Older age, severe coexisting diseases, and late hospitalization were the main causes of unfavorable outcomes of the management of incarcerated hernias.

Be aware also that compared with patients with aortoiliac occlusive disease, patients with an abdominal aortic aneurysm have a higher frequency of abdominal wall hernia and inguinal hernia, and are at significant increased risk for development of incision hernia postoperatively. The higher frequency of hernia formation in patients with abdominal aoritic aneurysms suggests the presence of a structural defect within the fascia. Further studies are needed to delineate the molecular changes of the aorta and its relation to the abdominal wall fascia. Gaining access to the peritoneal cavity for laparoscopic surgery may cause severe complications, most of which are related to the umbilical trocar. Although closed laparoscopy can be safely used, open laparoscopy is associated with a lower morbidity rate; therefore its utilization is recommended.

Patients who have had placement of a mesh graft can have lingering severe pain that may become disabling. Chronic inguinodynia or neuralgia after conventional inguinal herniorrhaphy is rare, and diagnosing the exact cause is difficult. Treatment has ranged from local injection to remedial surgery with variable results. The increasing popularity of prosthetic mesh repairs has not eliminated these pain syndromes from occasionally occurring. Complications that people are having with mesh surgeries occur. If you look back thru all of the posts here on Websites, you will see for yourself that there are many people who are having complications from these mesh products.

The FDA is aware of the post market complications, but have asked that everyone who is having complications regardless of how small they seem they are they should file an adverse event form with the Government. They have stated, that they feel these complications are well under reported and can not help until they feel a certain percentage is met.

It appears that coincident neurectomy affords better results than mesh removal alone. Relief with nerve block did not predict favorable outcomes. Despite the popularity and favorable outcomes of prosthetic mesh repairs, persistent postoperative pain still occurs in a small number of patients. This may become more evident with the rising interest in laparoscopy. Correcting this surgery problem, once presented, can be a formidable task. Remedial inguinal with mesh removal and neurectomy will provide relief in selected patients.

The secret appears to be that hernia repair, one of the most common surgeries, carries a high risk of chronic pain after surgery 30% of patients have restricted movement and chronic pain that can last a long time. On July 6, 2011 plaintiffs injured by the Composix Kugel Mesh hernia patch made by C. R. Bard received an offer for a $184 million settlement in 2,600 claims, most of those outstanding over the faulty hernia patch. The amount was negotiated with more than 100 law firms around the country representing plaintiffs who had suffered the effects of a broken plastic ring or defective mesh including infection, bowel perforation, fistulas, even death. C.R. Bard subsidiary Davol Inc. is based in Warwick, Rhode Island and manufactured the Kugel.

Female diseases may also cause abdominal pain. Endometriosis is a common and painful disorder in women where tissue that normally lines the inside of the uterus (the endometrium) becomes implanted on tissue outside the uterus such as the abdomen. This can cause women to have pain in their abdomen. However, organs that are part of your gastrointestinal system are usually the cause of your abdominal pain. If you have pain in your upper abdomen on the right side, you may have an inflamed gallbladder or an ulcer. Hepatitis can cause you to have pain. Pancreatitis, a painful inflammation of the pancreas, can cause pain in your mid abdomen that radiates to your back.

Renal stones and kidney stones on occasion can cause abdominal pain in addition to pain in your flanks. Kidney pain can arise from increased pressure in your kidney capsule or in your ureter. Pain you're your ureter can be referred to your sides (flanks) or to your groin. If your kidney is inflamed as from a stone or infection, a punch over the area of your kidney can cause pain. If you have blood in your urine, you may have a stone.

If you are a male and if your scrotum is painful and swollen, you need to see your doctor, as you may have twisting of your spermatic cord or torsion of your spermatic cord. You may need surgery. If your scrotum is infected, it is called an epididymitis. Interstitial cystitis is an inflammatory disease of your bladder that can cause you to have lower abdominal pain.

If your abdominal pain is associated with your menstrual cycle, keep a diary of how the pain is affected. Ovarian cysts can cause you to have pain in your lower abdomen. Abdominal pain is the pain that you feel in your abdominal area that is between your chest and groin. Another term for abdomen is your stomach or "belly." Always be aware that pain in your abdomen can originate from your chest or your pelvis (the area below your abdomen).

Interstitial cystitis is a painful pelvic pain from the bladder with a cause that is unknown. An examination using a cystoscope by an urologist may reveal ulcerations in the lining of your bladder. The exact cause may be your immune system. Many treatments have been proposed including surgery on your bladder. Psychological treatment may help as well as installation of various substances into your bladder. Blood vessels in your abdomen may also be a source of abdominal pain. For example, your aorta, which is a major blood vessel that comes off your heart, runs down through your abdomen and divides into major arteries that supply blood flow to your legs.

If you have an aneurysm, which is a defect in the wall of this great vessel, you can have pain in your abdomen. An aneurysm needs to be evaluated by your doctor. An aneurysm is a weakness in the wall of your aorta. If you have abdominal pain and are able to feel or palpate a strong pulse in your abdomen you should consult with your physician. This weak area could rupture, which could be fatal. If you can feel a palpable mass in your abdomen this may be an aneurysm. Ask your doctor if the mass that you feel is abnormal.

Your appendix, if it is inflamed, can cause you to have abdominal pain as well. Your appendix is part of your gastrointestinal system. If you have appendicitis, you will have pain in the right lower part of your abdomen. You will experience nausea and vomiting and may have a fever. It is important for you to see a doctor because an untreated appendicitis can rupture and cause peritonitis. Peritonitis can be fatal.

A viral infection in your intestine or gas in your intestine can cause you to have significant abdominal pain. As you probably know, this pain can be severe. This should alert you that the severity of the pain does not correlate with the severity of the disease. In other words, you can have cancer of your colon and have only mild pain. Causes of abdominal pain include gas, constipation, milk intolerance, stomach flu, an irritable bowel syndrome, indigestion, esophageal reflux, ulcers, gallstones, and diverticular disease.

Microorganisms can also be sources of abdominal pain. Parasites as well as bacteria like Helicobacter pylori can cause you to have abdominal pain. This bacterium is called in microbiological terms a gram-negative bacterium and can be found in the moist membrane lining of your stomach. It can cause you to develop a progressive gastritis (an inflammation of the lining of your stomach) as well as stomach cancer, heart disease, and gastric and duodenal ulcers. Antibiotic therapy will be effective. If your pain is severe, you may require narcotics for your pain management. If you have significant abdominal pain you should seek medical care immediately. Avoid belts over the counter medications etc.

44. THORACIC PAIN

Chest pain can be a frightful experience, as you probably know. Heart related pain requires immediate attention. However, not every chest pain is related to heart pathology. You have many structures in your chest that can be a cause of your chest pain. Shingles that is discussed in another chapter in this book can cause some chest pain. Even though minor medical conditions can cause you to have chest pain, if you are having a heart attack, it can be potentially fatal. For this reason, any chest pain should not be taken lightly.

Chest pain is difficult to diagnose. Chest pain is vague. There are many structures in your chest cavity. You have two lungs, a diaphragm, a heart and a larynx and an esophagus. Furthermore, these organs have wrappers around them. The organs are wrapped by a peritoneum. The peritoneum contains many pain fibers. If your peritoneum becomes inflamed you may experience chest pain.

The heart's function is to pump blood. The right side of the heart pumps blood to the lungs, where oxygen is added to the blood and carbon dioxide is removed from it. The left side pumps blood to the rest of the body, where oxygen and nutrients are delivered to tissues and waste products are transferred to the blood for removal by other organs. With respect to the chest pain example presented at the beginning of this chapter you need to realize that as people age, the heart tends to enlarge slightly, developing thicker walls and slightly larger chambers. These changes are usually not work related. The increase in heart size is mainly due to an increase in the size of individual heart muscle cells.

During rest, the older heart function in almost the same way as a younger heart except the heart rate in the older individual is slightly lower. However, during exercise, the older heart cannot increase the amount of blood pumped out as much as a younger heart. The walls of the arteries and arterioles become thicker as you age, and the space within the arteries expands slightly. Elastic tissue within the walls of the arteries and arterioles is lost. Together, these changes make your blood the vessels stiffer.

Because arteries and arterioles become less elastic as you get older, they cannot relax as quickly during the pumping of the heart. As a result, blood pressure increases in the older individual more when the heart contracts. High blood pressure during systole with normal blood pressure during diastole is very common among older people and this disorder is called isolated systolic hypertension. Many of the effects of aging on the heart and blood vessels can be reduced by regular exercise. Exercise helps you maintain cardiovascular fitness as well as muscular fitness. Exercise is beneficial regardless of the age at which it is initiated.

The arteries can become clogged over time. If one of your arteries that supplies blood to your heart muscle is deprived of oxygen, you will experience chest pain (angina). If the lumen of your artery is completely obliterated then your heart muscle can become damaged causing you to have a heart attack (myocardial infarction). These changes occurred over time.

Angina is pain in the center of your chest. Usually rest relieves angina. Anginal chest pain in men may spread to the jaws and arms. Pain that radiates from the left side of the chest into the left arm is especially characteristic of anginal pain in men. In women on the other hand, a decrease in oxygen to the heart muscle for some reason, causes anginal pain and pressure in the center of the chest accompanied by pain in the neck or arms. Angina or heart pain occurs when the demand for blood by the heart muscle exceeds the oxygen supply of the arteries. This why exercise like shoveling snow can cause angina.

A myocardial infarction (heart attack) or death of a segment of your heart muscle occurs following interruption of the blood supply to the heart muscle. This is more severe than angina. A heart attack can cause sudden severe chest pain. There is a danger that your heart could go into an irregular heartbeat called an arrhythmia. If you have a severe arrhythmia, your heart can stop, which is referred to as a cardiac arrest. If you have interruption of the blood flow going to your heart, you can have irreversible injury to your heart muscle. This injury usually begins within 20 minutes from the time of the loss of blood flow to your heart muscle. Therefore, if you think that you are having a heart attack, contact your local emergency room or your doctor. If your pain is severe, go directly to your emergency room by ambulance.

Angina pectoris is chest pain that results from decreased oxygen supply to your heart muscle. Angina pectoris is usually pain under your breastbone. You may perceive discomfort instead of pain or pressure. The pain, if it is present, or the pressure can radiate to your neck or arm that is usually your left arm. Shortness of breath may also be reported. Angina pectoris is usually elicited by physical exertion. Occasionally psychological stress can cause you to have angina pectoris. If you are worried about an impending job interview for example, you could develop angina.

Exposure to cold air can cause angina. Angina comes on quickly and can last for up to 15 minutes. It usually resolves with rest or with nitroglycerin.

Coronary artery disease can be a cause of angina. Over time coronary artery disease can also cause you to have a heart attack (myocardial infarction). Lifestyle changes such as diet, exercise, and stopping smoking tobacco can decrease the incidence of coronary artery disease. Atherosclerosis is a build-up of fat and other materials in the walls of arteries that causes them to become narrowed. This entity is caused by many factors. If you are hypertensive and have an elevated cholesterol and smoke, you are at a higher risk for developing atherosclerosis.

When you have a deposit of fat and calcium in your blood vessels, your heart will still pump blood through these vessels. It takes a decrease in the diameter of your blood vessels by approximately 70 percent to decrease your blood flow. Smoking is an important factor that can cause you to be at a high risk for developing coronary artery disease. When you smoke tobacco, the nicotine in the tobacco causes your coronary arteries to decrease in caliber. This action decreases blood flow to your heart muscles that decreases oxygen to your heart muscles. A decreased in heart muscle oxygen can cause a heart attack.

A high cholesterol blood level can increase your risk of developing coronary artery disease. If you have high levels of low-density lipoprotein cholesterol, you have an elevated chance of developing coronary heart disease. If your cholesterol is elevated, your doctor will help you reduce your cholesterol with both diet and with pharmacologic management. You must monitor your diet for fat intake. Cocaine can also contribute to heart disease. Cocaine use has become more and more prevalent in the United States. However, cocaine use can make the arteries in your heart to go into spasm. Cocaine can accelerate the deposition of fat and calcium in your blood vessels, which can cause you to have angina as well as a heart attack.

You will develop chest pain when your heart oxygen demand exceeds the supply of oxygen that your blood vessels are delivering to your heart. If your heart begins beating faster, the increase in oxygen demand is met by an increased blood flow in your arteries about your heart. The small arteries around your heart muscle will increase their diameter to provide your heart with more oxygenated blood. If your vessels cannot dilate, your heart will not receive enough oxygen and you will experience pain in your chest. Fat and calcium within your heart vessels will restrict the amount of blood that goes to your heart.

According to the American Heart Association, approximately 6.3 million men and 6.6 million women in the United States have heart attacks. In the year 2000, more than 500,000 people died from heart disease. Different types of angina have been described. Stable angina is angina that is chronic and is usually caused by physical activity or emotional stress. Stable angina is usually heart-related pain relieved by rest or nitroglycerin. Unstable angina, on the other hand, can increase with rest. Other types of unstable angina can occur at low activity levels. Unstable angina may not be responsive to nitroglycerin. Sometimes you can develop spasms of your arteries that supply your heart muscle. This type of spasm is called Pinzmetal's angina and can be relieved frequently with nitroglycerin.

Stable angina is a term used to describe pain that is predictably caused by narrowing of your coronary arteries and a given stress to your heart. Shoveling the snow off your steps can cause you to experience angina. The pain is predictable in terms of its severity, how long it lasts, and what brings about relief (such as a single tablet of nitroglycerin placed under the tongue). On the other hand, unstable angina describes a new pattern of pain not previously experienced, for example, pain previously felt after a flight of stairs is now suddenly experienced at rest. Unstable angina is a medical emergency that should be immediately evaluated by a doctor.

In many instances during an angina attack your EKG, (a tracing of the electrical activity of your heart) may show signs of cardiac injury. However, it is also possible that your EKG can be completely normal, and this finding does not rule out heart attack or angina. If you are having chest pain and your EKG appears normal, your doctor may do an echocardiogram or administer radioactive dye and do a heart perfusion study. Your doctor may take a sample of your blood to have it analyzed for any elevations of your heart enzymes.

If you have heart muscle damage, the injured tissue will release chemicals called iso-enzymes. If these heart isoenzymes are increased, this may be a sign that you are having a heart attack. If you have a history of risk factors for coronary artery disease and if your symptoms are stable, your doctor may do a pharmacologic stress test. A dobutamine echocardiogram study may be done. You will be given a drug that will increase your heart rate. You will be monitored with a continuous EKG to see if there are any changes on your EKG that suggest decreased perfusion to your heart muscles. Occasionally your cardiologist may want to do a coronary angiogram, which is a test that uses a dye to assess the extent of your coronary artery disease.

A chest pain syndrome that may be more prevalent in women is an entity called syndrome X. If you have this syndrome, you may have an exaggerated response of the small arteries that go to your heart muscles. This exaggerated response is constriction of the diameter of your arteries. When this happens, you have decreased blood flow going to your heart. Usually women that suffer from this illness have a generalized increase in their body pain overall. This disease is undergoing further research at present. The prevalence of the cardiac syndrome X is higher in women when compared to men. Estrogen deficiency has been shown to play a major role in the origin of cardiac syndrome X.

Aspirin can affect your blood's ability to clot and, if you are having angina or if you suspect that you are having a heart attack, aspirin can be lifesaving. Nutrients such as fish oils might be effective for the prevention of heart disease. Remember that angina (heart pain) is not a heart attack. Angina is your body's warning to you that something is wrong and only means that some of your heart muscle is not getting enough blood temporarily.

Angina does not mean that your heart muscle is suffering permanent damage. A heart attack, on the other hand, occurs when the blood flow to your heart muscle is suddenly and permanently cut off. This event will usually cause permanent damage to your heart muscle. If you have angina, you must assume that you have underlying coronary artery disease unless proven otherwise.

If you have unstable angina or chest pain at rest, you may need hospitalization for intensive medical therapy. Aspirin and heparin can be given to decrease the clotting factors of your bloodstream. If you have angina, these drugs can decrease the progression of angina to a heart attack.

If you suspect that you are having a heart attack, seek immediate medical attention. Most deaths associated with an acute heart attack occur during the first hours following the onset of the heart attack. Nitroglycerine and morphine might be administered to you through your veins. If your heart rate is abnormal, your cardiologist will treat your abnormal heart rate as well.

Your EKG can be sent by telemetry by your emergency medical technician to a local emergency room so that the emergency room doctor can make a diagnosis of your heart rhythm and recommend any treatments that may be immediately necessary. It is important that blood is restored to your heart muscle. Sometimes your blood flow to your heart muscles can be increased by administering therapy to you that will break up blood clots in your heart blood vessels. Streptokinase is one drug that can be used in this situation. You will be confined to bed for 24 to 36 hours. You will be placed in a cardiac care unit. Your activities will be gradually increased. There are enzymes that are released into your bloodstream when you have heart muscle damage.

Other medicines called as beta blockers can be used to slow your heart rate and decrease the contraction of your heart muscles. This maneuver will conserve oxygen. Propanolol (Inderal) is an example of a beta blocker. Calcium channel blockers (Verapimil) affect the calcium in your muscle cells. Calcium channel blockers such as Verapamil can decrease the incidence of you having angina as well as a heart attack.

If medication fails to control your angina, coronary artery bypass surgery is sometimes necessary. A blood vessel is grafted onto your blocked artery. This allows your blood flow to bypass the blockage so that blood can go to your heart muscle to provide your heart muscle with needed oxygen. Your surgeon can use an artery inside your chest or take a vein from your leg. Another treatment that can be used to increase your artery size is called balloon angioplasty. This involves insertion of a catheter that has a tiny balloon on the end of it into an artery either in your arm or your leg. The balloon is inflated briefly to widen your vessel in places where your arteries are narrow.

Another type of procedure that can increase your blood flow to your heart is called a stent. A stent is a surgical procedure, but it is a minor procedure compared to open-heart surgery. Stents are implanted through your veins with a catheter. The stent expands when it is placed. The stent will provide better blood flow at the location of your artery where the blood flow is decreased. The purpose of the stent is to permanently hold your artery open.

There are three other causes of non-cardiac chest pain that you should be familiar with; intercostal neuropathy, costochondritis and Tietze"s syndrome. Injury to your nerve under your rib bone can occur following a rib fracture, lung surgery or heart surgery or from an infection. This pain may be relieved by anticonvulsant and/or antidepressant drugs. In some instances, your intercostal nerve needs to be injected with a local anesthetic with a steroid. If this fails, freezing the nerve with a cryo probe can provide you with significant pain relief.

Tietze's syndrome usually occurs in individuals less than 40 years of age. Usually only one pain site is experienced by this syndrome. It occurs at the junction between your ribs and your breast-bone (sternum) at the level of your second rib. Costochondritis usually occurs in individuals over 40.

More than one area of pain is involved and is at the levels of your second to fifth ribs. Tietze's syndrome follows a respiratory infection while costochondritis follows a neck sprain or coronary heart disease. The treatment of these two pain syndromes is the same as the intercostals neuropathy with the exception that injection therapy is done at the location of the pain.. Chest pain must not be ignored. In most cases it is benign. However, in some instances, it is fatal. You must therefore seek medical attention if you experience chest pain.

About the Author

Dr. William Ackerman is a pain management who brings considerable pain management experience to the medical community. He is a clinician, academician, lecturer, author, researcher, and an expert witness in medical malpractice cases. He is Board certified in Pain Medicine and Anesthesiology, and is a Graduate of the University Of Louisville School Of Medicine, completed a Residency in Anesthesiology at the University of Kentucky, and was Chief Resident in anesthesiology and Critical Care Medicine he did a Fellowship in Pain Medicine at the Texas Tech Health Sciences Center in Lubbock, Texas.

Dr. Ackerman was: Nominated previously for the Southern Medical Society Medical Research Award, Bristol-Meyers Squibb award for distinguished achievement in Pain Research and was a recipient of the Karl Koehler research grant from the American Society of Regional Anesthesia and Pain Medicine. He has been a Guest speaker at Medical school department meetings and academic symposiums throughout the country and at international meetings. His research has been featured in the National media.

He has published books and coauthored chapters in multiple medical textbooks including the AMA best seller: The AMA Guides to Injury and Disease Causation (First and Second editions). He authored 135 scientific articles in prestigious medical journals such as: Anesthesia Analgesia, Canadian Journal of Anaesthesia, Regional Anesthesia and Pain Management, The Journal of Hand Surgery etc. His book, Gender Factor Pain Management for Males and Females is now archived at The Arkansas Studies Institute which is a branch of the Central Arkansas Library System.

This book: "Pain Treatment Fraud A Prescription for Disaster" was written because readers must realize that there can be considerable fraud in pain management.

www.ingramcontent.com/pod-product-compliance
Lightning Source LLC
Chambersburg PA
CBHW071410180526
45170CB00001B/39